Cognitive Rehabilitation for Neuropsychiatric Disorders

Cognitive Rehabilitation for Neuropsychiatric Disorders

Edited by

Patrick W. Corrigan, Psy.D.
Stuart C. Yudofsky, M.D.

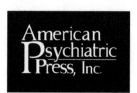

American Psychiatric Press, Inc.

Washington, DC
London, England

Copyright © 1996 American Psychiatric Press, Inc.
ALL RIGHTS RESERVED
Manufactured in the United States of America on acid-free paper
99   98   97   96   4   3   2   1

American Psychiatric Press, Inc.
1400 K Street, N.W., Washington, DC   20005

Library of Congress Cataloging-in-Publication Data
Cognitive rehabilitation for neuropsychiatric disorders / edited by
   Patrick W. Corrigan, Stuart C. Yudofsky.
        p.   cm.
   Includes bibliographical references and index.
   ISBN 0-88048-551-5 (cloth)
   1. Cognition disorders—Treatment.   2. Brain damage—Patients—
Rehabilitation.   I. Corrigan, Patrick W.   II. Yudofsky, Stuart C.
   [DNLM: 1. Cognition Disorders—rehabilitation.
2. Neuropsychology—methods.   3. Cognitive Therapy.   WM 204 C6767
1996]
RC553.C64C656   1996
616.8'046—dc20
DNLM/DLC
for Library of Congress   96-13648
                                                              CIP

British Library Cataloguing in Publication Data
A CIP record is available from the British Library.

Contents

Contributors

Hans Dieter Brenner, M.D., Ph.D.
Professor of Psychiatry and Chairman, Psychiatric University Services, Berne, Switzerland

Jeffrey E. Cassisi, Ph.D.
Assistant Professor, Department of Psychology, Illinois Institute of Technology, Chicago, Illinois

Caroline Clements, Ph.D.
Assistant Professor, Finch University of Health Sciences/The Chicago Medical School, North Chicago, Illinois

Michael J. Cohen, Ph.D.
Chief, Behavioral Medicine Research, Veterans Affairs Medical Center, Long Beach, California, and Adjunct Professor, Departments of Neurology and Psychiatry and Human Behavior, College of Medicine, University of California, Irvine, California

Peter E. Cook, M.D.
Executive Director, Hamilton Program for Schizophrenia, and Associate Clinical Professor, Department of Psychiatry, McMaster University, Hamilton, Ontario, Canada

Patrick W. Corrigan, Psy.D.
Associate Professor of Psychiatry and Director, University of Chicago Center for Psychiatric Rehabilitation, Chicago, Illinois

Joseph M. Cunningham, Ph.D.
Neuropsychology Postdoctoral Fellow, Department of Neurology, Medical College of Wisconsin, Milwaukee, Wisconsin

George Ellis, M.A.
Adjunct Professor of Psychology, Fairleigh Dickinson University, Madison, New Jersey

Michael D. Franzen, Ph.D.
Associate Professor, Medical College of Pennsylvania/Hahneman University, Allegheny Campus, Pittsburgh, Pennsylvania

Elizabeth L. Glisky, Ph.D.
Associate Professor, Department of Psychology, The University of Arizona, Tuscon, Arizona

Joel O. Goldberg, Ph.D.
Clinical Director, Hamilton Program for Schizophrenia, and Assistant Professor, Department of Psychiatry, McMaster University, Hamilton, Ontario, Canada

Shirley Hartlage, Ph.D.
Assistant Professor, Departments of Psychiatry, Psychology, and Social Sciences, Rush-Presbyterian-St. Luke's Medical Center, Rush Medical College, Chicago, Illinois

Daniela Heimberg, M.A.
Research Fellow, Department of Theoretical and Evaluative Psychiatry, Psychiatric University Clinic, Berne, Switzerland

Robert K. Heinssen, Ph.D.
Director of Behavior Therapy and Director of Partial Hospitalization, Chestnut Lodge Hospital, Rockville, Maryland

Anita Hirsbrunner, M.A.
Research Fellow, Department of Theoretical and Evaluative Psychiatry, Psychiatric University Clinic, Berne, Switzerland

Pamela S. Klonoff, Ph.D.
Clinical Director, Adult Day Hospital for Neurorehabilitation, Barrow Neurological Institute, St. Joseph's Hospital and Medical Center, Phoenix, Arizona

Thomas V. Merluzzi, Ph.D
Associate Professor of Psychology, University of Notre Dame, Notre Dame, Indiana

James Petrick, Ph.D.
Clinical Neuropsychologist, Behavioral Neuropsychology Associates, Pittsburgh, Pennsylvania

Neil H. Pliskin, Ph.D.
Assistant Professor of Psychiatry and Neurology and Director of Neuropsychology, University of Chicago Hospitals, Chicago, Illinois

Jeffrey Poland, Ph.D.
Visiting Assistant Professor of Philosophy, Department of Philosophy, University of Nebraska—Lincoln, Lincoln, Nebraska

George P. Prigatano, Ph.D.
Chairman, Neuropsychiatry, Barrow Neurological Institute, St. Joseph's Hospital and Medical Center, Phoenix, Arizona

Dorie Reed, Ph.D.
Research Assistant Professor of Psychology, Department of Psychology, University of Nebraska—Lincoln, Lincoln, Nebraska

John E. Roberts, Ph.D.
Assistant Professor of Psychology, State University of New York at Buffalo, Buffalo, New York

Steven L. Schandler, Ph.D.
Professor, Division of Psychology, Chapman University, Orange, California, and Chief, Addiction Research Laboratory, Veterans Affairs Medical Center, Long Beach, California

William D. Spaulding, Ph.D.
Professor of Psychology, Department of Psychology, University of Nebraska—Lincoln, Lincoln, Nebraska

Daniel M. Storzbach, Ph.D.
Postdoctoral Fellow in Neuropsychology, Department of Psychology, Portland VAMC, and Oregon Health Sciences University, Portland, Oregon

Shirley F. Szekeres, Ph.D.
Associate Professor and Chair, Department of Speech-Language Pathology, Nazareth College of Rochester, Rochester, New York

Jacqueline Remondet Wall, Ph.D.
Graduate Student, Illinois Institute of Technology, Chicago, Illinois

Judith Waters, Ph.D.
Professor of Psychology, Fairleigh Dickinson University, Madison, New Jersey

Mark Ylvisaker, Ph.D.
Assistant Professor, Department of Communication Disorders, College of Saint Rose, Albany, New York

Stuart C. Yudofsky, M.D.
Professor of Psychiatry and Chairman, Department of Psychiatry, Baylor College of Medicine, Houston, Texas

Foreword

The history of psychiatry has been marked by significant paradigmatic shifts in the locus, focus, and modus of treatment. Moral therapy emphasized the role played by the individual's social environment and designed asylums to counteract putative toxic effects of urban crowding and poverty. Psychoanalysis postulated unconscious psychological conflicts as the root of psychopathology and sought to neutralize those conflicts by insight achieved in office-based treatment. The development of psychotropic agents has focused attention on the biological underpinnings of the major mental disorders and has enabled most patients to receive treatment in the community outside of hospitals.

More recently, these approaches have been replaced by a more integrative biopsychosocial model. Proponents of the biopsychosocial approach articulate the need for a multidimensional understanding of multifactorial disease processes, such as those discussed in *Cognitive Rehabilitation of Neuropsychiatric Disorders*. The authors of each chapter of this text have taken great pains to emphasize the biological, psychological, and environmental factors that contribute to the assessment and intervention strategies for each disorder.

Superimposed on the biopsychosocial perspective, another paradigm is evident in this text. The rehabilitation model (modus) directs attention to the functional capabilities (focus) and community adaption (locus) of the mental health consumer. The editors of this volume, Corrigan and Yudofsky, insist that we no longer be content with the amelioration of symptoms or control of dysfunctional behaviors. Instead, emphasis and resources should be given toward identifying and building on patients' strengths—facilitating the acquisition of the cognitive-behavioral skills needed to improve quality of life.

Rehabilitation of central nervous system disorders gains its impetus from the growing realization of the plasticity of the brain. Brain functioning is determined by genes and by experience, with the genetic code laying down the limits and opportunities for the brain's responsiveness to life experiences. In a very real sense, the biological basis of the brain's structure and function contains the seeds for its own growth and development through interactions with the environment. Behavior, including emotional, cognitive, intellectual, social, and instrumental modes of personal functioning, is the reflection of the interactions between brain and environment; as such, it becomes the proper target for therapeutic, biobehavioral interventions. Because the interactions among the brain, behavior, and environment are dynamic and represent an open system, therapeutic interventions can derive from one or a combination of the interacting domains and can also affect one or more of these domains.

Hence, cognitive rehabilitation in schizophrenia can be achieved through social interventions such as social skills training (Liberman and Green 1992) and pharmacological treatments (Lee et al. 1994), as well as through direct training of cognitive functions by improving a patient's performance on neuropsychological tests such as the Wisconsin Card Sorting Test or the Span of Apprehension Task (Kern et al. 1995). It is far too early to identify the most cost-effective approaches to cognitive rehabilitation. We do not know whether "top-down" treatments that start with broadly conceived psychosocial programs of services will be more or less efficacious than "bottom-up"–type interventions that start with discrete training of cognitive functions in the laboratory with the hope that these functions, once improved or remediated, will have generalized impact on the individual's clinical status and wider psychosocial performance. The current state of the field calls out for a broad array of initiatives that explore the boundaries of the feasible and the possible—from "macro" interventions involving in vivo amplified skills training (Wallace and Liberman 1995) to "micro" laboratory-based training of elementary cognitive functions such as attention and memory (Green 1993).

As we explore the universe of treatments aimed at cognitive rehabilitation, we must retain the scientific modesty that comes from our limited knowledge of the brain. Neuroscientists estimate that our brains contain 100 billion to 1 trillion neurons, each of which contains 10,000 interconnections with other neurons. These neurons are constantly forging new connections and unraveling old ones in response to signals through our sense organs that originate in the environment and from other parts of our body. Investigators have discovered more than 150 neurotransmitters that provide the signal transductions throughout the brain, but only a small amount is known about less than a dozen of these chemical messengers. Although we believe that many cognitive, emotional, intellectual, social, and instrumental behaviors are controlled or determined by combinations of neurotransmitters operating within specific neural circuits, almost nothing is known about the way these systems actually work. Somehow, the brain connects neuron to neuron, forming circuitry that in some way corresponds to patterns in the outside world.

Cognitive rehabilitation is not likely to become a practical therapeutic science until we have achieved a greater understanding of the functioning of the brain. However, just as the control of infectious diseases through public health measures did not have to wait for the discovery of the germ theory and bacteria, progress in cognitive rehabilitation does not have to wait for more fundamental discoveries in brain function. In this text, Corrigan and Yudofsky have assembled an expeditionary force of scientist-practitioners who have begun a therapeutic assault on the still obscure interrelations among brain, behavior, and environment. The extent of their success will be measured, not by the limited evidence of therapeutic progress and generalization of clinical improvement currently available, but rather by the stimulation of work in this field that they generate.

In this volume, Corrigan and Yudofsky have edited state-of-the-art overviews of what has been termed "cognitive rehabilitation." The first chapter provides a thorough discussion of "normal" cognitive functioning, which grounds the book in sound neuropsychiatric principles. The second chapter introduces the concept of cognitive rehabilitation and elaborates on four models that serve as frameworks for organizing and developing treatment strategies. The succeeding three chapters in the first section summarize what is known about the cognitive deficits in depression, psychotic disorders, and social anxiety, respectively. The second and third sections describe cognitive rehabilitation interventions for a variety of neuropsychiatric disorders. The final section covers specific subjects relevant to a comprehensive approach to cognitive rehabilitation.

Corrigan and Yudofsky have brought us up-to-date on a relatively young and quickly changing field. Their concern with the rehabilitation potential of their patients, and their scrupulous attention to the therapeutic strategies that may aid these difficult-to-treat populations, should bring renewed hope and confidence to many clinicians, researchers, administrators, third-party payers, patients, and families. Further developments in this field, possibly built on the foundations laid in these chapters, may overcome the therapeutic nihilism that is regrettably pervasive in the treatment of neuropsychiatric disorders and usher in a truly enlightened era of psychiatry.

Alex Kopelowicz, M.D., and Robert Paul Liberman, M.D.

References

Green MF: Cognitive remediation in schizophrenia: is it time yet? Am J Psychiatry 150:178–187, 1993

Kern RS, Green MF, Goldstein MJ: Modification of performance on the span of apprehension, a putative marker of vulnerability to schizophrenia. J Abnorm Psychol 104:385–389, 1995

Lee MA, Thompson PA, Meltzer HY: Effects of clozapine of cognitive functioning in schizophrenia. J Clin Psychiatry 55(Sept suppl B):82–87, 1994

Liberman RP, Green MF: Whither cognitive-behavioral therapy for schizophrenia? Schizophr Bull 18:27–35, 1992

Wallace CJ, Liberman RP: Psychiatric rehabilitation, in Treatment of Psychiatric Disorders. Edited by Gabbard GO. Washington, DC, American Psychiatric Press, 1995, pp 1019–1038

Preface

When clinicians consider functional deficits that occur as a consequence of neuropsychiatric conditions, they frequently conceptualize these deficits as irreversible. Moreover, neuropsychiatric conditions are often misperceived as unremittingly degenerative with the consequent progressive loss of function. In this context, therapeutic remediation of function may be viewed as unrealistic or even impossible. The unfortunate result of these misconceptualizations is a therapeutic nihilism that is particularly pervasive when applied to the rehabilitative potential of those who suffer from cognitive deficits secondary to neuropsychiatric disorders. The purpose of this book is to present an overview—from the theoretical to the clinically applicable—of the current knowledge of cognitive function and dysfunction, as well as the therapeutic strategies used to restore function that is lost as the result of central nervous system disorders. It is our hope that this book will provide a knowledge base that will aid the clinician in choosing treatment options that are relevant, respectful, and effective for their patients with cognitive disorders that occur as the result of central nervous system disorders. This book also will inform the reader about which therapies to avoid because they are expensive, frustrating, and ineffective for the patients we serve.

Syndromes and symptoms that are associated with brain disorders may emerge rapidly and dramatically, such as those that occur subsequent to stroke or traumatic brain injury, or they may have subtle and insidious onsets, as often occur with central nervous system illnesses such as schizophrenia. With both types of onset, clinicians frequently fail to consider cognitive rehabilitation. In the case of the sudden and dramatic onset of a neuropsychiatric disorder, the cognitive aspects of this condition are frequently neglected with the emphasis being placed on the sensorimotor sequelae. In cases of neuropsychiatric conditions that advance gradually, cognitive conditions are often not recognized or are misdiagnosed. A clinical example is Mr. W., who was referred to the neuropsychiatric inpatient service at Columbia Presbyterian Medical Center for treatment of major depression with suicidal preoccupations. Eighteen months prior to admission, Mr. W. became sad, suffered insomnia, and had decreased energy, reduced motivation, reduced ability to concentrate, and diminished self-esteem. Extensive trials of various antidepressants, combined with psychotherapy and family therapy, did not ameliorate his condition. Neuropsychiatric evaluation, including magnetic resonance imaging of his brain and lumbar puncture with analyses of Mr. W.'s spinal fluid, confirmed a diagnosis of multiple sclerosis. Neuropsychological testing revealed extensive cognitive dysfunctions including calculating ability, abstracting, and a variety of memory functions. Although Mr. W.'s depression remitted after treatment with a combination of a monoamine oxidase inhibitor and a heterocyclic antidepressant, repeated testing revealed only minor improvements in his cognitive functioning. The neuropsychologists determined that the cognitive impairments were not mood related but were more likely associated with the multiple sclerosis. Mr. W.'s profession was a materials engineer for a large contractor for the space program. Interviews with his supervisors and co-workers revealed that Mr. W. had been experiencing performance-related problems at work for approximately 2 years. Although specialized neuropsychological assessment showed that Mr. W. was not able to perform his previous occupational functions, many cognitive skills remained. Working closely with a cognitive therapist, a clinical psychologist, and his supervisor from work, Mr. W. successfully returned to occupational functions, which subsequently engendered a sense of satisfaction and increased self-esteem.

Consistent with important changes that appear in DSM-IV (American Psychiatric Association 1994), in this text we do not distinguish cognitive impairments associated with the "traditional" organic mental disorders (e.g., traumatic brain injury, cerebral vascular accidents, toxins, etc.) from those that occur with what had previously been viewed as "functional illnesses" such as schizophrenia and major depression. As indicated in DSM-IV, there are always important psychological factors in so-called organic illnesses and important biological factors in so-called psychological disorders. We also take a broad view of cognitive rehabilitation strategies that incorporate 1) biological therapies to enhance recovery or repair of the central nervous system; 2) the use of medications to treat the full range of mood, behavioral, and cognitive impairments; 3) relevant psychotherapies, family and couples counseling, and occupational counseling; 4) Alcoholics Anonymous and other advocacy and support groups; and 5) the wide variety of behavioral and cognitive-rehabilitation therapeutic approaches that will be described in this book.

This book has been divided into four sections to facilitate description of cognitive rehabilitation models and therapeutic strategies. In Part I, the form and impact of cognitive deficits on neuropsychiatric disorders are discussed. Corrigan begins Part I by summarizing various psychological models that might be adopted to describe, categorize, and conceptualize cognitive deficits. Corrigan and Yudofsky discuss the nature of cognitive rehabilitation, given the various models by which cognitive deficit is explained. The section then presents two chapters designed to orient the reader to fundamental issues in cognition and knowledge derived from experimental psychology. Schandler and Cohen discuss the manner in which cognitive deficits are affected by psychophysiological functions. Part I also includes chapters that address specific cognitive deficits of three neuropsychiatric populations: depression, schizophrenia, and anxiety. Hartlage and Clements discuss structural models of depression; Spaulding and his colleagues review process-oriented models of schizophrenia and other psychoses; and Merluzzi presents the psychological literature on cognitive deficits related to social anxiety.

Parts II and III review various rehabilitation programs for neuropsychiatric disorders. The chapters in Part II address the rehabilitation of deficits associated with neuropsychiatric disorders. Pliskin and his colleagues delineate communicative and cognitive programs for treating the cognitive deficits of cerebrovascular accident and Alzheimer's disease. Prigatano, Glisky, and Klonoff review their research on treatment of traumatic brain injury; Franzen and Petrick present the limited literature on behavior treatments of seizure disorder. Cognitive rehabilitation of children is discussed by Ylvisaker and Szekeres.

Part III includes chapters that discuss rehabilitation strategies for disorders that are conventionally conceptualized as psychiatric. Roberts and Hartlage review cognitive therapies for depression, whereas Storzbach and Corrigan summarize the more process-oriented rehabilitation strategies for schizophrenia. Brenner and his colleagues have developed a comprehensive rehabilitation program for severe mental disorders called integrated psychological therapy; they present this program in Chapter 12. Goldberg and Cook discuss a broad range of cognitive treatments for the negative symptoms of psychiatric disorders. In Part IV, Heinssen summarizes environmental requirements for setting up rehabilitation programs, and Waters and Ellis review uses and potential of video and computer equipment for these purposes.

Many chapters in this book describe various strategies for remediating the broad range of cognitive deficits associated with neuropsychiatric disorders. Ironically, several authors have concluded that the early excitement about the potential for correcting cognitive deficit through rehabilitation should be tempered by more sober findings from research. Thus, it is our belief that this text is balanced and will not only be helpful by defining the strengths but also the weaknesses of rehabilitation interventions, as well as the opportunities afforded by future research. It is our hope that this book will be a useful tool for clinicians who strive to help patients overcome cognitive disabilities associated with neuropsychiatric conditions.

Reference

American Psychiatric Association: Diagnostic and Statistical Manual of Mental Disorders, 4th Edition. Washington, DC, American Psychiatric Association, 1994

Part I

Cognitive Deficits and Neuropsychiatric Deficits

Chapter 1

Models of "Normal" Cognitive Functioning

Patrick W. Corrigan, Psy.D.

Before we can describe strategies for rehabilitating neuropsychiatric populations of their various cognitive deficits, the nature of these deficits needs to be fairly well understood. Sufficient explanation of these deficits is best accomplished when built on empirically based models of "normal" cognitive functioning. Several such models have been developed and tested in cognitive and social psychology, many of which have been useful for investigators of experimental psychopathology and cognitive rehabilitation. Some of the most relevant models are presented in this chapter with their significance for cognitive rehabilitation highlighted.

The essential question of this chapter then, is "What is normal cognition?" Answers to this question vary significantly depending on the perspective of the investigator making the inquiry. A broad spectrum of models is outlined in Figure 1–1 and is presented for their heuristic value; the boundaries of what might normally be considered cognition or rehabilitation are enlarged considerably to include intelligence, information processing, cognitive schema, and problem solving and decision making. *Intelligence* is the most molar construct discussed in this chapter, resting on the oldest body of literature. In part, discussion of intelligence is included as a historical orientation to cognition, showing from where theorizing in this area originated, as well as discussing more recent strengths and limitations of the view. Moreover, the predictive utility of models of intelligence, especially regarding educational and vocational achievement, yield some useful questions for cognitive rehabilitation.

Models of *information processing* and *cognitive schema* are presented because they represent a distinguished dichotomy in cognitive science: How do we think? (cognitive components) versus, What do we think about? (cognitive content) (R. J. Sternberg 1985). Information processing approaches have been appealing because they organize various cognitive functions into an

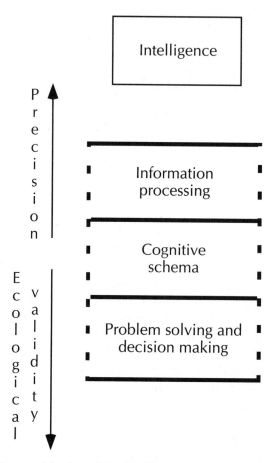

Figure 1–1. Four models of cognition. Intelligence is put at the apex because it has set the scope for many cognitive questions. The three other models differ from each other in terms of precision and ecological validity.

interactive process. The cognitive schema viewpoint has been especially useful for explaining social cognition. There are also "cognitive" models that have largely developed outside of cognitive science but are especially relevant to rehabilitation. *Problem solving* and *decision making*, in real-life, provide for more cognitive-behavioral models of functioning and rehabilitation strategies.

Models reviewed in this chapter are not mutually exclusive; many methodological and conceptual constructs overlap. Moreover, this is not an exhaustive discussion of cognitive models of normalcy but rather a sample of important paradigms.

Information processing, cognitive schema, and problem solving and decision making differ in terms of their methodological precision and ecological validity. Investigations of information processing constructs occur in the laboratory and typically include computerized apparatus to collect and transform data. The internal validity of well-prepared studies in this area is among the best. Cognitive schema studies have adapted various information processing research strategies, frequently from memory studies, but without the same methodological rigor.

Precision and generalizability are inversely related. Although studies of problem solving and decision making do not demonstrate the elegant algorithms or intricate apparatus of laboratory-bound research, findings from these disciplines tend to be applied more easily to settings in the real world. As Spaulding (1992) recently pointed out, the question of generalizability is more complex than whether the content of rehabilitation programs includes social information. Laboratory-based information processing tasks that improve a patient's ability to attend to social skills training modules are worth their weight in ecological validity.

Costs and benefits to precision versus ecological validity exist. Laboratory research is not easily interpreted in terms of the everyday experiences of our patients. Conversely, internal validity from highly generalizable research can also have its limitations. Interestingly, investigators of experimental psychopathology, with their interest in nosology and description, seem to be drawn to the more precise methods of information processing. Rehabilitation researchers, on the other hand, are more attracted to problem solving and communication models because these findings seem to translate more readily into treatment techniques. The investigator and clinician who have an understanding of cognitive science are in a better position to foresee new developments in neuropsychology, experimental psychopathology, and cognitive rehabilitation.

Intellectual Deficits

The study of intelligence has as long a history as the discipline of psychology itself and represents the first attempts of behavioral scientists to measure the manner in which humans know the world. Intelligence, as a forebear of cognitive science, has defined many of the original assumptions that still direct research in this area. These assumptions include the following:

1. Relatively private acts related to knowing and cognition can be measured through performance on in-the-world tasks.
2. Generalizations about overall cognitive functioning can be derived from performance on these discrete tasks.
3. Specific cognitive functions are adaptive; individuals who manifest these functions are expected to be more skillful in meeting their needs.

4. Predictions about the individual's functioning in the future, not only in academic settings, but also in most areas of behavior can be made from individuals adaptive functioning in the present.
5. Cognitive functioning has trait-like characteristics that remain relatively immutable over time and evolving qualities that correspond with key developmental phases.[1]

These issues are important not only for understanding intelligence but also are fundamental to the other models discussed in this chapter.

Models of Intelligence

Investigators who represent the second and third generation of the study of intelligence have begun to develop evaluative models of the construct, summarizing strengths and weakness of the theory and outlining future research directions. For example, R. J. Sternberg (1985) proposed a triarchic theory looking at three relevant questions: 1) What is the relationship of intelligence to the internal world?, 2) What is the relationship of intelligence to the external world?, and 3) What is the relationship of intelligence to experience? The triarchic model is used in this chapter to outline important issues in intelligence.

Intelligence and the internal world. Classic models of intelligence have attempted to map the inner world in terms of overall versus specific intellectual functions. Some of the earliest models were based on overall descriptors of intelligence. Binet and Simon (1916) labeled intelligence "judgement, otherwise called good sense, practical sense, initiative, the faculty of adapting one's self to circumstances" (p. 42). Forty years later, Wechsler (1958) talked about intelligence as "the aggregate or global capacity of the individual to act purposefully, to think rationally, and to deal effectively with his environment" (p. 7). Intelligence represents an individual's proclivity for success in conducting adaptive functions.

An intrinsic quality of the internal world theory is that intelligence has trait-like characteristics that can be identified at an early age; intelligence has at least a partial organizing effect on subsequent developmental tasks. Therefore, measurements of this intelligence trait will predict functioning and achievement later in life. In fact, the predictive aspect of intelligence became essential to research dedicated to psychometric strategies that measure the construct. The development of tests and theories paralleled the evolution of multivariate, statistical procedures. As depicted in Figure 1–2,

---

[1] Although developmental models are essential for full comprehension of the dynamic qualities of cognition, space limitations prevent any significant discussion of these models in this chapter.

test theorists have varied in their conceptualization of intelligence, with some proposing an overall "g" factor accounting for performance on all intellectual tasks and others suggesting more than a hundred independent factors accounting for intelligence.

Spearman (1927) discussed two factors of intelligence: a "g" factor that describes overall intelligence plus a specific intelligence factor relevant to the verbal or nonverbal ability necessary to score well on various tests. Alternatively, Cattell (1963) distinguished between two types of intelligence, crystallized and fluid. Fluid intelligence refers to nonspecific, culture-free abilities that tend to underlie many cognitive tasks, whereas crystallized intelligence refers

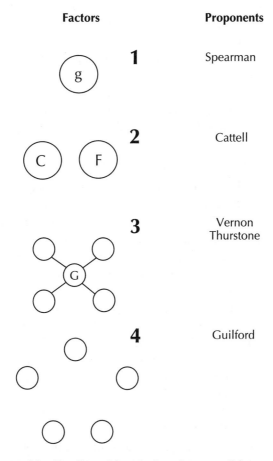

Figure 1–2. Models of intellectual functioning. 1) An overall factor accounting for all intellectual functioning, "g"; 2) Small multifactor theories such as Cattell's distinction between crystallized (C) and fluid intelligence (F); 3) Combination of "G" and multifactor theories; 4) Multiple independent factors.

to acquired knowledge and school learning. Vernon (1950) elaborated on Spearman's two-factor perspective by proposing a hierarchical theory of intelligence. According to Vernon, an overall "g" factor is divided into two major factors—verbal-educational and spatial-mechanical. Major factors are further divided; for example, the verbal-education factor includes creative abilities, verbal fluency, and numbers.

Others have argued that the "g" factor theories are inaccurate representations of intelligence that do not portray the multifaceted and relatively independent nature of human abilities (Thorndike 1927). For example, Thurstone (1938) used relatively crude factor analytic methods to show that Thurstone's factors were significantly interrelated, suggesting a single superordinate factor. Guilford (1967) generated the most prominent multifactor theory. He uncovered more than 100 independent factors of intelligence using a series of factor analyses of several tests of intellectual abilities. These eight primary factors varied over three dimensions: the kind of mental operation used, the content of the mental operation, and the product of the operation. Each dimension was, in turn, divided into major factors; for example, operations include evaluation, convergent production, divergent production, memory, and cognition. Permutations of dimensional factors defined 120 unique cells, each with a distinct cognitive function.

Intelligence and the external world.   Several psychologists, sociologists, and anthropologists have defined intelligence as it is described by culture. "In order to understand the invention, one must first understand the culture and why it would invent intelligence in a particular way" (R. J. Sternberg 1985, p. 1115). Sternberg listed several variations of this theme that diverge in terms of intelligence existing independently from the investigators and the culture that define it. At one extreme are the radical culturalists who argue that intelligence cannot stand outside of the society that defines it (Berry 1974). If intelligence denotes adaptive functioning, then it depends on the (cultural) setting in which individual behavior occurs. Therefore, Western views of intellectual functioning, as measured by IQ tests, have little value outside a narrow cultural sphere. It is conceivable, according to this perspective, that adaptive skills (and hence a high IQ) in one culture might be irrelevant or ineffectual in another and therefore result in a low IQ.

At the opposite end of the external world spectrum is the contextualist view (Jenkins 1974; Keating 1984). According to this model, the focus of investigation is the manner in which the internal world of intelligence is mediated by cultural and other temporal factors. Proponents of contextualist models seek universal representations of achievement that are mitigated by culture.

Statements embodied in varying models of intelligence and models of the external world sum up many of the clinical criticisms of measures of intellectual functioning. IQ tests such as the Wechsler Adult Intelligence Scale—Revised (Wechsler 1981) have been repeatedly criticized as overrepresenting left brain, verbal skills while being relatively less sensitive to right brain, mechanical skills (Sattler 1982). Similarly, IQ predicts school learning fairly well but does not suggest the creative potential of an individual. IQ tests frequently are not culturally fair, misrepresenting the intellectual abilities of many ethnic groups (Flaugher 1978).

Intelligence and experience. Finally, R. J. Sternberg's (1985) triarchic theory looks at the interaction between the internal and the external world of intelligence and how experience mediates the relationship between these two worlds. Sternberg refers to two models of this interaction: Piaget's (1972) biological model, which represents intelligence as an evolving system, and Vygotsky's (1978) sociological model, which represents intelligence as an internalization of social processes. Piaget's model embraces evolutionary perspectives—survival requires internal adaptation to the external world. As the individual discovers that certain behaviors and cognitions do not meet all the person's needs, the individual becomes open to, and may actually seek out, alternative cognitive skills. Adaptation occurs as a complex interaction between assimilating information into existing knowledge structures and accommodating or creating new structures when existing knowledge bases are insufficient. Key periods of assimilation and accommodation are defined developmentally.

Unlike Piaget, who believed that cognitive development is biologically driven, Vygotsky postulated that development of intelligence originates in one's interactions with other people. Hence, individuals are able to internalize social information, and later perform cognitively, only what they have been guided to do as children (by their parents or other caretakers). Internalized information comes out only after this information has been acted on in the world.

Relevance of Intellectual Models for Cognitive Rehabilitation

The influence of intelligence on development and evaluation of rehabilitation strategies can be understood using the triarchic model. Study of the internal world suggests that cognitive deficits reside in the individual organism. Given the psychoeducational characteristics of rehabilitation, intelligence test scores that predict patients' capacity for learning may be invaluable. For example, a description of intellectual impairments may suggest that patients are not ready for rehabilitation. Studies have shown that severely mentally ill patients with high verbal IQs are better able to acquire interpersonal skills (trained during psychosocial rehabilitation modules) than patients with lower IQs (Aylward et al. 1984; Corrigan et al. 1991). Hence, IQ may be a useful variable for planning treatment. This kind of planning is apparent with mentally retarded patients, the DSM-IV (American Psychiatric Association 1994) population that is defined, in large part, by intelligence scores. Generally, interventions for this patient population are based on the management of reinforcers and punishers rather than cognitive strategies, especially when the developmental disability is more severe (Madle and Neisworth 1990).

Multifactor theories of the internal world of intelligence expand the predictive possibilities vis-à-vis cognitive rehabilitation even more. For example, adoption of Guilford's (1967) perspective on divergent intellectual operations, products, and contents would suggest several functions that predict success in rehabilitation programs. The five factors comprising Guilford's mental operations dimension suggest distinct rehabilitation foci and interventions. Depending on the deficit, clinicians would have to target memory, evaluation, cognition, divergent productions, or convergent productions. A multifaceted model also suggests that the effects of rehabilitation may be discrete; a large set of intervention strategies is needed to address the range of possible deficits.

Despite the predictive benefits of the internal world models of intelligence, these constructs have an immutable quality that makes for strange bedfellows with cognitive rehabilitation. The training strategy or environmental manipulation cannot affect an individual's cognitive abilities because of the individual's genetic and developmental predispositions. If the immutable quality of cognitive abilities were supported in the literature, without controversy, then the predictions of who can and cannot succeed at rehabilitation would be valuable. Given the choices that cost-conscious administrators must make about program development, rehabilitative possibilities for low-IQ populations would be limited. However, measures of intelligence have been shown to be prejudicial representations of the "g" factor with the relative invariable nature of intelligence in doubt. Research shows that when students participate in strategic enrichment programs, learning disabilities (which may deflate IQ scores), as well as performance on achievement tests, have been shown to improve (McIntyre 1989; Scruggs and Wong 1990).

Models of intelligence and of the external world raise questions about what should be the focus of cognitive rehabilitation. Contrary to classical assumptions about universal qualities defining intelligence, cultural relativists have outlined the manner in which history and society affect these qualities. Therefore, rehabilitation strategies that attempt to remediate deficits need to assess the cultural aspects of cognition.

How can the culturally unique aspects of cognition and cognitive rehabilitation be assessed? Goldfried and D'Zurilla (1969) discussed a survey method to assess culturally specific situations in which subjects identify behavioral (or in this case, cognitive) problems and solutions to these problems. The procedure comprises three steps:

1. *Situational analysis:* Subjects are asked to list problem situations relevant to the social issue of interest. For example, "I have a hard time understanding my father's requests."
2. *Response enumeration:* After a list of situations is generated, subjects are instructed to name effective responses to each problem. "I could ask Dad what he's trying to say" or "I could ask Mom what Dad is trying to say."
3. *Response evaluation:* Individual responses are evaluated by subjects to determine consensually whether or not each coping behavior is effective.

This procedure has been used to effectively assess the repertoire of skill deficits in severely mentally ill patients (Corrigan and Holmes 1994; Goldsmith and McFall 1975). This method might be used to identify the content of cognitive rehabilitation programs. How do neuropsychological problems affect everyday life? Findings from such surveys seem more relevant to social cognitive questions (What skills are essential for understanding and reacting to interpersonal situations?) than to laboratory-based measures of cognition (What functions are necessary to learn a list of nonsense syllables?). Ironically, however, the cognitive problems that neuropsychiatric patients are supposed to report may prevent insight into the problem. Can patients be expected to remember the manner in which recall problems affect their life? Studies on patients who have suffered traumatic brain injury suggest that almost one-half the group demonstrated a significant lack of awareness of problems related to their injuries some time after injury (Oddy et al. 1985; Prigatano and Altman 1990; Sunderland 1983). Conversely, another study shows that severely mentally ill adults were not impaired by their thought disorder or intellectual limitations (Corrigan and Holmes 1992). More than likely, the abilities of neuropsychiatric patients to participate in surveys such as this will vary depending on their illness and course. Cognitive surveys need not be limited to patients. Family members and others may be reliable sources for outlining relevant skill areas for a cognitive rehabilitation program.

What implications do models of intelligence that combine internal and external worlds have for cognitive rehabilitation? Piaget's (1972) biological model suggests that rehabilitation, like cognition, is highly dependent on developmental stages. This suggestion has obvious implications for individuals at key stages in the life course. Cognitive rehabilitation models must account for the developmental tasks of children and adolescents as well as the unique developmental issues of elderly persons. Programs will fall short if a specific strategy tries to target a deficit that is not biologically wired for individuals in that age group.

Information Processing Models

The fundamental assumption of information processing paradigms is that the macro aspect of sensory input is divided into discrete information bytes (e.g., visual stimuli can be described in terms of color, contrast, depth, location, and size) and that the macro experience of human cognition can be divided into composite functions (such as attention, memory, and response selection). These composite functions interact in some meaningful order (e.g., serial or parallel distribution). Hence, the process of knowing can be understood by studying the various components of the information processing, individually and together. From a methodological standpoint, breaking down information and cognition into theoretical elements greatly enhances the study of these phenomena. The range of research questions increases geometrically with the number of defined elements. Similarly, methodological precision is enhanced as the questions of cognitive research narrow from "How does a person know?" to "How does a person attend, recall, recognize, or react?"

An information processing paradigm has several advantages for the clinical investigator's understanding of cognitive functioning (Ingram and Kendall 1986; Merluzzi et al. 1981). The specificity and organization of this approach facilitates the identification of cognitive deficits. Findings about specific cognitive functions seem to coincide with biological research suggesting putative correspondences between information processing and central nervous system (CNS) structure. Moreover, measurement strategies used in defining information processing have been easily adapted for assessment of cognitive deficits. Variations of these assessment strategies have been used as rehabilitative tools.

An extensive body of literature exists on models of information processing, the typical investigation of these models having been completed in rigorous laboratory settings. Unfortunately, the laboratory rigor of most information processing studies underscores the primary criticism of the model (Neisser 1976, 1980, 1985); namely, much of the paradigm has poor ecological validity. What does being able to attend to an array of letters flashing on a screen have to do with listening closely to a conversation at a cocktail party? The ecological validity of the information processing models is a point that will come up throughout this chapter. The holistic nature of the human enterprise seems to challenge the reductionist aspects of a processing model (Lachman and Lachman 1986). Hence, the use of information processing models for cognitive rehabilitation needs to be tempered by the insights garnered from a social cognitive approach.

Stage Theory

Many of the early information processing theories, such as serial-search models of cognition (Sternberg 1966, 1967), worked their way from the bottom up

(Figure 1–3). Information processing is a serial process in that it manipulates information in a stepwise fashion, one byte at a time; functions include information intake and encoding, storage and retrieval, transformation and conceptualization, and response selection and action. These models are "bottom-up" in that processing is initiated by attention to incoming information. Let's take a closer look at these models beginning with attention.

As represented in Figure 1–3, the relative infinite amount of information in the subject's environment is significantly reduced by an attentional filter. Broadbent (1958, 1977) believed that this filter was a selective process enabling individuals to focus attention on only a few channels of incoming information. For example, subjects in a study might attend to a complex auditory message while ignoring the written message on a computer screen. Information from the visual channel typically dominates attentional processing (Posner et al. 1976).

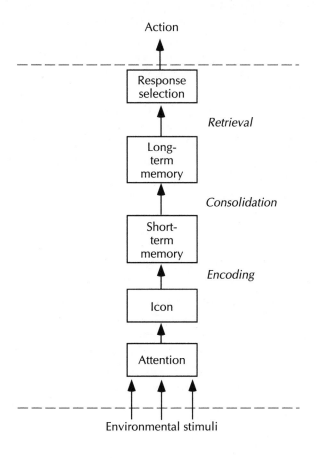

Figure 1–3. Bottom-up model of information processing that is initiated by selective attention to environmental stimuli.

Attended information then becomes the figural "snapshot" that is available in iconic memory for a very short time (Averbach and Coriell 1961; Sperling 1960). Most of this information is lost as the icon decays or is replaced by subsequent incoming information and only a few bytes of the original information remain. This information is encoded vis-à-vis extant memory traces so that information has meaning beyond its stimulus qualities. For example, the stimulus of a conglomeration of lines and curves and shades and hues is perceived to be the image of a human being.

The amount of information that can be held in short-term memory is relatively limited and decays quickly (G. A. Miller 1956). Short-term memory is often called *working memory* and refers to an individual's ability to report "what is currently on his or her mind." Depending on the individual's previous experience with incoming information, his or her mental set, and environmental conditions, some information in short-term memory will be consolidated into long-term memory (Atkinson and Shiffrin 1968). Investigators believe that information in long-term memory is sorted into categories, memory structures that are defined by a set of unique and descriptive attributes. Glass and Holyoak (1986) distinguished among three kinds of attributes: *physical properties* (e.g., "The **BALL**[2] category includes all things that are round."), *functional definitions*, in which a category is described in terms of the way it is used (e.g., **WEAPONS** are for fighting), and *relational attributes*, in which a category is defined by its relationship to other categories (e.g., an **ORPHAN** is a **CHILD** without **PARENTS**). Categories with similar attributes are proximal to each other in long-term memory storage.

Information in long-term memory may be retrieved in the future; two forms of retrieval have been described: *recognition* and *recall* (Mandler 1972; Rabinowitz et al. 1977). In terms of recognition, individuals may compare incoming information to categories in memory storage, thereby recognizing the data: "Oh, I know you, you're **MR. JONES**." Alternatively, the executive function (internal decision) of an individual may initiate a more active and cognitively demanding memory search to recall a perceptual instance. "Let's see. In the past, I've seen Mr. Jones and Ms. Smith at the street corner." Categories in long-term memory storage are frequently represented as nodes; the nodes vary in terms of activation level (Neely 1977; Neely et al. 1983). As the activation level of particular cues surpasses the activation level for a category, information in that category enters consciousness. Several variables influence activation level including *familiarity* (**CATS** and **DOGS** have higher activation

---

[2] Examples of information traces (i.e., unobservable cognitive phenomena such as visual stimuli, specific situational features, or categories in long-term memory) will be printed in **BOLD CAPS** throughout this chapter.

than **HYENAS** and **KOALAS** in the United States), *relationship to other categories* (it's easier to recall the state of **PENNSYLVANIA** if I am already thinking about **NEW JERSEY**), and *number of cues* (it's easier to recall a situation if more descriptors are provided) (Brown 1968).

The recall process also suggests the manner in which motoric responses are generated. A response may be elicited in reaction to an external stimulus (comparison function) or to an internal decision (executive function). The generated response may come from several motor actions that are arranged hierarchically in long-term memory storage (Broen and Storms 1966; Hull 1952). Positions in the response hierarchy vary in arousal level; the positions in long-term memory are determined based on past learning history and present situational demands. In highly familiar situations, the arousal of certain reactions exceeds most others, and individuals tend to respond automatically (i.e., with little conscious consideration of response alternatives and with little cognitive effort) (Hasher and Zacks 1979, 1984; Schneider and Shiffrin 1977). In less familiar situations, conscious consideration is necessary when arousal of a range of responses exceeds a response-strength ceiling. Individuals will select a response from these alternatives or, if unsatisfied with the options, search their memory again for other alternatives.

The cognitive processes in bottom-up models, and their juxtaposition to neighboring processes, readily suggest the possibility for cognitive problems. For example, according to Figure 1–3 cognitive deficits may result from 1) an overly restrictive attentional filter that results in patients missing key information or being bombarded by data, 2) sensory icons that are quickly disrupted by subsequent information, 3) inaccurate encoding of incoming information, 4) rapid decay of information from short-term memory, 5) diminished consolidation to long-term memory, 6) an inability to retrieve information in long-term storage, 7) impoverished set of responses available for selection, and 8) a random selection of responses from the response hierarchy. Similarly, these problem areas suggest specific rehabilitation strategies. For example, remediation of attentional deficits may include self-instruction strategies in which patients tell themselves to focus their attention on narrow stimulus bands, practice attentional tasks repeatedly, and use differential reinforcement for attention to targeted stimuli.

Much of the research from neuropsychology has tried to find CNS correlates to specific information processes. Milner (1966) provided a cogent example of this by showing, in several classic reports, that lesions in the hippocampus lead to significant diminutions in consolidating information from short- to long-term memory. Similarly, research in experimental psychopathology has attempted to demonstrate the specificity of processing deficits across nosological groups; for example, patients with traumatic injury to the frontal lobes are thought to have deficits in complex cognitive functions such as conceptual flexibility (Heaton 1981). If this body of research is fruitful, algorithms may be developed for prescribing cognitive rehabilitation strategies depending on the patient's CNS disturbance or pattern of psychopathology.

Bottom-up models suggest that information processing is both initiated at and controlled by environmental input. Attentional filters (and hence, the information processing system itself) are "turned on" after environmental stimuli impinge on the organism. Top-down processing might influence cognition as well; higher cognitive functions affect the performance of lower information processes. In fact, some of the serial stages listed above imply a top-down effect. For example, the long-term memory category that occurs higher up in Figure 1–3 affects the selection and encoding of incoming information. A serial information processing model actually includes complex feedback loops in which lower processes and higher cognitive functions influence one another.

Limits to Serial Processing

Serial models successfully present the complex phenomena related to cognition in a comprehensible model that consists of readily examinable, component processes. This model has generated a large body of important research for understanding the cognitive deficits of neuropsychiatric patients and strategies to ameliorate these deficits. However, subsequent research programs have identified limits to serial processing models. These alternative views have implications for development of rehabilitation strategies.

Modularity. The serial nature of information processing suggests that individual cognitive functions are significantly interrelated with other cognitive functions. Accordingly, measures of attentional functioning are expected to correlate with memory measures that in turn should be associated with conceptualization measures. A directional relationship is implied in this model. Deficits in attention, conceived as a primary information process, would significantly inhibit subsequent encoding and consolidation functions. However, discrete lesions that might impede consolidation of new information should have little effect on earlier information processes such as attention. Investigators have used the primacy of attentional deficits to account for all other cognitive deficits that patients with schizophrenia might show (Venables 1964).

Research, however, has suggested that cognitive functions have a greater degree of independence than that presumed by a serial model of processing. According to the theory of *modularity*, cognitive functions describe isolable subsystems that are domain specific; for example, domains may represent discrete cognitive functions such as attention, memory, conceptualization, and language (Fodor 1983; Marr 1982; Posner 1978; Shallice 1988; Tulving 1983). Predictions from modularity would suggest that deficits in attentional functioning would be relatively unrelated to memory functioning. These subsystems are present at birth and exist as hard-wired entities. Theorists vary on the degree of independence between cognitive modules; Fodor (1983) asserted that modules are "computationally autonomous," whereas Marr (1982) believed that modules varied in their degree of independence from subsystems.

A modularity model of information processing has significant implications for cognitive rehabilitation. Strategies that target attentional deficits should have little effect on memory problems. Hence, patients that show a profile of discrete deficits may need to participate in a series of different cognitive rehabilitation programs.

Capacity theory.   Serial models suggest that information processing begins with selecting targeted information and filtering out extraneous data. Contrary to this view, however, attention has been conceptualized as a limiting capacity that is allocated to multiple cognitive processes in the series (Kahneman 1973). According to this perspective, individual information processes require a finite cognitive capacity that is drawn from a capacity reservoir. Multiple functions, the sum of which does not exceed available capacity, can occur simultaneously (implying parallel processing, which is discussed in the next section). Kahneman believed that capacity demand increases as cognitive functions move from information-intake stages to more complex cognitive stages; hence, an individual may be able to attend to multiple sensory inputs more easily than recall various memory traces. In addition, tasks, or a combination of tasks, that exceed an individual's capacity limits will not be completed successfully. For example, most people easily attend to a chess game or to a television drama but find that watching both simultaneously exhausts their cognitive capacity.

One implication of capacity theory is that cognitive deficits in neuropsychiatric disorders may not be related to deficits in discrete cognitive functions. Rather, factors that diminish capacity level may trickle down to hamper several discrete information processes. Nuechterlein and Dawson (1984) completed an elegant review of the cognitive literature in which they showed that the various deficits of schizophrenia may be efficiently explained by capacity limits.

Kahneman (1973) identified several factors that affect capacity levels in Figure 1–4; these include psychophysiological arousal and processing capacity. Using a Yerkes Dodson model, the relationship between arousal and processing capacity is described by an inverted U. Available capacity, and hence processing efficacy, are minimal during periods of low and high arousal. The capacity reservoir is at its greatest level during moderate arousal levels. Patient populations with tonic hypo- or hyperarousal should have diminished cognitive functioning. For example, Gjerde (1983) has argued that the aberrant arousal levels characteristic of schizophrenia account for diminished capacity and hence impeded processing. The relationship between arousal and capacity has implications for development of rehabilitation strategies (Spaulding et al. 1986). Rehabilitation interventions that teach patients to moderate arousal level will help patients increase available capacity. Such strategies can be proactive, wherein patients avoid stressful situations that may lead to overarousal, or reactive where they might learn coping skills that can be helpful for future, potentially overwhelming situations.

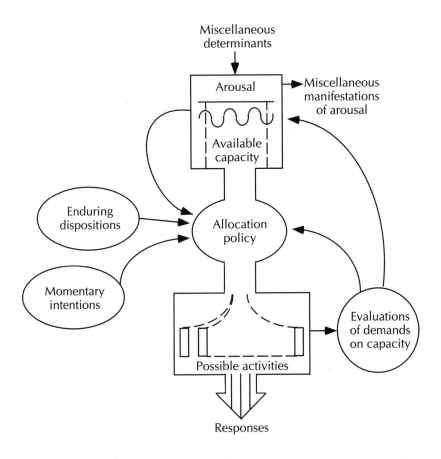

Figure 1–4.   Daniel Kahneman's model of processing capacity that outlines factors affecting available capacity. *Source.* Kahneman D: *Attention and Effort.* Englewood Cliffs, NJ, Prentice-Hall, 1973, p. 10. Reprinted by permission of Prentice-Hall, Inc. Copyright 1973.

Processing capacity also diminishes as an individual gains experience with a task. Novel tasks are relatively effortful and demand substantially more capacity than tasks that have been practiced multiple times in the past and are relatively automatic (Hasher and Zacks 1979, 1984; Schneider and Shiffrin 1977). Fitts and Posner (1967) outlined a two-phase process that helps a cognitive task or behavioral skill move from effortful to automatic processing. During the cognitive phase, the learner must consciously and actively rehearse the new task; for example, as individuals learn to decipher a secret code they must continuously repeat decoding strategies to themselves aloud. Functioning at this step is slow and awkward. During the associative phase, conscious mediation of the task is no longer necessary. The individual can now quickly decode the message without having to rehearse each step.

Because cognitive capacity is allocated to effortful processes (that have not become automatic), neuropsychiatric deficits may occur. Alternatively, cognitive deficits might be specific to high-demand effortful tasks. For example, research suggests that depressed persons have significant difficulty on effortful tasks, whereas automaticity of performance on tests that require automatic responses remains intact (Hartlage et al. 1993). Beck's (1967, 1976) assertions that the role automatic negative thinking plays in developing and maintaining depressive symptoms are supported by the idea that automaticity remains intact. This problem seems to be uniquely descriptive of depressed populations compared with patients with anxiety disorders, schizophrenia, or senile dementia.

Clinicians can facilitate capacity retrieval for brain-damaged patients by helping them to automatize effortful tasks. Repeated practice and mnemonic strategies help to reduce the cognitive demand of novel tasks. Dividing an effortful task into steps that require less capacity also can be helpful.

Parallel distributed processing.   Serial processing models, which represent cognition as a step-by-step event with one information byte in the processing unit at a time, provide an inefficient representation of cognition; this representation does not correspond with data about the manner in which information is actually processed. For example, given the time constraints of the functioning nervous system, perhaps only a hundred processing steps can be accomplished serially in the half-second between perceiving and responding to an environmental stimulus (Feldman 1981). In actuality, however, this simple cognitive event probably requires hundreds or thousands of steps to complete. Parallel processing models, like the one implied by the capacity theory, suggest that several cognitive events occur simultaneously during simple tasks.

McClelland and Rumelhart (1985) diagrammed the general case of the parallel distributed processing (PDP) model reproduced here in Figure 1–5, *A*.

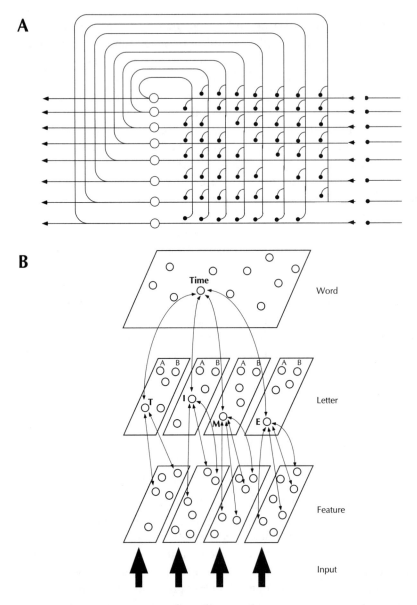

Figure 1–5. The parallel distributed processing model. *A*: Outline of the general case. *B*: Restricted model as applied to word recognition. *Sources. A*: Reprinted from McClelland JL: "Putting Knowledge in Its Place: A Scheme for Programming Parallel Processing Structures on the Fly." *Cognitive Science* 9:113–146, 1985. Used with permission. *B*: Reprinted from McClelland JL, Rumelhart DE: "Distributed Memory and the Representation of General and Specific Information." *Journal of Experimental Psychology General* 114:159–188, 1985. Copyright 1985 by the American Psychological Association. Reprinted by permission.

In PDP models, cognitive events consist of multiple interconnected units; in the general case, all units are interconnected, receive input from the environment, and send output to the environment. In the simplest models, connections between units are excitatory or inhibitory (on-off switches). In more restricted examples of the general case, some units may receive no input from, nor give output to, the environment and may be unconnected to other units. A PDP model of word recognition is provided in Figure 1–5, *B* as an example of the restricted model (McClelland 1985; McClelland and Rumelhart 1981). Units represent hypotheses about sensory input that are arranged in three levels: *feature level, letter level,* and *word level.* Interconnections between unit levels may be excitatory or inhibitory. For example, the horizontal crossbar of the T will excite the appropriate unit at the feature level and inhibit features representing curves. The combined features are interconnected and excite the T unit at the letter level; similar letters like X will be inhibited. The combination of letter units will excite the **TIME** unit at the word level.

PDP models have been helpful for the development and testing of several components of cognition including active representation of information processing, knowledge, and learning; interested readers should review texts by McClelland, Rumelhart, and the PDP Research Group (1986) and, more recently, by Morris (1989b). Discussion of cognitive events, à la PDP, is significantly different than discussion of other information processing models because it avoids reliance on the multitude of *hypothetical* constructs assumed to underlie specific processes. For example, instead of the construct of active representation requiring "encoding," "consolidation," "categorization," and "retrieval," the manner in which information is represented and subsequently recalled can be modeled by the interconnected network of units and the changing pattern of graded excitation and inhibition represented by those connections. Therefore, models of the entire cognitive process can be conceived and all components of the model can be measured. The huge number of units and connections in PDP models resemble the billions of somas and dendrites in the CNS. In fact, PDP models have an intimate history with neurobiology such that investigators from that discipline have described neurological and cognitive events in terms of the network of units and connections (Morris 1989a). Unlike neuropsychologists who attempt to define discrete information functions in terms of CNS organs, PDP investigators are attempting to describe finite cognitive events in terms of the interaction of discrete neural mechanisms. New forms of computational modeling have been derived to address stochastic issues related to the exceedingly large number of interconnected units (Jordan 1986; Williams 1986).

Although PDP models have more than a 15-year history of representing cognitive processes, transposition of these models to understand neuropsychiatric deficits has, as of yet, been a limited enterprise. For example, PDP models have only recently been used to describe the myriad of cognitive deficits found in schizophrenic patients (Cohen and Servan-Schreiber 1990). PDP models may redirect the focus of understanding cognitive deficits. Rather than trying to identify the structural foci or the processing module that suggests a cognitive deficit, understanding breakdowns at the level of units, connections, and patterns may provide better description of processing deficit.

Signal Detection and Information Processing

Performance on many of the information processing functions discussed in this section is measured using indices such as correct identification (the frequency in which an individual says a target stimulus is present when it in fact was) and false-positive rate (the frequency in which a stimulus is reported as observed when it was not present). For example, in an attention task in which subjects are to report when they see the number 0 flash in a series of single digits, hit rate is the number of 0s correctly identified; false-positive rate is the number of digits other than 0 reported as 0. Unfortunately, correct identification and false-positive rates are biased measures of the subject's true sensitivity to the cognitive function of interest.

For example, a subject's report of seeing a flashing light depends not only on the individual's actual sensory experience, but also on the perceived payoff for correct versus incorrect responses. Subjects who are told that they will be paid $1 each time they report seeing a light stimulus (when the light was present) will respond more freely than peers who are told that they will lose $1 for each stimulus report that does not correspond with the presence of the light. Other factors have been found to affect rate of correct identification: the frequency of previous experience with the vigilance task, task instructions and performance feedback, and the ratio of test stimuli to distractor noise in the task (Davies and Parasuraman 1982). Therefore, measures of information processing that report rate of correct identification as the index of performance, in fact, are presenting a variable representing the individual's decision criteria based on the cognitive task.

Signal detection theory (SDT) has sought nonbiased parameters of an individual's sensitivity to cognitive tasks; original work in this area was limited to the subject's sensitivity to vigilance tasks (Broadbent and Gregory 1963; Green and Swets 1966; Swets 1964). According to SDT, two normal distributions—much like the ones in Figure 1–6—that represent the probability of deciding either "signal" or "noise" are presented and show the subject's response to a simple vigilance task. Assuming equal variance in noise and signal distributions, the detectability index, d', equals the difference between the means of the two distributions. For a vigilance task in which it is difficult to discriminate signal from noise, such as hearing a voice in a noisy room, the two distributions will greatly overlap and the difference between distribution means will be small. Conversely, vigilance tasks where signal and noise are grossly divergent, such as hearing a gunshot in a quiet meadow, will result in two distributions with no overlap and d' will be large. As an unbiased parameter of vigilance, d' is unaffected by decision payoffs. So, although correct identification will increase and decrease with changing rewards for hits, d' will remain constant.

Regardless of d', individuals might choose a criterion level on the decision axis that yields a set probability for correct identification, x_k, in Figure 1–6. Observed stimuli greater than this criterion would be reported "present," and stimuli below the cutoff would be reported "not present." The criterion value for x_k, called *beta*, moves to the left as the individual wants to maximize correct identifications (but also risks false-positives) and to the right as the individual chooses a more conservative response set with less false-positives and less correct identifications.

Derivations of d' and *beta* for vigilance tasks require that signal and noise distributions be normal and have equal variance. Unfortunately, many experimental tests of vigilance do not meet such rigorous criteria, thereby necessitating nonparametric measures of sensitivity and response criterion. Davies and Parasuraman (1982) discussed ways to calculate estimates of d' and *beta* without meeting these rigorous requirements. Many of these indices are algebraic combinations of correct identification and false-positive rates.

SDT assumptions derived from vigilance tasks also may be violated when applying this model to cognitive tasks such as recognition or recall memory (Banks 1970; Lockhart and Murdock 1970). Vigilance assumptions include the following: 1) signal and noise are externally generated, 2) probability of occurrence of

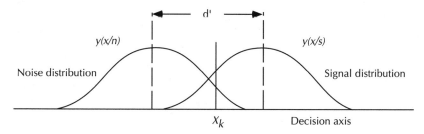

Figure 1–6. Signal detection model of auditory stimulus perception. Perceived brightness is plotted on the *x* axis and the probability of perceiving brightness is plotted on the *y* axis. *Source.* Reprinted from Davies DR, Parasuraman R: *The Psychology of Vigilance.* New York, Academic Press, 1982. Used with permission.

signal and noise conditions are under experimenter control, and 3) range of decision options is presented in a forced choice format (e.g., "Yes or no: Did you see the light?"). During memory tasks, however, both signal and noise are internally generated such that a priori memory distributions and noise traces are not solely under the experimenter's control. Furthermore, during recall tasks, the range of responses is much larger than in the forced-choice paradigm found in many vigilance tasks. Keeping these problems in mind, Banks (1970) concluded that nonparametric indices may accurately represent subjects' sensitivity to recognition memory tasks. However, he believed that measures of recall-memory sensitivity challenge SDT assumptions significantly and therefore need to be interpreted more cautiously. Despite this caveat, investigators have been able to use nonparametric SDT indices to significantly enhance understanding of memory functioning in psychiatric populations (Corrigan and Green 1991; Sahgal 1987; Snodgrass and Corwin 1988).

SDT principles have methodological implications for studying cognitive deficits of neuropsychiatric populations. Cognitive measures that report correct identification rate as the index of performance may be representing a processing deficit in terms of response biases (that depend on the situation), rather than in terms of a subject variable reflecting the disease course. For example, a hit rate of 50% on a vigilance task may represent the patient's current motivation level given his or her perceptions of the payoff for responses. Identification rate would change as the patient's perception of external payoffs changes or as the individual's experience with the task increases. SDT sensitivity measures are unaffected by these factors, are relatively unchanged as a result, and therefore are more uniquely representative of a patient's performance on the task in question.

SDT also has interesting implications for the use of reinforcement and punishment in cognitive rehabilitation. Several studies have investigated the effects of using reinforcing contingencies as a strategy to improve performance on vigilance or memory tasks. For example, schizophrenic subjects in a reaction-time task were given 5¢ (reinforcement) each time they accurately key-pressed after a test stimulus (e.g., a light) was presented and they did not react to a distractor stimulus (a tone) (Meiselman 1973). Subjects in this study improved their correct-identification rate; they correctly key-pressed in response to lights more often. However, given the manner in which false-positives are linked to correct identification rate—and assuming that correct-identification and false-positive rates vary for patient populations as suggested in SDT—subjects' error rates probably increased as well; that is, they incorrectly key-pressed at a higher rate to tones. Hence, patients' sensitivity to the task did not improve. This is not to deny the usefulness of improving correct-identification rates. Investigators merely need to be aware of the manner in which these findings are confounded.

Cognitive Schemata

Information processing models describe the cognitive functions that external information passes through as it is encoded, adapted, transposed, and stored; models also describe how internal information is retrieved, modified, and reacted to. A parallel theoretical body of literature has developed that describes the complicated manner in which information is represented and the effects these representations have on an individual's cognition and behavior. This body of literature was alluded to in the discussion of information processes where representation of knowledge was presented via principles of categorization. Categories are groups of perceived phenomena and cognitive constructs that vary in terms of abstraction (from the concrete chair to the abstract sitting implement). Categories are arranged hierarchically. Linnaeus's zoological taxonomy is a good example: kingdom, phylum, class, order, family, genus, and species. For example, superordinate **ANIMALS** include **MAMMALS, BIRDS**, and **REPTILES. BIRDS** include **DUCKS, CANARIES**, and **PARROTS**. Categorical membership is determined by inclusion and exclusion criteria with some criteria being central (**BIRDS FLY AND HAVE WINGS, BIRDS DO NOT BREAST-FEED THEIR YOUNG**), whereas others are extraneous (**A FEW BIRDS SING**).

Categories introduce economy and efficiency into the cognitive process. As cognitive schema, categories provide the templates through which new or incoming information is encoded and comprehended (Mandler 1967; Tulving 1962). For example, the influence of schema in comprehending textual material can be seen in the following test item from a study by Bransford and Johnson (1972). Subjects were instructed to read the following passage:

> The procedure is actually quite simple. First you arrange things into different groups. Of course, one pile may be sufficient depending on how much there is to do. If you have to go somewhere else due to lack of facilities that is the next step, otherwise you are pretty well set. It is important not to overdo things. That is, it is better to do too few things at once than too many. In the short run, this may not seem important but complications can easily arise. A mistake can be expensive as well. At first the whole procedure will seem complicated. . . . (p. 722)

After completing the paragraph, subjects were told to recall as much of the text as possible. The control group had a very difficult time recalling significant chunks of this text. The experimental group, however, was told before reading the passage that it was about "Doing the Laundry." The addition of this orienting schema resulted in significantly better recall.

Generally, categories are thought to be mutually exclusive; for example, the **ANIMAL** exemplar is either a **BIRD** or a **MAMMAL**; the person is either

DOING THE LAUNDRY or MAKING DINNER. However, rather than having firm boundaries, there are perceptual and cognitive phenomena that tend to blend categories. For example, traditional principles of categorization would predict that stimulus colors are divisible into discrete categories. However, research suggests that a continuum of categories would be more appropriate (Berlin and Kay 1969). Even the most rigid of categories can have its fuzzy bounds. As an example, stimulus items 15 through 19 in Figure 1–7 seem to stretch the limits of the CUP category. In addition, there also are many objects that may earn membership in multiple categories at the same level of the hierarchy BATS ARE MAMMALS THAT FLY.

There exist frequently used concepts in the vernacular for which definition of categorical criteria is difficult. For example, Wittgenstein (1953) posed the question, "What is a game?" Most people would sort baseball, poker, tag, dancing, and checkers into the game category. However, characteristics cannot be easily defined to describe each exemplar. GAME is an especially pertinent example of a "fuzzy concept" for human behavior. Would individuals group some of the games people play identified in Berne's book *Games People Play* (1964) with other recreational activities above?

Some investigators have argued that information is stored in terms of family resemblances and prototypes rather than distinctive categories (Rosch et al. 1976). Prototypes represent the central tendencies of the categories of information. The *similarity* of exemplars to the prototype defines the exemplar's membership into the category. For example, stimulus item 15 in Figure 1–7 might be considered the prototype of CUP, and membership into this category would depend on the exemplar similarity to this item. Several studies have shown that subjects consensually agree on the typicality of prototypes vis-à-vis a set of exemplars (Rips et al. 1973; Rosch 1974, 1975a, 1975b; Rosch and Mervis 1975). Limitations in the categorical approach to knowledge structures are diminished by changing the focus away from defining boundaries between groups to defining the central tendencies of these groups. Although limits to the prototype theory also exist (Glass and Holyoak 1986), the model has produced useful strategies for studying the manner in which social information is represented.

Social Schemata

Just as there are categories and prototypes that define objects, knowledge structures that describe key interpersonal constructs also exist. Social schemata are the templates by which social information is encoded as well as the blueprints that guide interpersonal responses. Research has focused on three sets of schemata—knowledge structures that represent situations, persons, and self.

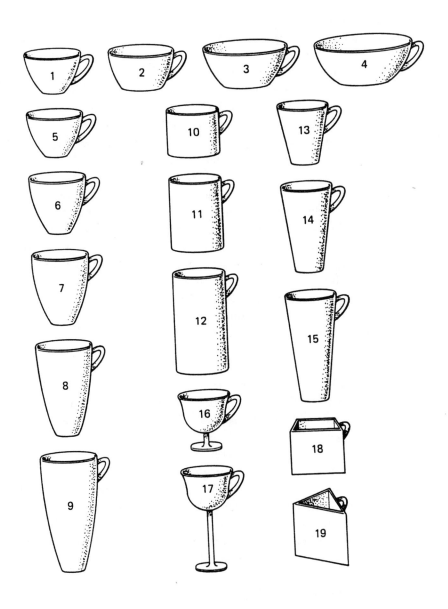

Figure 1–7. Objects in a cup category from Labov (1973). Notice how objects 18 and 19 would not meet standard definitions of **CUP**. *Source.* Reprinted from Glass AL, Holyoak KJ: *Cognition*, 2nd Edition. New York, Random House, 1986. Used with permission of McGraw-Hill.

Situational schema.   Research on situational schemata, also called scripts by some investigators (Galambos et al. 1986; Schank and Abelson 1977), is especially germane to rehabilitation because performance of social skills has been shown to be directly related to perception and processing of situational cues (Forgas 1983; Trower 1986). Hence, investigators have sought to outline the relationship between skill acquisition and *performance of cues* and processing of situational schema (Corrigan and Green 1993b). Several features have been identified that make up the schematic descriptions of situations (Argyle 1986; Avedon 1971). Examples of some common situational features are provided in Table 1–1. These features are related hierarchically (i.e., definition of certain features restrict the range of subordinate features). For example, goals defined by a specific situation narrow the set of rules that define the social interaction. The goals implied by driving into a hamburger joint—TO GET SANDWICHES FAST—preclude rules about social banter between waitress and customer that might be found at a coffee shop. Similarly, the role a person assumes in a situation defines the actions he or she may try: CHEFS COOK AT THE RESTAURANT; HOMEMAKERS EAT AT THE RESTAURANT AND COOK AT HOME.

Situational features have been further defined by several descriptors that help to distinguish among features. Galambos (1986) outlined three such descriptors: distinctiveness, standardness, and centrality. *Feature distinctiveness* refers to whether the goal, rule, role, action, or setting occurs in one or many different situations. For example, Galambos pointed out that seeing the head waiter is distinctive of GOING TO THE RESTAURANT because it is found in few, if any, other situations. *Standardness* refers to the frequency with which the feature occurs in a situation. HOSTS greet most people in restaurants, whereas having a WINE STEWARD is more characteristic of the fanciest of eating establishments. The first role is high and the second low in standardness.

The *centrality* of a feature represents how important that goal, rule, role, action, and setting is to the situation. In one study, Galambos found that subjects could arrive at a consensus regarding which of several actions—SEE HEAD WAITER, TIP THE WAITER, ASK FOR MENU, or EAT MEAL—are important when in the situation. The four actions listed above are arranged in ascending centrality. Similarly, WAITER, COOK, and CUSTOMER, are more central roles of EATING AT A RESTAURANT than PASTRY CHEF and BUSINESS MANAGER.

Galambos (1986) has described a fourth feature descriptor that is specific to situational actions, *sequence*. Actions in many situations have a sequential relationship to other actions. For example, restaurant patrons would expect the four actions in the preceding example to be in a set sequence: SEE HEAD WAITER, ASK FOR MENU, EAT MEAL, and TIP THE WAITER. Schank and

Table 1–1. Features that comprise situational schemata

Feature	Example EATING OUT AT A RESTAURANT
Goals: Individuals enter social situations to pursue certain needs or drives.	"To satiate my hunger." "To visit with friends."
Rules: Cognitive prescripts that govern interactions.	"Wait at the door to be seated." "Pay the waiter after you receive the check."
Settings: The physical environments in which the situation occurs.	"We went out to eat at a fancy café." "The hamburgers were picked up at McDonald's."
Roles: The positions individuals assume in situations defined by distinct patterns of behavior.	"Bartender, Waitress, Chef, Busboy, and Customer."
Actions: The repertoire of motor behaviors from which persons in the role might draw.	"Customers might order food, eat food, make small talk, and pay the bill." "Waitresses might review what's on the menu, take the order, serve the food, and clear the table."

Note. Examples in the table represent situational schema that describe **EATING OUT AT A RESTAURANT.**

Abelson (1977) pointed out that the strength of sequencing effects varies across situations. Order of actions is poorly prescribed in weak situations such as a work day in an office setting. The business executive may start with paperwork one day, a breakfast meeting another day, or a conference call the third day. There is little predictability regarding what will happen in situations such as these. Conversely, action sequence can be highly prescribed in ceremonial situations such as church services or college graduations. The sequential order of actions is so compelling that individuals quickly notice when actions are out of step in strong situations (Schank and Abelson 1977) and are more likely to remember the out of order element when recalling the situation in the future (Graesser et al. 1980).

In a particularly elegant test of the effects of sequencing and centrality on retrieval of information from memory, Galambos and Rips (1982) had subjects respond "yes" or "no" to whether a series of actions were part of an activity, as in the following example:

CHANGING A FLAT
RAISE THE CAR
REMOVE THE TIRE

Stimulus actions varied in their order in the situational sequence (early versus late) and in their centrality (low versus high). Results summarized in Figure 1–8 suggest that centrality significantly affected speed of retrieval, whereas situational sequence did not.

Person schema.   Personality theorists presume that individuals have enduring traits that explain current functioning as well as predict future behavior across multiple situations. Personality traits, however, may be epiphenomena that result from the prototypic manner in which individuals perceive others. Whether or not an individual acts consistently across situations, they are perceived to do so because their actions are understood in terms of various person schema (Cantor and Mischel 1979). For example, an **EXTROVERTED** schema defines individual exemplars as outgoing, chatty, and personable. If a person is perceived by others to be outgoing, then he or she would be expected to be chatty and personable. Information that diverges from schema-congruent expectations stands out clearly against the background schema and is more likely to be recalled in the future (Cantor and Mischel 1977). People are more likely to remember incidents when an extravert was shy than when that person was outgoing.

Our understanding of other persons, therefore, is encoded in terms of a large taxonomy of personality schemata (Cantor and Mischel 1979; Mischel, 1976). Elements in these taxonomies may relate hierarchically as outlined in Figure 1–9. Superordinate descriptors are the most abstract and subtend the greatest number of attributes. For example, the emotionally unstable person in Figure 1–9 includes descriptors specific to both mid-level categories. Mid-level and subordinate descriptors are more concrete and represent specific instances of the superordinate class.

Cantor and Mischel (1979) identified several characteristics of person schema including richness, differentiation, and concreteness. *Richness* of person schema subtend larger sets of attributes. Generally, more abstract, superordinate schema have larger sets of attributes. *Differentiation* refers to the amount of attributional overlap between two-person schemata. A **PLEASANT PERSON** and an **EXTROVERT** share many attributes and therefore have low differentiation. Prototypical opposites such as introverts and extroverts have

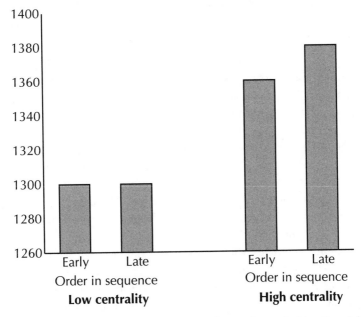

Figure 1–8. The interaction of sequence order and centrality on decision time. Adapted from data by Galambos JA, Rips LJ: Memory for routines. *Journal of Verbal Learning and Verbal Behavior* 21:260–281, 1982.

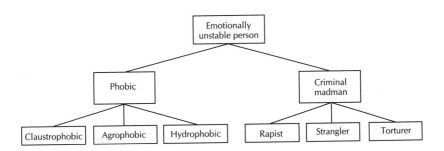

Figure 1–9. Person schema that represent conceptualizations of people with mental illness. Note that the superordinate concept of emotionally disturbed contains many familiar subordinates. Adapted from Cantor N, Mischel W: Prototypes in person perception, in *Advances in Experimental Social Psychology*, Vol 12. Edited by Berkowitz L. New York, Academic Press, 1979, pp. 4–52.

little overlap and high differentiation. Person schema also vary in terms of quality of content or *concreteness*. Personal ttributes have been divided into four groups: physical appearance or possessions, socioeconomic status, traits (e.g., happy or gloomy), or behavioral attributes (e.g., runs to the train, is sloppy).

Self-schema.   There are prototypes that affect persons' perception and comprehension of themselves; these prototypes help individuals make some sense of the pattern of thoughts, emotions, and behaviors they exhibit. A schema view of self reframes a psychodynamic construct as an abstract representation of past experiences and present data. The presence and effects of self-schemata have been inferred from one study where the self-statements of subjects were observed to go from overly generalized comments (e.g., I'm open minded) to conditional statements based on the situation (e.g., I'm a hard worker when I'm at the office) (Jones et al. 1974). Cantor and Mischel (1979) called this pattern "linguistic hedges" and found it to be characteristic of schematized statements. Self-reference is envisioned as a process involving the interaction between previous experience with personal data and new stimulus input.

Self-schema are extremely powerful agents in organizing information. For example, the effects of self-schema on recall memory have been shown in two studies. Rogers et al. (1977) instructed subjects to encode stimulus adjectives according to one of four strategies: *structural* (Stimulus word has big letters?), *phonemic* (Stimulus word rhymes with xxxx?), *semantic* (Stimulus word means same as yyyy?), or *self-referent* (Stimulus word describes you?). Craik and Lockhart (1972) had previously argued that subjects encode information in hierarchical levels such that information encoded at deeper levels will be recalled better at later times. Craik and Tulving (1975) showed that the levels of processing vary for structural, phonemic, and semantic encoding with rate of eventual recall corresponding with the ascending order of these three conditions. Rogers et al. (1977) showed that self-referent encoding yielded the best recall scores of all four levels.

In a second study, self-schemata were shown to result in more false alarms in a recall task, a finding consistent with schema theory (Rogers et al. 1979). Subjects in the study incorrectly identified nontest words as stimuli in a test list more frequently when these words had been previously self-rated as similar to the individual. This finding is similar to conclusions from research on situational schema (Galambos et al. 1986); namely, actions are more likely to be recalled as having occurred in a situation (when they actually did not) if the actions are consistent with schematized portrayals of the events.

Kuiper (1981) mapped out the effects of self-schema on reaction time. Subjects were instructed to key-press "yes" or "no" in response to whether or not several adjectives varied in similarity to the individual; subjects rated the adjective's similarity to themselves on a 9-point scale in a separate task. Results showed that the relationship between adjective similarity and reaction time was defined by an inverted U-curve, with reaction times being shortest for adjectives rated as very similar or very dissimilar.

Mood influences the processing of self-schemata (Hartlage et al. 1993; Matt et al. 1992). Research has shown that individuals with "normal" moods display superior recall for positive self-referent adjectives (e.g., loyal, organized) than negative adjectives (e.g., bleak, dismal) (Kuiper and Derry 1981; Kuiper and MacDonald 1982). However, individuals with a depressed mood show equal recall for positive and negative self-referent adjectives. If the functioning of nondepressed subjects is viewed as baseline, depressed mood may be viewed as causing the effects of negative self-schemata to be more pronounced.

Mood and Cognitive Representation

These models have been described, for the most part, as cold cognition models of knowledge representation. The effects of mood and affect—hot cognition—was alluded to briefly in discussing information processing and arousal. Ability to recognize and recall information depends on the learner's affect when acquiring the information and when retrieving it. Simply put, this phenomenon would suggest that words learned under one mood (e.g., happy) would be recalled at a higher rate under the same mood (happy) than under a different mood (sad). This hypothesis has not been consistently supported, however (Bower et al. 1978), leading Bower (1989) to hypothesize a more complex crossover effect to explain mood-congruent learning. A study describing this assumption is outlined in Figure 1–10.

In Trial 1, subjects were instructed to learn word list A under either sad or happy mood-induction conditions. In Trial 2, they were asked to learn list B under the same or a different mood condition. Finally, during Trial 3, they were asked to recall list A under mood conditions that were the same as or different from the moods in Trial 1. Results, as shown in Figure 1–10, illustrate the crossover effect. Subjects recalled significantly more words when in the same mood as when they originally learned the words. Moreover, there was no main effect for mood. In other words, subjects who learned the words "sad" did no better nor worse than subjects who learned "happy."

Mood-congruent memory has been shown in other studies as well. For example, subjects in another study by Bower (1989) were instructed to keep copious diaries about their week's experiences, rating individual incidents on a pleasantness scale. At the end of the week, pleasant or unpleasant moods were hypnotically induced in subjects after which they were instructed to recall

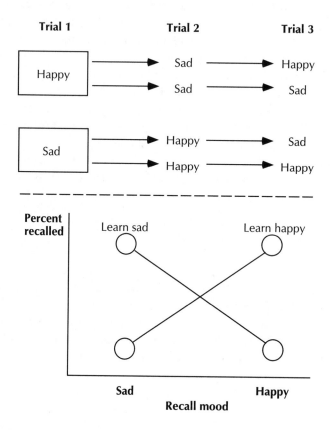

Figure 1–10.   Subjects who recalled test words in a mood that was congruent with the learning mood scored significantly higher than subjects who learned the items in one mood (e.g., sad) and recalled in another (happy). Adapted from Bower GH: "Mood and Memory." *Am Psychol* 36:129–148, 1989.

as many incidents from the list as they could. Results showed a crossover effect once again. Individuals in the pleasant state recalled more pleasant incidents, whereas subjects in the unpleasant mood recalled unpleasant events.

Does this mood and memory relationship appear in affective disorders? In one study, the number of free associations to stimulus words were counted as manic patients cycled into depression (Henry et al. 1973). Results showed that the number of "euphoric" associations decreased significantly as the patient normalized and then became depressed. These findings suggest that patients' mood and agitation must be considered when attempting to affect their knowledge structures using rehabilitation strategies.

Relevance of Cognitive Schemata for Cognitive Rehabilitation

Models of cognitive schemata and interpersonal prototypes are in many ways relatively more ecologically valid representations of thinking. Rather than describing remote processes such as attention and iconic memory, schema theorists describe the manner in which real-world information is understood and stored. Note, however, that as the generalizability of cognitive models increases—as the assumptions of situational schema apply more directly to everyday information—the generalizability of specific corollaries ironically diminishes. For example, situational schema describe information specific to interpersonal circumstances and are relatively extraneous to understanding other domains of knowledge. On the other hand, the construct of attention applies to a primary cognitive function in all domains of knowledge: attending to math homework, attending to the action at the neighborhood hamburger joint, attending to the personality characteristics of one's spouse, and attending to the mood variations in one's self.

In terms of rehabilitation strategies, if the effects of interventions from information processing models generalize, then targeting discrete processing functions such as attention, memory, and conceptual flexibility should lead to enhanced functioning in all knowledge domains. However, if rehabilitation strategies based on information processing models do not effectively generalize, then clinical investigators should develop more discrete training strategies. Perhaps patients need to be differentially trained to attend to, and encode, the features of a situation versus the characteristics of a personality or the fluctuations of the self.

Findings from schema theory also provide productive heuristics for experimental psychopathology. Qualitative differences between specific schema may account for differential deficits in various neuropsychiatric populations. For example, research suggests that content of situational and person schemata affect patient processing. Depressed populations have been shown to be more sensitive to the negative rather than to the positive content of schema (Blaney 1986; Matt et al. 1992). Similarly, patients with schizophrenia are better able to identify negative facial affect (e.g., angry, depressed, or worried) than more pleasant facial emotions (Morrison et al. 1988).

Neuropsychiatric patients also are more likely to blur the boundaries between social schema, thereby confusing informational groups. Research suggests that patients with severe and chronic mental illness show over-inclusive thinking (Payne 1966). That is, the set of rules these patients use to define categories is much larger than the normal categorical criteria. As a result, the schema used to encode and understand information do not reflect the neat categories of nondepressed people; situations and people are perceived incorrectly.

Features that define situations and persons vary in level of abstraction. For example, goals and rules (e.g., the man yelled because he was angry) that define a social situation require more abstract processing than the more fundamental actions and roles (e.g., the man cooked an egg because he is a chef). Therefore, schizophrenic and depressed-patient populations with demonstrated deficits in abstraction tasks that require high-capacity demand (Hartlage et al. 1993; Nuechterlein and Dawson 1984) should identify the abstract features of social schema less effectively. This hypothesis has been supported by a recent study on schizophrenic patients (Corrigan and Green 1993b).

Cognitive, psychophysiological, and neurochemical processes alone may not cause the diminished social schema found in neuropsychiatric populations. Development of social schema depends on an individual's experience with exemplars of various situations and persons. Individuals with impoverished lifestyles will have less opportunity to interact with different settings and persons and, therefore, should have a narrower range of social schema. This fact suggests that neuropsychiatric patients with chronic histories of illness, or whose onset of illness was at an early age, may have experienced a variety of institutionalized impoverishment that impeded acquisition of various schemata. Research that supports this hypothesis suggests that environmental-enrichment programs, which expose patients to a vast array of events, may facilitate cognitive rehabilitation goals.

Problem Solving and Decision Making

The last cognitive model discussed in this chapter is problem solving and decision making. Social interactions represent "puzzles" that need to be figured out and acted on. According to problem-solving models, social information is processed sequentially such that output from early stages (e.g., identification of a problem situation) becomes the input for subsequent stages (e.g., generation of solutions to the situation). Problem-solving models yield a means-end analytic paradigm of social situations. Human beings are perceived to be rational agents who select means (various interpersonal and coping skills) that help them satisfy their social ends (instrumental or affectional goals) (Trower 1982).

Investigators have divided problem solving into several cognitive steps or stages (McFall 1982; Wallace 1982; Wallace et al. 1980). Wallace (1982) divided problem solving into three sets of cognitive skills: receiving, processing, and sending skills. The relationship between these skills and the serial stages of linear information processing is evident. *Receiving skills* include processes by which patients identify the content of interpersonal messages as well as the concomitant emotions and intents communicated by another. *Processing skills* define the situational goals toward which individuals strive as well as plans for achieving these ends.

Sending skills include observable behaviors that follow from goals and plans; these are skills people actually implement to resolve the problem.

Behavior therapists have listed several steps that make up interpersonal problem solving (D'Zurilla 1986; D'Zurilla and Goldfried 1971); an example of social problem solving in seven steps is illustrated in Table 1–2. According to this outline, problem solving begins with a confident "problem-solving" attitude. Individuals must believe that their attempts at understanding and acting on interpersonal difficulties will end successfully. Bandura (1977) has shown that individuals who expect their efforts to be successful are more likely to carry out an innovative behavioral agenda.

People begin to resolve their individual problems by defining difficulties in terms of the specific situation and people involved. In Table 1–2, Frank is angry because John does not keep the kitchen clean. The problem also involves their roommate, Harry, who uses the kitchen. Problem solving works best when all relevant parties are included, so Frank needs to ask John and Harry to join him in fixing the problem. Individuals are then encouraged to generate solution alternatives and are instructed not to censor alternatives at this stage of problem solving. Costs and benefits to each alternative are then considered and, based on the resulting ratio, individuals select the alternative that best addresses the problem at that time. The involved parties as a group plan out the chosen solution, making sure to specifically address when and where the alternative will be implemented and what resources are needed to complete the solution. Problem solving includes a feedback loop. Some time after the plan is implemented, involved parties should get together again and discuss the plan's success.

Problem-solving skills have been shown to be significantly lacking in psychiatric populations (Platt and Spivack 1972a, 1972b). More than likely, research on patients with neuropsychological deficits would find similar limitations in problem-solving skills. Individual strengths in receiving, processing, and sending skills that make up problem solving have been shown to be significantly correlated with verbal intelligence (Corrigan and Toomey 1995; Donahoe et al. 1990). Hence, patients with higher verbal intelligence are more likely to learn and subsequently use problem-solving skills; however, mentally retarded individuals may require some adjunctive training procedures to facilitate acquisition of these skills.

Critics challenge whether the means-end analysis implied in social problem solving represents the real-world manner in which people understand and resolve interpersonal difficulties (Bellack et al. 1989). Many interpersonal problems cannot be dissected into neat components that become the targets of behavioral responses. Instead, problems are frequently experienced as "ill-structured" such that individuals are unable to define the problem or, even more pointedly,

Table 1–2.   Steps of social problem solving

Step 1:	**Adopt a problem-solving attitude.**
	"I think this problem can be solved."
	"I've had success with similar difficulties in the past."
Step 2:	**Identify the problem.**
	"My roommate, John, messes up the kitchen each morning."
Step 3:	**Brainstorm solutions.**
	"Tell John it bothers me."
	"Ignore it; it's John's only flaw."
	"Clean it up myself."
	"Mess up something of John's and hope he gets the message."
	"Ask our other roommate, Harry, to tell him."
Step 4:	**Evaluate the solutions and pick one.**
	"If I tell John, he might get mad at me."
	"I can't ignore it. It really bothers me."
	"I don't want to clean it up myself."
	"Messing up something of his won't help. It will only make John mad."
	"I shouldn't ask Harry to do the dirty work."
	"Although it's got its risk, I think I'll tell John myself."
Step 5:	**Plan out the implementation of the chosen solution.**
	"Monday night, just after we clean up the dinner dishes, I will ask John to sit down with me over the kitchen table to discuss this issue. It will probably be a good idea to have some kind of clean-up plan already thought out. Perhaps we could have a rule that all dishes must be clean before leaving the house."
Step 6:	**Try it out.**
	"Monday night I met with John. He felt that he did not need to keep the kitchen clean because Harry did not make a sincere effort to keep the living and dining rooms clean."
Step 7:	**Reevaluate the solution and try another if the chosen one did not work.**
	"I decided to have a similar Monday night meeting with all roommates present. At this time, we would discuss cleaning rules for the entire house."

are unaware that a problem exists (Kitchener 1983, 1986). In fact, the ease of problem definition is frequently overestimated (Arlin 1986). Even when problems can be adequately described, formal brainstorming of solutions does not parallel the manner in which individuals effectively respond to problems (Rogoff 1984). Rather than systematically listing and evaluating a range of solutions to the indexed problem, individuals tend to respond more intuitively. Implementation of solutions tends to be a dynamic process with individuals adjusting responses as the environment reacts to their behaviors (Kitchener 1983). These combined findings suggest that "real-life" problem solving does not occur as a stepwise logical event. Hence, training procedures presenting such views are a disservice to the patient.

Whether or not problem solving is a stepwise process in healthy individuals has not been resolved empirically. However, as a technique, the multiple steps of problem solving may be a useful "prosthesis" that guides patients with social disorders in resolving interpersonal difficulties (Gazzaniga 1978; Liberman et al.1995). This prosthesis may not totally approximate normative problem solving, but then, artificial limbs do not always look like arms and legs. However, the clearly specified steps of problem solving assist patients with cognitive limitations in better understanding their problems and in figuring out solutions.

Social Decision Making and Judgment Heuristics

Attribution theorists have written extensively about the decision-making process related to social functioning and problem solving, specifically focusing on attempts that ordinary people make to comprehend the causes and implications of events they observe (Ross 1977). Kelley (1967, 1972) likened individuals to rational scientists in the world. Much like problem solving, attributions are governed by logical and empirical rules; examples of two such rules are the covariance and the discounting principles (Ross 1977). Attributions based on the covariance principle conform to rules of inferential logic in which causality is judged from several occurrences of like events. For example, an individual who experiences a co-worker as sullen day after day is likely to attribute a hostile interaction about the office car pool as a varied recurrence of this pattern. "You've got to excuse Joe; he's always kinda down." The discounting principle yields attributions that arise from single occurrences in which causality is evaluated from the individual's previous knowledge of the actor's disposition, goals, etc. Hence, the sullen co-worker may be judged differently by employees who know that he is depressed because of a recent death in the family.

Many attributions are not dictated by the laws of inference and may lead to erroneous conclusions (Kahneman et al. 1982). Tversky and Kahneman (1974) challenged the notion that individuals are rational scientists in the world by identifying several judgment heuristics that bias perception of interpersonal situations. One of these interpersonal situations, misconception of regression to the mean, can lead to inaccurate conclusions about social events. For example, Bonnie is an excellent athlete who usually runs 3 seconds faster than her peers on the track team. Last week, her times were a half-second slower because she had a cold; her coach called her lazy because he now perceived Bonnie to be running slower than her teammates. Inattention to previous probabilities and ignorance of base rates also lead to misattributions. A parole officer at the county jail noticed the large number of sex offenders in the female prison population. The officer concluded that women in general have a higher likelihood of perpetrating sexual assaults than men. Illusory correlations can guide people to odd behaviors. For example, Betty noticed that older women at work received greater praise from their superiors. Thinking that the praise was related to appearance, she dyed her hair gray.

Social psychologists have identified several attribution errors that may lead to misconceptions about social situations. Because of the fundamental attribution error, individuals are likely to describe actions of other people in terms of disposition; in contrast, individuals are likely to describe their own responses in terms of situational factors (Ross 1977). For example, individuals are more likely to label the "character" of a hostile co-worker as intrinsically flawed, whereas they may attribute their own angry transgressions to momentary hassles from the boss. Alternatively, the self-serving attributional bias suggests that individuals are likely to ascribe their achievements to personality factors and failings to environmental influences (D. T. Miller and Ross 1975). Both attribution errors may lead to overestimation of dispositional factors and relative ignorance of situational factors.

Narrower attribution errors have been defined as well; for example, belief in a just-world hypothesis can lead to miscomprehension of social interactions (Lerner 1970). An unfortunate consequence of this hypothesis has been the derogation of innocent victims of crime (Lerner and D. T. Miller 1978): "that woman was probably raped because she dresses like a floozy." By finding fault with the victim's character or behaviors, individuals are able to hold on to their assertions that the world is a safe place to live.

Implications for Rehabilitation

We have assumed that attribution errors challenge basic suppositions of problem-solving models and, therefore, undermine the intervention's efficacy in rehabilitating social cognitive deficits in patient populations. To our knowledge, however, there is little research investigating the form these errors take in neuropsychiatrically disordered populations. Future research needs to determine whether attribution errors in neuropsychiatric populations approximate normal manifestations and whether they vary across diagnostic groups.

Research also must determine the effects that patient judgment errors have on social functioning. The efficacy of problem-solving approaches need not be threatened even if research suggests that attribution errors are potentiated or amplified in patient populations. Research continues to show the problem-solving approach to be useful for patients that are brain damaged (Corrigan and Jakus 1994) or severely mentally ill (Coche and Flick 1975; Hansen et al. 1985; Wallace and Liberman 1985). Perhaps findings will show that the "prosthetic" nature of social problem solving obviates the confounds of attribution errors. The artificial means of understanding and responding to social information leads to improved clinical outcomes.

What should clinicians do if attribution errors are shown to be a significant factor in the social-information processing of patient populations? Theories that explain attribution errors may result in important heuristics for the development of rehabilitation strategies. For example, attribution models have been divided into cool and hot (D. T. Miller and Porter 1988). *Cool models* depict judgment errors in terms of the natural, cognitive rules that control social attributions. These models suggest that cognitive rehabilitation strategies (such as those developed for information processing) that help patients ameliorate misperceptions and misunderstandings may be fruitful for challenging these errors. *Hot models* define these errors in terms of the more subtle (unconscious) motivations that govern interpersonal relationships. For example, by manipulating the subjects' ego involvement, D. T. Miller (1976) influenced the self-serving attribution bias in response to success and failure experiences. This finding suggests that support and social-reinforcement therapies that manipulate interpersonal motivation may alter the effect of attribution biases.

Summary

Meehl and Cronbach (1955) recommended that clinical practices be built on strong theoretical foundations providing a network of descriptions and predictions. These foundations should have withstood numerous empirical tests. Four divergent models of normal cognition that meet these criteria were reviewed in this chapter. Models of intellectual functioning provide a developmental and personological view of human cognition. R. J. Sternberg's (1985) triarchic theory of intelligence concentrates on not only the trait-like characteristics of intellectual functioning, but also on the manner in which the internal cognitive world meets the external world's formulation of knowing. Alternatively, information processing models provide a micro approach to cognition, describing "macro" knowing in terms of discrete functions and processes. The serial stage model of information processing has been an important heuristic for understanding human cognition. However, limitations of this model have been augmented by more recent theories of modularity, limited capacity, and parallel distributed processing.

Models of cognitive schema focus more on the manner in which information is represented than processed. Much of this work has been completed by social psychologists and focuses on more clinically relevant phenomena such as situations, persons, and self. Clinical investigators also have developed problem-solving models that represent the most ecologically valid cognitive paradigm. According to this view, humans are rational agents who perceive and interact with their world in logical fashion. Unfortunately, the stepwise approach to interpersonal situations has not been shown to correspond with the more intuitive manner in which individuals approach their world. Several biased-judgment heuristics have been identified that govern some interpersonal decisions.

Models reviewed in this chapter reflect only a small sample of relevant theories. Several other models also might be helpful for describing cognitive deficits of patient populations and for developing rehabilitation strategies for these deficits; for example, language and communication models focus on the form in which cognitive deficits are presented to the world. Patterns of both verbal and nonverbal communication have been investigated in patient populations (Coulthard 1977, 1984; Rosenthal et al. 1975). This viewpoint is especially germane to understanding psychoses where formal thought disorder—which is observed by clinicians as disorganized speech—is pathognomonic of the disorders and to understanding the aphasias common to neuropsychological disorders.

Cognitive models differ significantly in methodological precision and ecological validity. Information processing models have been developed, for the most part, in laboratory settings and offer rigorous methodological strategies. Problem-solving models are less experimentally robust. However, constructs from this (problem-solving) viewpoint seem more ecologically meaningful. Cognitive models might be evaluated by other values. Cognitive models are useful in terms of rehabilitation when they provide rich descriptions of deficit patterns or when they provide practical strategies for remediating these deficits. The clinical investigator who is familiar with the range of cognitive models of normal functioning is best equipped for development and evaluation of models of rehabilitation in the future.

References

American Psychiatric Association: Diagnostic and Statistical Manual of Mental Disorders, 4th Edition. Washington, DC, American Psychiatric Association, 1994

Argyle M: Social skills and the analysis of situations and conversations, in Handbook of Social Skills Training, Vol 2. Edited by Hollin CR, Trower P. New York, Pergamon, 1986, pp 185–216

Arlin PK: Problem finding and young adult cognition, in Adult Cognitive Development: Methods and Models. Edited by Mines RA, Kitchener KS. New York, Praeger, 1986, pp 22–32

Atkinson RC, Shiffrin RM: Human memory: a proposed system and its control processes, in The Psychology of Learning and Motivation, Vol 2. Edited by Spence K, Spence J. New York, Academic Press, 1968, pp 90–197

Avedon EM: The structural elements of games, in The Study of Games. Edited by Avedon EM, Sutton-Smith B. New York, Wiley, 1971, pp 306–350

Averbach E, Coriell AS: Short-term memory in vision. Bell Systems Technical Journal 40:309–328, 1961

Aylward E, Walker E, Bettes B: Intelligence in schizophrenia: meta-analysis of the research. Schizophr Bull 10:430–459, 1984

Bandura A: Social Learning Theory. Englewood Cliffs, NJ, Prentice-Hall, 1977

Banks WP: Signal detection theory and human memory. Psychol Bull 74:81–99, 1970

Beck AT: Depression: Clinical, Experimental, and Theoretical Aspects. New York, Harper & Row, 1967

Beck AT: Cognitive Therapy and the Emotional Disorders. New York, International Universities Press, 1976

Bellack AS, Morrison RL, Mueser KT: Social problem solving in schizophrenia. Schizophr Bull 15:101–116, 1989

Berlin B, Kay P: Basic Color Terms: Their Universality and Evolution. Berkeley, University of California Press, 1969

Berne E: Games People Play. New York, Grove Press, 1964

Berry JW: Radical cultural relativism and the concept of intelligence, in Culture and Cognition: Readings in Cross-Cultural Psychology. Edited by Berry JW, Dasen PR. London, Methuen, 1974, pp 225–230

Binet A, Simon T: The Development of Intelligence in Children. Baltimore, MD, Williams & Wilkins, 1916

Blaney PH: Affect and memory: a review. Psychol Bull 99:229–246, 1986

Bower GH: Mood and memory. Am Psychol 36:129–148, 1989

Bower GH, Monteiro KP, Gilligan SG: Emotional mood as a context of learning and recall. Journal of Verbal Learning and Verbal Behavior 17:573–585, 1978

Bransford JD, Johnson MK: Contextual prerequisites for understanding: some investigations of comprehension and recall. Journal of Verbal Learning and Verbal Behavior 11:717–726, 1972

Broadbent DE: Perception and Communication. London, Pergamon Press, 1958

Broadbent DE: The hidden preattentive process. Am Psychol 32:109–118, 1977

Broadbent DE, Gregory M: Vigilance considered as a statistical decision. Br J Med Psychol 54:309–323, 1963

Broen W, Storms L: Lawful disorganization: the process underlying a schizophrenic syndrome. Psychol Rev 73:265–279, 1966

Brown J: Reciprocal facilitation and impairment of free recall. Psychonomic Science 10:41–42, 1968

Cantor N, Mischel W: Traits as prototypes: effects on recognition memory. J Pers Soc Psychol 35:38–48, 1977

Cantor N, Mischel W: Prototypes in person perception, in Advances in Experimental Social Psychology, Vol 12. Edited by Berkowitz L. New York, Academic Press, 1979, pp 4–52

Cattell RB: Theory of fluid and crystallized intelligence: a critical experiment. J Educ Psychol 54:1–24, 1963

Coche E, Flick A: Problem solving training groups for hospitalized psychiatric patients. J Psychol 91:19–29, 1975

Cohen JD, Servan-Schreiber D: A parallel distributed processing approach to behavior and biology in schizophrenia. Technical Report AIP-100. Washington, DC, Office of Naval Research, 1990

Corrigan PW, Green MF: Signal detection analysis of short term recall in schizophrenia. J Nerv Ment Dis 179:494–497, 1991

Corrigan PW, Green MF: The situational feature recognition test: a measure of schema comprehension for schizophrenia. International Journal of Methods in Psychiatric Research 3:29–36, 1993b

Corrigan PW, Holmes EP: Behavioral analysis of street smarts and schizophrenia. Paper presented at the Annual Meeting of the Association for the Advancement of Behavior Therapy, November 1992

Corrigan PW, Holmes EP: Patient identification of "street skills" for a psychosocial training module. Hosp Community Psychiatry 45:273–276, 1994

Corrigan PW, Jakus MR: Behavioral treatment, in Psychiatric Aspects of Traumatic Brain Injury. Edited by Silver JM, Yudofsky SC, Hales RE. Washington DC, American Psychiatric Press, 1994, pp 733–770

Corrigan PW, Tommey RM: Interpersonal problem solving and information processing in schizophrenia. Schizophr Bull 21:395–404, 1995

Corrigan PW, Wallace CJ, Green MF, et al: Cognition and social functioning in schizophrenia. Paper presented at the Annual Meeting of the American Psychiatric Association, New Orleans, May 1991

Coulthard M: An Introduction to Discourse Analysis. London, Longman, 1977

Coulthard M: Conversation analysis and social skills training, in Radical Approaches to Social Skills Training. Edited by Trower P. New York, Methuen, 1984, pp 37–64

Craik FI, Lockhart RS: Levels of processing: a framework for memory research. Journal of Verbal Learning and Verbal Behavior 11:671–684, 1972

Craik FI, Tulving E: Depth of processing and the retention of words in episodic memory. J Exp Psychol Gen 104:268–294, 1975

D'Zurilla TJ: Problem Solving Therapy: A Social Competence Approach to Clinical Intervention. New York, Springer, 1986

D'Zurilla TJ, Goldfried MR: Problem solving and behavior modification. J Abnorm Psychol 78:107–126, 1971

Davies DR, Parasuraman R: The Psychology of Vigilance. New York, Academic Press, 1982

Donahoe CP, Carter MJ, Bloem WD, et al: Assessment of interpersonal problem-solving skills. Psychiatry 53:329–339, 1990

Feldman JA: A connectionist model of visual memory, in Parallel Models of Associative Memory. Edited by Hinton GE, Anderson JA. Hillsdale, NJ, Erlbaum, 1981, pp 314–344

Fitts PM, Posner ML: Human Performance. Belmont, CA, Brooks/Cole, 1967

Flaugher RL: The many definitions of test bias. Am Psychol 33:671–679, 1978

Fodor JA: The Modularity of the Mind. Cambridge, MA, MIT Press, 1983

Forgas JP: Social skills and the perception of interaction episodes. Br J Clin Psychol 22:195–207, 1983

Galambos JA: Knowledge structures for common activities, in Knowledge Structures. Edited by Galambos JA, Abelson RP, Black JB. Hillsdale, NJ, Lawrence Erlbaum, 1986, pp 21–48

Galambos JA, Rips LJ: Memory for routines. Journal of Verbal Learning and Verbal Behavior 21:260–281, 1982

Galambos JA, Abelson RP, Black JB (eds): Knowledge Structures. Hillsdale, NJ, Lawrence Erlbaum, 1986

Gazzaniga MS: Is seeing believing: notes on clinical recovery, in Recovery from Brain Damage: Research and Theory. Edited by Finger S. New York, Plenum Press, 1978, pp 76–102

Gjerde PF: Attentional capacity dysfunction and arousal in schizophrenia. Psychol Bull 97:57–72, 1983

Glass AL, Holyoak KJ: Cognition, 2nd Edition. New York, Random House, 1986

Goldfried MR, D'Zurilla TJ: A behavioral-analytic method for assessing competence, in Current Topics in Clinical and Community Psychology. Edited by Spielberger CD. New York, Academic Press, 1969, pp 147–163

Goldsmith JB, McFall RM: Development and evaluation of an interpersonal skill training program for psychiatric patients. J Abnorm Psychol 84:51–58, 1975

Graesser AC, Woll SB, Kowalski DJ, et al: Memory for typical and atypical actions in scripted activities. J Exp Psychol Learn Mem Cogn 6:503–515, 1980

Green DM, Swets JA: Signal Detection Theory and Psychophysics. New York, Wiley, 1966

Guilford JP: The Nature of Human Intelligence. New York, McGraw-Hill, 1967

Hansen DJ, St. Lawrence JS, Christoff KA: Effects of interpersonal problem-solving training with chronic aftercare patients on problem-solving component skills and effectiveness of solution. J Consult Clin Psychol 53:167–174, 1985

Hartlage S, Alloy LB, Vazquez CV: Automatic and effortful processing in depression. Psychol Bull 113:247–278, 1993

Hasher L, Zacks RT: Automatic and effortful processes in memory. J Exp Psychol Gen 108:356–388, 1979

Hasher L, Zacks RT: Automatic processing of fundamental information: the case of frequency of occurrence. Am Psychol 39:1372–1388, 1984

Heaton RK: Wisconsin Card Sorting Test Manual. Odessa, FL, Psychological Assessment Resources, 1981

Henry GM, Weingartner H, Murphy DL: Influence of affective states and psychoactive drugs on verbal learning and memory. Am J Psychiatry 130: 966–971, 1973

Hull CL: A Behavior System. New Haven, CT, Yale University Press, 1952

Ingram RE, Kendall PC: Cognitive clinical psychology: implications of an information processing perspective, in Information Processing Approaches to Clinical Psychology. Edited by Ingram RE. New York, Academic Press, 1986, pp 3–21

Jenkins JJ: Remember that old theory of mind? well, forget it. Am Psychol 29: 785-795, 1974

Jones RA, Sensenig J, Haley JV: Self-descriptions: configurations of content and order effects. J Pers Soc Psychol 30:36–45, 1974

Jordan MI: An introduction to linear algebra in parallel distributed processing, in Parallel Distributed Processing: Explorations in the Microstructure of Cognition: Vol I, Foundations. Edited by McClelland JL, Rumelhart DE, PDP Research Group. Cambridge, MA, Bradford Books, 1986, pp 365–422

Kahneman D: Attention and Effort. Englewood Cliffs, NJ, Prentice-Hall, 1973

Kahneman D, Slovic P, Tversky A (eds): Judgment Under Uncertainty: Heuristics and Biases. Cambridge, England, Cambridge University Press, 1982

Keating DP: The emperor's new clothes: the "new look" in intelligence research, in Advances in the Psychology of Human Intelligence, Vol 2. Edited by Sternberg RJ. Hillsdale, NJ, Lawrence Erlbaum, 1984, pp 1–46

Kelley HH: Attribution theory in social psychology, in Nebraska Symposium on Motivation. Edited by Levine D. Lincoln, NE, University of Nebraska Press, 1967, pp 192–238

Kelley HH: Causal schemata and the attribution process, in Attribution: Perceiving the Causes of Behavior. Edited by Jones EE, Ebersol AJ, Franklin T. Morristown, NJ, General Learning Press, 1972, pp 151–174

Kitchener KS: Cognition, metacognition, and epistemic cognition: a three-level model of cognitive processing. Hum Dev 26:222–232, 1983

Kitchener KS: The reflective judgment model: characteristics, evidence, and measurement, in Adult Cognitive Development: Methods and Models. Edited by Mines RA, Kitchener, KS. New York, Praeger, 1986, pp 76–91

Kuiper NA: Convergent evidence for the self as a prototype: the "inverted-U RT effect" for self and other judgments. Personality and Social Psychology Bulletin 7:438–443, 1981

Kuiper NA, Derry PA: The self as a cognitive prototype: an application to person perception and depression, in Cognition, Social Interaction, and Personality. Edited by Cantor N, Kihlstrom J. Hillsdale, NJ, Lawrence Erlbaum, 1981

Kuiper NA, MacDonald R: Self and other perception in mild depressives. Social Cognition 1:223–239, 1982

Labov W: The boundaries of words and their meanings, in New Ways of Analyzing Variation in English. Edited by Baily CJN, Shuy RW. Washington, DC, Georgetown University Press, 1973, pp 220–276

Lachman R, Lachman JL: Information processing psychology: origins and extensions, in Information Processing Approaches to Clinical Psychology. Edited by Ingram RE. New York, Academic Press, 1986, pp 23–49

Lerner MJ: The desire for justice and reactions to victims, in Altruism and Helping Behavior. Edited by Macaulay J, Berkowitz L. New York, Academic Press, 1970, pp 57–84

Lerner MJ, Miller DT: Just world research and the attribution process: looking back and ahead. Psychol Bull 85:1030–1051, 1978

Liberman RP, Vaccarro JV, Corrigan PW: Psychiatric rehabilitation, in Comprehensive Textbook of Psychiatry, 6th ed. Edited by Kaplan HI, Sadock BJ. Baltimore, MD, Williams & Wilkins, 1995, pp 2696–2718

Lockhart RS, Murdock BB: Memory and the theory of signal detection. Psychol Bull 74:100–109, 1970

Madle RA, Neisworth JT: Mental retardation, in International Handbook of Behavior Modification and Therapy, 2nd ed. Edited by Bellack AS, Hersen M, Kazdin AE. New York, Plenum Press, 1990, pp 731–762

Mandler G: Organization and memory, in The Psychology of Learning and Motivation, Vol 1. Edited by Spence KW, Spence JT. New York, Academic Press, 1967, pp 461–503

Mandler G: Organization and recognition, in Organization of Memory. Edited by Tulving E, Donaldson W. New York, Academic Press, 1972, pp 146–160

Marr DC: Vision: A Computational Investigation into the Human Representation and Processing of Visual Information. San Francisco, CA, Freeman, 1982

Matt GE, Vazquez C, Campbell WK: Mood congruent recall of affectively toned stimuli: a meta-analytic review. Clinical Psychology Review 12:227–255, 1992

McClelland JL: Putting knowledge in its place: a scheme for programming parallel processing structures on the fly. Cognitive Science 9:113–146, 1985

McClelland JL, Rumelhart DE: An interactive activation model of context effects in letter perception, I: an account of basic findings. Psychol Rev 88:375–407, 1981

McClelland JL, Rumelhart DE: Distributed memory and the representation of general and specific information. J Exp Psychol Gen 114:159–188, 1985

McClelland JL, Rumelhart DE, PDP Research Group (eds): Parallel Distributed Processing: Explorations in the Microstructure of Cognition: Vol II, Psychological and Biological Models. Cambridge, MA, Bradford Books, 1986

McFall RM: A review and reformulation of the concept of social skills. Behavioral Assessment 4:1–33, 1982

McIntyre T: A Resource Book for Remediating Common Behavior and Learning Problems. Boston, MA, Allyn & Bacon, 1989

Meehl PE, Cronbach LJ: Construct validity in psychological tests. Psychol Bull 52:3–31, 1955

Meiselman KC: Broadening dual modality cue utilization in chronic nonparanoid schizophrenia. J Consult Clin Psychol 41:447–453, 1973

Merluzzi TV, Rudy TE, Glass CR: The information processing paradigm: implications for clinical science, in Cognitive Assessment. Edited by Merluzzi TV, Glass CR, Genest M. New York, Guilford Press, 1981, pp 148–192

Miller DT: Ego involvement and attributions for success and failure. J Pers Soc Psychol 34:901–906, 1976

Miller DT, Porter CA: Errors and biases in the attribution process, in Social Cognition and Clinical Psychology: A Synthesis. Edited by Abramson LY. New York, Guilford Press, 1988, pp 3–30

Miller DT, Ross M: Self-serving biases in the attribution of causality: fact or fiction? Psychol Bull 82:213–225, 1975

Miller GA: The magical number seven, plus or minus two: some limits on our capacity for information processing. Psychol Rev 63:81–97, 1956

Milner B: Amnesia following operation on the temporal lobes, in Amnesia. Edited by Whitty CWM, Zangwill OL. London, Butterworth, 1966, pp 347–398

Mischel W: Introduction to Personality, 2nd ed. New York, Holt, Rinehart & Winston, 1976

Morris RGM: Introduction: computational neuroscience: modelling the brain, in Parallel Distributed Processing: Implications for Psychology and Neurobiology. Edited by Morris RGM. Oxford, England, Clarendon Press, 1989a, pp 216–289

Morris RGM (ed): Parallel Distributed Processing: Implications for Psychology and Neurobiology. Oxford, England, Clarendon Press, 1989b

Morrison RL, Bellack AS, Mueser KT: Deficits in facial-affect recognition and schizophrenia. Schizophr Bull 14:67–84, 1988

Neely JH: Semantic priming and retrieval from lexical memory: role of inhibitionless spreading activation and limited capacity attention. J Exp Psychol Gen 106:226–254, 1977

Neely JH, Schmidt SR, Roediger HL: Inhibition from related primes in recognition memory. J Exp Psychol Learn Mem Cogn 9:196–211, 1983

Neisser U: Cognition and Reality: Principles and Implications of Cognitive Psychology. San Francisco, CA, Freeman, 1976

Neisser U: On "social knowing." Personality and Social Psychology Bulletin 6:601–605, 1980

Neisser U: Toward an ecologically oriented cognitive science, in New Directions in Cognitive Science. Edited by Shlechter TM, Toglia MP. Norwood, NJ, Ablex, 1985, pp 108–175

Nuechterlein KH, Dawson ME: Information processing and attentional functioning in the developmental course of schizophrenic disorders. Schizophr Bull 10:160–203, 1984

Oddy M, Coughlan T, Tyerman A, et al: Social adjustment after closed head injury: a further follow-up seven years after injury. J Neurol Neurosurg Psychiatry 48:564–568, 1985

Payne RW: The measurement and significance of overinclusive thinking and retardation in schizophrenic patients, in Psychopathology of Schizophrenia. Edited by Itoch P, Zubin J. New York, Grune & Stratton, 1966, pp 114–156

Piaget J: The Psychology of Intelligence. Totowa, NJ, Littlefield, Adams, 1972

Platt JJ, Spivack G: Problem-solving thinking of psychiatric patients. J Consult Clin Psychol 39:148–151, 1972a

Platt JJ, Spivack G: Social competence and effective problem-solving thinking in psychiatric patients. J Clin Psychol 28:3–5, 1972b

Posner MI: Chronometric Explorations of Mind. Hillsdale, NJ, Lawrence Erlbaum, 1978

Posner MI, Nissen MJ, Klein RM: Visual dominance: an information processing account of its origins and significance. Psychol Rev 83:157–171, 1976

Prigatano GP, Altman IM: Impaired awareness of behavioral limitations after traumatic brain injury. Arch Phys Med Rehabil 71:1058–1064, 1990

Rabinowitz JC, Mandler G, Patterson KE: Determinants of recognition and recall: accessibility and generation. J Exp Psychol Gen 106:302–329, 1977

Rips LJ, Shoben EJ, Smith EE: Semantic distance and the verification of semantic relations. Journal of Verbal Learning and Verbal Behavior 12:1–20, 1973

Rogers TB, Kuiper NA, Kirker WS: Self-reference and the encoding of personal information. J Pers Soc Psychol 35:677–688, 1977

Rogers TB, Rogers PJ, Kuiper NA: Evidence for the self as a cognitive prototype: the "false alarms effect." Personality and Social Psychology Bulletin 5:53–56, 1979

Rogoff B: Introduction: thinking and learning in social context, in Everyday Cognition: Its Development in Social Context. Edited by Rogoff B, Lave J. Cambridge, MA, Harvard University Press, 1984, pp 173–224

Rosch E: Linguistic relativity, in Human Communication: Theoretical Perspectives. Edited by Silverstein A. New York, Halsted Press, 1974

Rosch E: Cognitive representations of semantic categories. J Exp Psychol Gen 104:192–233, 1975a

Rosch E: The nature of mental codes for color categories. J Exp Psychol Hum Percept 1:303–322, 1975b

Rosch E, Mervis CB: Family resemblances: studies in the internal structure of categories. Cognit Psychol, 7:573–605, 1975

Rosch E, Simpson C, Miller RS: Structural bases of typicality effects. J Exp Psychol Hum Percept 2:491–502, 1976

Rosenthal R, Hall JA, DiMatteo MR, et al: Sensitivity to Nonverbal Communication: The PONS Test. Baltimore, MD, Johns Hopkins University Press, 1975

Ross L: The intuitive psychologist and his shortcomings: distortion in the attribution process, in Advances in Experimental Social Psychology, Vol 10. Edited by Berkowitz L. New York, Academic Press, 1977, pp 174–221

Sahgal A: Some limitations of indices derived from signal detection theory: evaluation of an alternative index for measuring bias in memory tasks. Psychopharmacology (Berl) 91:517–520, 1987

Sattler JM: Assessment of Children's Intelligence and Special Abilities, 2nd Edition. Boston, MA, Allyn and Bacon, 1982

Schank RC, Abelson RP: Scripts, Plans, Goals, and Understanding. Hillsdale, NJ, Lawrence Erlbaum, 1977

Schneider W, Shiffrin RM: Controlled and automatic human information processing, I: detection, search, and attention. Psychol Rev 84:4–66, 1977

Scruggs TE, Wong BYL: Intervention Research in Learning Disabilities. New York, Springer-Verlag, 1990

Shallice T: From Neuropsychology to Mental Structure. New York, Cambridge University Press, 1988

Snodgrass JG, Corwin J: Pragmatics of measuring recognition memory: applications to dementia and amnesia. J Exp Psychol Gen 117:34–50, 1988

Spaulding WD: Design prerequisites for research on cognitive therapy for schizophrenia. Schizophr Bull 18:39–42, 1992

Spaulding WD, Storms L, Goodrich V, et al: Applications of experimental psychopathology in psychiatric rehabilitation. Schizophr Bull 12:560–577, 1986

Spearman C: The Abilities of Man. New York, Macmillan, 1927

Sperling GA: The information available in brief visual presentations. Psychol Monogr 74, 1960 (Entire issue)

Sternberg RJ: Human intelligence: the model is the message. Science 230: 1111–1118, 1985

Sternberg S: High-speed scanning in human memory. Science 153:652–654, 1966

Sternberg S: Two operations in character recognition: some evidence from reaction time measurements. Percept and Psychophys 2:45–53, 1967

Sunderland A, Harris JE, Baddeley AD: Do laboratory tests predict everyday memory? a neuropsychological study. Journal of Verbal Learning and Verbal Behavior 22:341–347, 1983

Sunderland A, Harris JE, Gleave J: Memory failures in everyday life following severe head injury. J Clin Neuropsychol 6:127–142, 1984

Swets JA: Is there a sensory threshhold? Science 134:168–177, 1964

Thorndike EL: The law of effect. Am J Psychol 39:212–222, 1927

Thurstone LL: Primary Mental Abilities. Chicago, IL, University of Chicago Press, 1938

Trower P: Toward a generative model of social skills: a critique and synthesis, in Social Skills Training: A Practical Handbook for Assessment and Treatment. Edited by Curran JP, Monti PM. New York, Guilford Press, 1982, pp 399–428

Trower P: Social skills training and social anxiety, in Handbook of Social Skills Training, Vol 2. Edited by Hollin CR, Trower P. New York, Pergamon, 1986, pp 39–66

Tulving E: Subjective organization in free recall of "unrelated" words. Psychol Rev 69:344–354, 1962

Tulving E: Elements of Episodic Memory. London, Oxford University Press, 1983

Tversky A, Kahneman D: Judgment under uncertainty: heuristics and biases. Science 185:1124–1131, 1974

Venables PH: Input dysfunction in schizophrenia, in Progress in Experimental Personality Research, Vol 1. Edited by Maher BA. New York, Academic Press, 1964, pp 1–48

Vernon PE: The Structure of Human Abilities. New York, Wiley, 1950

Vygotsky L: Mind in Society. Cambridge, MA, Harvard University Press, 1978

Wallace CJ: The social skills training program of the Mental Health Clinical Research Center for the Study of Schizophrenia, in Social Skills Training: A Practical Handbook for Assessment and Treatment. Edited by Curran JP, Monti PM. New York, Guilford Press, 1982, pp 57–89

Wallace CJ, Liberman RP: Social skills training for patients with schizophrenia: a controlled clinical trial. Psychiatry Res 15:239–247, 1985

Wallace CJ, Nelson CJ, Liberman RP, et al: A review and critique of social skills training with schizophrenic patients. Schizophr Bull 6:42–63, 1980

Wechsler D: The Measurement and Appraisal of Adult Intelligence, 4th Edition. Baltimore, MD, Williams & Wilkins, 1958

Wechsler D: Manual for the Wechsler Adult Intelligence Scale—Revised. New York, Psychological Corporation, 1981

Williams RJ: The logic of activation functions, in Parallel Distributed Processing: Explorations in the Microstructure of Cognition: Vol I, Foundations. Edited by McClelland JL, Rumelhart DE, PDP Research Group. Cambridge, MA, Bradford Books, 1986, pp 423–443

Wittgenstein L: Philosophical Investigations. New York, Macmillan, 1953

Chapter 2

What Is Cognitive Rehabilitation?

Patrick W. Corrigan, Psy.D., and Stuart C. Yudofsky, M.D.

In a subsequent chapter, cognitive functioning is subcategorized into intelligence, information processing, cognitive schema, problem solving, and decision making. When any of these functions are impaired by disorders of the central nervous system (CNS), cognitive rehabilitation should be considered to recover the function. In this chapter, we review models and theories of recovery of cognitive function, as well as those theories and models of therapeutic strategies that enhance recovery of cognition. In this fashion, we hope to provide a philosophical and theoretical foundation to approach answering the question, "What is cognitive rehabilitation?" The manner in which rehabilitation strategies ameliorate patients' problems depends not only on the nature of the cognitive deficit, but also on the natural process of recovery of brain function. Although we recognize that most conventionally conceptualized psychiatric conditions have important organic underpinnings, for the purpose of explication, we have dichotomized patient populations into those with neurological lesions and those with what were previously called "functional" psychiatric illnesses such as schizophrenia and bipolar disorder.

Theories of Recovery in Patients With Neurological Impairment

Kertesz (1985) identified several characteristics of the CNS that may predict recovery in patients with neuropsychological disorders. For example, research has shown that, contrary to theories of a one-to-one correspondence between brain system and function, destruction of certain areas of the brain does not result in total loss of the corresponding cognitive function. According to the theory of *equipotentiality* (Lashley 1938), other areas of the CNS might assume a function lost to a specific lesion. Pribram (1971) used the concept of a hologram—a transparent three-dimensional photograph of an object—as a metaphor to explain this phenomenon. In particular, he adopted a unique aspect of holograms to explain brain function: individual pieces of a cut-up hologram contain the same information as the complete photo; in other words, each fragment shows the entire three-dimensional object. Extrapolating to the brain, Pribram reasoned that each section of the CNS has sufficient architecture to represent the cognitive functions of the entire functioning brain. Hence, cognitive functions that reside in damaged brain tissue may be assumed by holographic images of the function elsewhere.

Another example of the equipotential phenomenon is *substitution;* that is, functions specific to a damaged hemisphere may transfer to the undamaged hemisphere. This phenomenon has been shown in language functions, when some verbal skills are assumed by the right hemisphere after hemispherectomies (Smith 1966) or callosal sections (Gazzaniga 1970). Research suggests, however, that the extent to which the nondominant hemisphere picks up a previously absent function is limited. For example, right-handed patients with a severely damaged left hemisphere are not expected to become verbally fluent. In fact, substitution may represent an accentuation of subtle functions that always were present in the nondominant hemisphere (e.g., primitive right-hemisphere speech) rather than transfer of function from the damaged area (Kinsbourne 1971). This phenomenon may occur because of *hierarchical rerepresentation* (Geschwind 1974), wherein higher brain centers (such as the left hemisphere) control and, perhaps, inhibit some functions in lower brain centers. Thus, suppression of the influence of the higher center frees up the dormant functions of the lower center.

An alternate theory to equipotentiality is *diaschisis.* Von Monakow (1914) believed that areas of the brain may experience temporary shock, or diaschisis, when these areas are suddenly deprived of normal stimulation from neighboring, severely damaged regions. On occasion, the undamaged tissue receives sufficient stimulation from intact proximal regions so that the absent function returns. Diaschisis seems to be more pronounced after acute injuries such as infarcts and trauma rather than insidious processes such as dementia of the Alzheimer's type. Physiological research supporting this phenomenon seems to be equivocal, however (Kertesz 1985; Meyer et al. 1970, 1974); additional research examining the validity of this concept is required.

Recovery also depends on the *plasticity* of damaged tissues. Traditionally, it was thought that damaged neurons were irreplaceable in the CNS. However, research in different patient populations challenges this assertion. Structural components of the CNS of children may be relatively more dynamic than those of adults; for example, neuronal growth and branching of the dendrites continue during early childhood, so that compensatory structures might develop if traumatic insult occurs during this time. Animal research has shown that lesions in immature organisms have minimal effects compared with similar damage in mature organisms (Kennard and McCulloch 1943). Similarly, damage to the speech area does not seem to limit functioning in children as profoundly as it does in adults (Hecaen 1976). Research also suggested that some neuronal tracts in the brain may *regenerate* in a manner similar to patterns of growth that have been demonstrated in the peripheral nervous system. For example, Schneider (1973) found axonal regrowth in catecholaminergic fibers after lesion. Additionally, neurons proximal to damaged tissue may sprout synapses to vacant terminals (Liu and Chambers 1958). This regrowth can result in a muted return of functioning.

Some neuronal tracts that lose stimulation from neighboring damaged areas become hypersensitive to the action potential of remaining axons (Stavraky 1961). This hypersensitivity may diminish loss of function related to the damaged area. Interestingly, research has suggested that recovery functions related to *denervation hypersensitivity* may interact with other restorative processes. For example, research suggests that *collateral sprouting* may reduce the effects of denervation (Goldberger 1974).

Clinicians developing rehabilitation plans need to be mindful of the restorative processes that are "hard wired" within the CNS. Before drawing conclusions about the extent of a particular dysfunction associated with a particular lesion, clinicians should wait several months for diaschisis to remit and to determine the transfer effects related to substitution and hypersensitivity. The pattern of spontaneous remission that is observed during this period may suggest specific deficits in a profile of dysfunctions that are more amenable to intervention.

Case Example

Ms. J. presented to the emergency room with acute delirium after being exposed to toxic chemicals during an industrial accident. Although the extreme disorientation and disturbed thinking commensurate with delirium had, for the most part, remitted soon after admission, results of a neuropsychological exam during her first week in the hospital showed that she was having difficulty paying attention and scored poorly on measures of recall and recognition memory. The treatment team decided to put off rehabilitation planning for several more weeks to determine whether these cognitive deficits remitted further. Subsequent testing showed that Ms. J.'s vigilance and recognition memory returned to normal levels. Although recall memory was still diminished, recollection was enhanced when she was instructed on how to use retrieval strategies.

Theories of Recovery in Psychiatric Patients

Researchers also outlined characteristics of patients with severe mental illness that suggest their rehabilitative course. For the most part, these studies described subject characteristics that affect social and adaptive functioning. These patterns of change also have implications for cognitive rehabilitation. For example, research showed that males with schizophrenia had a more severe prodrome as well as a more tortuous clinical course than females (Angermeyer et al. 1990; Childers and Harding 1990). Similarly, patients with schizophrenia who abuse drugs or alcohol have far more severe interpersonal disabilities than patients who do not use these substances (Turner and Tsuang 1990). Hence, among severely mentally ill individuals, female patients who do not abuse drugs or alcohol should have better prognoses and may also be more responsive to rehabilitation strategies.

Contrary to Kraepelin's (1896/1987) contention that schizophrenia-spectrum disorders have a progressively dementing course, recent longitudinal studies suggest that some severely mentally ill patients do not show inevitable deterioration. Harding (1988) defined eight course types that vary in prognosis (see Figure 2–1).

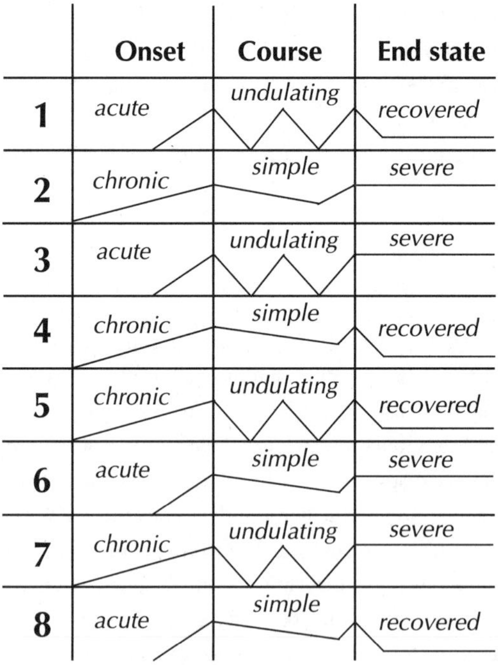

	Onset	Course	End state
1	acute	undulating	recovered
2	chronic	simple	severe
3	acute	undulating	severe
4	chronic	simple	recovered
5	chronic	undulating	recovered
6	acute	simple	severe
7	chronic	undulating	severe
8	acute	simple	recovered

Figure 2–1.   Course types of schizophrenia. The eight course types depend on whether onset is abrupt or insidious, course is variable or static, and outcome leads to remission or severely compromised functioning.

Results from several longitudinal studies showed that between 25% and 50% of patients with schizophrenia had poor outcomes (Bleuler 1978; Ciompi 1980; Harding et al. 1987). However, subgroups of patients with schizophrenia showed undulating patterns in which acute episodes were interspersed with periods of complete remission. Identification of the course of a patient's illness can provide useful information for rehabilitation planning (Corrigan 1992).

Demographic, legislative, and fiscal necessity dictate that most inpatient psychiatric programs limit treatment to patients in one or two course types. For example, because of caps on insurance policies, freestanding, for-profit hospitals treat a preponderance of patients with acute illnesses of relatively recent onset, and state hospitals treat patients with more long-standing conditions and poorer prognoses. Programs of units that primarily treat patients who have few acute episodes should feature rehabilitation strategies that help patients quickly return to the community. In this circumstance, interventions for cognitive problems might include goal setting and strategic reinforcement to facilitate return to prehospital levels of functioning. Conversely, units that treat patients with chronic, deteriorated course types should use more intensive, behaviorally focused interventions. Strong incentive programs such as the token economy must be incorporated into the treatment plan to encourage patients to participate.

Models of Rehabilitation

Several models of cognitive and behavioral rehabilitation have been developed; these contribute a framework for developing comprehensive intervention programs specific to various patient problems (Corrigan and Jakus 1994; Diller and Gordon 1981; Horton and Wedding 1984). Some of these models are summarized in Table 2–1. For the most part, these models have not been rigorously tested in terms of treatment outcome. Rather, they serve as heuristic guidelines for the development and future evaluation of rehabilitation programs.

The *integrative* model frames behavioral rehabilitation vis-à-vis a combination of relatively disparate professional perspectives: the neurologist's definition of the insult in terms of neuroanatomical foci and physiological sequelae; the neuropsychologist's perspective on test description of the behavioral and cognitive deficits associated with the injury; and the behaviorist's treatment plans targeting the profile of behavioral problems requiring remediation (Diller and Gordon 1981). This view developed out of a professional consensus regarding the need for blending what had previously been the independent domains of each profession (Horton and Miller 1984; Horton and Sautter 1986; Horton and Wedding 1984).

Information about the neuroanatomical focus of a problem may reveal cognitive deficits that remain after recovery from other, less subtle dysfunctions.

Table 2–1.   Conceptual models of rehabilitation

Model	Strengths
Integrative	Combines strategies of neuropsychological assessment, neurological lab tests, and behavior intervention
Evaluative	Uses neuropsychological data to develop and evaluate behavioral treatment plans
Prosthetic	Defines impact of behavioral rehabilitation in terms of neurological models of recovery
Process	Bases interventions on processes that might cause behavioral deficits and excesses

Knowledge of physiological sequelae may provide insight into the dynamic characteristics of cognitive deficits. The combination of neuroanatomical and psychophysiological aspects of each disorder will guide the neuropsychologist in selecting an assessment battery aimed at defining the specific cognitive deficit associated with a lesion or disorder. An important component of the test report is a description of the manner in which deficits discovered during the neuropsychological examination translate into limitations in the real-life functioning of the individual assessed.

Behavior therapists have developed a therapeutic armamentarium to aid patients in learning new skills to overcome life problems after brain damage or disorders. Guided by the neuropsychologist's recommendations, the behavior therapist can prescribe various reinforcement and skills-training interventions to address the patient's current life problems. The following case example illustrates the manner in which this diverse information is integrated:

Case Example

Results of a neurological assessment indicated that Mr. P. suffered permanent structural damage to the parietal and temporal regions of his left hemisphere after a severe car accident. Despite his injuries, he was alert and attentive throughout his postinjury course. Expecting dysfunctions commensurate with lesions in left temporal-parietal regions of the brain, the neuropsychologist selected tests for the assessment battery that would be sensitive to deficits in language and memory. The neuropsychologist did not burden the patient with a shotgun battery of tests that were likely to reveal little that could be used in the treatment plan. Test results showed that the patient experienced a relatively mild expressive and receptive aphasia.

The behavior therapist used findings from the test report to develop a treatment plan that included teaching Mr. P. semantic elaboration (a strategy in which encoding of new information is facilitated by restating the information in the patient's own words) and recall strategies (e.g., free-associating cues to the task question). The patient was also encouraged to use external organizers to keep track of day-to-day information. He was shown how to post notes in his work area in organized fashion and to develop daily and hourly lists of things to do to guide his actions.

Lewinsohn and colleagues (Glasgow et al. 1977; Lewinsohn et al. 1977) developed a model of behavioral rehabilitation similar to the integrative model. According to their *evaluative* model, information from the neuropsychological assessment is used as a template for developing behavioral plans. Subsequent evaluations then serve as feedback information to help determine successes and failures of the behavioral plan based on this template and to titrate individual strategies accordingly. The behavioral plan and evaluative feedback loop begin in a well-controlled "laboratory" setting and are later transferred to the real world as applications of the strategies are worked out. Usually, the treatment plan is initiated in well-controlled, inpatient settings where the resources of an ample staff are available. As the cognitive deficit is improved in this setting, the behavioral program is amended so that it can be implemented by family members and friends in the patient's real-world setting.

Both the integrative and evaluative models were developed to treat patients with what are conventionally conceptualized as neurological disorders such as stroke or traumatic brain injuries. For example, both models reflect the neuropsychological assumption that cognitive deficit is somehow related to focal damage in the CNS. Nevertheless, these models also are useful for rehabilitation planning for psychiatric patients. Gjerde (1983) posited that the cognitive deficits of schizophrenia can be understood better when information about psychophysiological arousal is added. Alternatively, the integrative and evaluative models suggest that patients show idiosyncratic patterns of cognitive deficit regardless of the commonalities in biological causes underlying the disorder. Spaulding and his colleagues (1989) maintained that each patient shows a distinctive cognitive profile that must be identified to develop a specific and individualized rehabilitation plan for that patient.

The work of Gazzaniga (1974, 1978) led to a third rehabilitative model: behavioral *prosthetics*. Gazzaniga believed that some behavioral strategies augment remaining neural and cognitive processes that lead to the individual's recovery. In this way, behavioral strategies can act as prosthetics that patients might adopt to improve cognitive skills. Just as patients without a leg are able to walk with the assistance of artificial limbs and crutches, so persons with cognitive deficits might be able to rectify these deficits by adopting a behavioral strategy or external aid. For example, patients might be taught to control vigilance deficits using self-instructional strategies, discriminative signals, and contingent reinforcers (Meichenbaum 1969; Meichenbaum and Cameron 1973). These strategies do not cure the deficit any more than a hearing aid cures deafness. However, once mastered, prosthetics provide tools that patients might repeatedly call on to meet future life challenges.

Case Example

> Mr. L., a person with schizophrenia, was unable to attend to a social skills training program for longer than a few minutes at a time. The problem did not seem to remit after he participated in a repeat-practice, computer-based attention recovery program. Therefore, his rehabilitation counselor decided to help him learn a behavioral prosthetic that would facilitate focusing his attention. Mr. L. was given a watch that beeped every 5 minutes during the class. On each beep, he was instructed to say, "If I pay attention to the class, I will learn things that will help me get out of the hospital." This message was written on the back of his counselor's business card as a reminder.

Unlike the other models, which are derived from rehabilitation strategies based on descriptive paradigms of neurology and neuropsychology, the *process* model was first developed to explain behavioral deficits in severely mentally ill populations (Corrigan et al. 1988, 1990). However, elements of the component processes of the model are relevant for understanding the etiology of a deficit, as well as factors maintaining the problem. A process model tends to view deficits as absence of a skill; for example, a patient has poor memory because of diminished recall and reduced recognition skills. The model, presented here as it applies to cognitive rehabilitation, includes component processes that address three essential questions:

1. *Acquisition.* Why has the patient not acquired certain fundamental skills? The answer to this question varies, depending on the psychopathological category. Developmental disorders such as mental retardation and autism imply that certain cognitive capacities have been missing since birth or early developmental periods. Similarly, it is possible that cognitive deficits of certain psychiatric disorders may be predetermined, albeit in dormant fashion, since infancy. Conversely, cognitive deficits of patients with conventionally conceptualized neurological disorders such as stroke and brain tumors represent recent loss rather than lack of acquisition. Implicit in

acquisition is the belief that some cognitive skills might be acquired that can replace or augment cognitive deficiencies. Of course, there are biological and behavioral limits to learning certain cognitive skills.

2. *Performance.* Why doesn't the patient use certain cognitive skills that apparently exist in his or her repertoire? Could it be that incentive affects the patient's cognition? Patients who are not motivated to recall an event will not do so. Lashley illustrated this point in a poignant example (reported in Kertesz 1985). He bet a patient, who in 900 trials had failed to learn the alphabet, 100 cigarettes that he could *not* learn the letters. Ten trials later the patient recalled them perfectly. Findings such as these suggest that reinforcement strategies are necessary adjuncts to rehabilitation programs.

3. *Generalization.* Why does improved performance in one treatment milieu not generalize to other situations? All too often, little change is observed at the home of a patient even though significant improvement is noted in the treatment setting. Successful changes accomplished in the treatment setting often do not generalize to other environments. Clinicians must include strategies such as homework to help patients transfer newly (re)acquired cognitive skills from the treatment setting into their family, social, and occupational environments.

The process model is useful for rehabilitation of cognitive deficits because treatment strategies are clearly wedded to the specific deficient process in question—that is, to the phenomena that brought about the behavioral excess and deficit and to the phenomena that maintain these disabilities. When combined with the neuropsychiatrist's and neuropsychologist's perspectives, the process model yields a potent programmatic approach to the treatment of the behavioral excesses and deficits of neuropsychiatric patients.

Case Example

Ms. D. continued to exhibit cognitive and behavioral deficits 6 months after her cerebral vascular accident. In particular, she was frequently inattentive, showed poor recognition and recall memory, and performed poorly on measures of conceptual ability. Moreover, she was no longer completing activities of daily living (ADLs) and had poor interpersonal skills.

Results of a careful behavioral analysis showed that basic attentional and recognition memory functions seemed to be intact, but that the patient was not motivated to use these cognitive skills. Similarly, she was able to recount the components of her morning hygiene, but she expressed little desire to complete the regimen. Therefore, her rehabilitation team designed a reinforcement program in which Ms. D. received tokens each time she was found to be paying attention during the daily social skills training groups.

Moreover, she was rewarded for showering, brushing her teeth, and dressing each morning. These tokens could be turned in for cigarettes and coffee, two commodities that she frequently consumed. The treatment team observed that her attentional functioning and ADLs soon returned to normal levels.

On the other hand, recall memory was not affected by reinforcement strategies. No matter how many tokens she was promised for performing better on learning tasks, Ms. D. could not increase her recollection from baseline. Therefore, she was taught some basic semantic encoding skills to help improve retrieval of information. In particular, she was instructed to put the learning points of the skills training groups into her own words. The quality of her participation in the training classes was soon observed to improve, as did the quality of her interpersonal skills.

Even though many of Ms. D.'s attentional, memory, and behavioral problems improved at the rehabilitation center, her family reported little change at home. Therefore, the rehabilitation staff decided to train the family in reinforcement strategies to generalize the patient's improvement outside of the training milieu. Ms. D.'s parents were instructed on the benefits of a reinforcement program and shown how to reward Ms. P. for completing her ADLs each morning at home. Daily hygiene was soon enhanced at home.

Criteria for Evaluating Cognitive Rehabilitation Strategies

The four models of rehabilitation provide a framework for evaluating the efficacy of individual intervention programs. Rehabilitation models generate specific outcome hypotheses that might be the focus of pre- and posttesting. Unfortunately, treatment strategies derived from the aforementioned theoretical foundations are poorly supported by outcome research (Gordon et al. 1989). Perusal of the literature on treatment methodology suggests that program evaluation of cognitive rehabilitation must address three criteria to assess clinical efficacy: comprehensiveness, scientific rigor, and relevance.

Comprehensive research requires broad assessment of the construct of cognition. Distinct theoretical perspectives have developed that require unique strategies for measuring deficits; examples of these measures are included in Table 2–2. The domains of measurement in Table 2–2 are diverse, multifaceted, and, in some instances, relatively independent. For example, assessment of an information-processing deficit is a distinctly different task from documenting a formal thought disorder.

Comprehensive research programs that evaluate psychosocial rehabilitation approaches include many domains of functioning, of which cognitive deficits and thought disorder are only two (Corrigan 1989). Dependent measures included in cognitive rehabilitation research need to be broadened beyond

Table 2–2. Examples of cognitive measures that might be used for evaluating cognitive rehabilitation programs

Perspective of cognition	Sample measure
Information processing	
Attention	Continuous Performance Test (Kornetsky 1972)
	Subtracting serial sevens
	Trail Making (Army Individual Test Battery 1944)
Memory	Auditory Verbal Learning Test (Rey 1964)
	Wechsler Memory Scales (Wechsler 1945)
	Babcock Story Recall Test (Babcock 1930)
	Complex Figure Test (Osterreith 1944)
Verbal functions	Controlled Oral Word Association (Benton and Hamsher 1976)
	Wide Range Achievement Test, Revised (Jastak and Wilkinson 1984)
	National Adult Reading Test (Nelson and O'Connell 1978)
Conceptual functions	Proverbs Test (Gorham 1956)
	Abstract Words Test (Tow 1955)
	Category Test (Halstead 1947)
	Wisconsin Card Sorting Test (Heaton 1981)
	Object Sorting Test (Goldstein and Scheerer 1941)
Intelligence	Stanford-Binet (Terman and Merrill 1973)
	Wechsler Intelligence Tests (Wechsler 1981)
	Raven's Progressive Matrices (Raven 1960)
Formal thought disorder	Thought, Language, Communication Scale (Andreasen 1986)
	Thought Disorder Index (Solovay et al. 1986)
	Bizarre idiosyncratic responses (Marengo et al. 1986)
	Exner's Rorschach Criteria (Exner et al. 1978)
Aphasic communication	Aphasia Screening Test (Halstead and Wepman 1959)
	Token Test (Boller and Vignolo 1966)
Social perception	Perception of Nonverbal Stimuli (Rosenthal et al. 1975)
	Facial Affect Recognition (Ekman and Oster 1979)
	Social Cue Recognition Test (Corrigan and Green 1993a)
	Situational Feature Recognition Test (Corrigan and Green 1993b)

Note. Many of the information processing and aphasia measures were selected from Lezak MD: *Neuropsychological Assessment,* 2nd Edition. New York, Oxford, 1983.

discrete cognitive changes. Other measurement domains might include social competence (i.e., how the person's interpersonal skills change with improved cognition), family burden (i.e., what impact the patient's cognitive deficits and rehabilitation have on his or her family), and patient satisfaction (i.e., whether the patient finds his or her treatment satisfactory).

Comprehensive research does not assure *rigorous* study (Carpenter et al. 1981; Corrigan 1989; Luborsky et al. 1975; May 1968). Common confounds to cognitive rehabilitation research jeopardize this rigor. In a "true" experimental test of cognitive rehabilitation strategies, subjects are randomly assigned to either the rehabilitation condition or an appropriate control group. However, the effects of random assignment are greatly diminished when samples are as small as the patient groups commonly available for cognitive rehabilitation studies (Kraemer et al. 1987). Difficulties with small sample size can be averted by matching treatment and comparison groups on key subject variables. Similarities and differences in these variables should be checked after all the data have been collected.

Appropriate comparison treatments should be equally valued by the therapists who carry them out. Waiting list control groups and poorly organized treatments do not provide notable contrasts that allow the investigator to conclude that significant effects resulted from the cognitive intervention itself, rather than from nonspecific variables like prolonged treatment with an empathic therapist. Comparison treatments might include occupational or art therapies that actively involve patients and foster close interpersonal relationships.

The amount of treatment and the quality of the therapists should be equal across conditions as well. Investigators also should take steps to ensure that cognitive and control treatments are implemented faithfully. Treatment manuals that specify the clinician's role and actions with respect to the intervention in question should be written before the initiation of a study. Manuals are especially necessary in highly prescribed cognitive interventions. Staff fidelity to the intervention can be determined by regular observations conducted by an independent rater using a fidelity checklist. Patient samples should be well described. Diagnoses should be independently determined with structured clinical interviews and neurological technology.

Research investigating cognitive strategies also must be *relevant* (Carpenter et al. 1981); that is, the applicability, generalizability, and limitations of new strategies should be reported. Frequently, the implications drawn from research findings are overzealous; assertions regarding the success of specific interventions are overgeneralized to other patient populations. Characteristics of neuropsychiatric subjects who respond to cognitive rehabilitation strategies need to be reported. For example, some patients have been ruled out of psychotherapeutic treatments because of telltale personality traits (Gunderson and

Mosher 1975). Poorly motivated patients and patients with grossly labile affect would be inappropriate candidates for certain cognitive rehabilitative interventions.

Treatment also should be evaluated in light of patients' perception of its effects. In terms of cognitive interventions, do individuals with neuropsychiatric disorders report different experiences with real-world information? The effects of cognitive approaches on patients' quality of life help determine their value.

Summary

What is cognitive rehabilitation? The answer to that question depends on the clinician's opinion about what comprises a cognitive deficit and what rehabilitation is. Subsequent chapters of this book provide divergent perspectives on the definition of cognitive dysfunction. In this chapter, we described four models of rehabilitation as frameworks for organizing and developing strategies to remediate these deficits. Integrative and evaluative models suggest that a mix of findings from the physician, psychologist, and behaviorist will lead to treatment plans that address the unique deficits of the patient. The prosthetic model posits that rehabilitation programs are significantly enhanced when intact cognitive strengths are identified and used as a "crutch" for the patient to regain or circumvent deficient functions. The process model identifies three processes relevant to the acquisition and maintenance of cognitive deficits. Each process suggests specific rehabilitation strategies that might lead to remediating the deficit.

References

Andreasen NC: Scale for the assessment of thought, language, and communication (TLC). Schizophr Bull 12:473–496, 1986

Angermeyer MC, Kuhn L, Goldstein JM: Gender and the course of schizophrenia: differences in treatment outcomes. Schizophr Bull 16:293–308, 1990

Army Individual Test Battery: Manual of Directions and Scoring. Washington, DC, War Department, Adjutant General's Office, 1944

Babcock H: An experiment in the measurement of mental deterioration. Arch Psychol 117:105, 1930

Benton AL, Hamsher KS: Multilingual Aphasia Examination. Iowa City, IA, University of Iowa, 1976

Bleuler M: The Schizophrenic Disorders: Long Term Patient and Family Studies. Translated by Clemens SM. New Haven, CT, Yale University Press, 1978

Boller F, Vignolo LA: Latent sensory aphasia in hemisphere-damaged patients: an experimental study with the Token Test. Brain 89:815–831,1966

Carpenter WT Jr, Heinrichs DW, Hanlon TE: Methodologic standards for treatment outcome research in schizophrenia. Am J Psychiatry 138:465–471, 1981

Childers SE, Harding CM: Gender, premorbid social functioning, and long-term outcome in DSM-III schizophrenia. Schizophr Bull 16:309–318, 1990

Ciompi L: Catamnestic long-term study on the course of life and aging of schizophrenics. Schizophr Bull 6:606–618, 1980

Corrigan PW: Rehabilitation research methods for schizophrenia. Schizophr Res 2:425–437, 1989

Corrigan PW: Behavior therapy and the course of schizophrenia. The Behavior Therapist 15:61–65, 1992

Corrigan PW, Green MF: Schizophrenic patients' sensitivity to social cues: the role of abstraction. Am J Psychiatry 150:589–594, 1993a

Corrigan PW, Green MF: The situational feature recognition test: a measure of schema comprehension for schizophrenia. International Journal of Methods in Psychiatric Research 3:29–36, 1993b

Corrigan PW, Jakus MR: Behavioral treatment, in Psychiatric Aspects of Traumatic Brain Injury. Edited by Silver JM, Yudofsky SC, Hales RE. Washington, DC, American Psychiatric Press, 1994, pp 733–770

Corrigan PW, Davies-Farmer RM, Lome HB: A curriculum based, psychoeducational program for the mentally ill. Psychosocial Rehabilitation Journal 12:71–73, 1988

Corrigan PW, Davies-Farmer RM, Lightstone R, et al: An analysis of the behavior components of psychoeducational treatment of persons with chronic, mental illness. Rehabilitation Counseling Bulletin 33:200–211, 1990

Diller L, Gordon WA: Rehabilitation and clinical neuropsychology, in Handbook of Clinical Neuropsychology. Edited by Filskov SB, Boll TJ. New York, Wiley, 1981, pp 702–733

Ekman P, Oster H: Facial expressions of emotion. Annu Rev Psychol 30: 527–554, 1979

Exner JE, Weiner IB, Schuyler W: A Rorschach Workbook for the Comprehensive System. Bayville, NY, Rorschach Workshops, 1978

Gazzaniga MS: The Bisected Brain. New York, Appleton, 1970

Gazzaniga MS: Determinants of cerebral recovery, in Plasticity and Recovery of Function in the Central Nervous System. Edited by Stein DG, Rosen JJ, Butters N. New York, Academic Press, 1974, pp 106–142

Gazzaniga MS: Is seeing believing: notes on clinical recovery, in Recovery from Brain Damage: Research and Theory. Edited by Finger S. New York, Plenum Press, 1978

Geschwind N: Late changes in the nervous system: an overview, in Plasticity and Recovery of Function in the Central Nervous System. Edited by Stein D, Rosen J, Butters N. New York, Academic Press, 1974, pp 86–115

Gjerde PF: Attentional capacity dysfunction and arousal in schizophrenia. Psychol Bull 93:57–72, 1983

Glasgow RE, Zeiss RA, Barrera M, et al: Case studies on remediating memory deficits in brain damaged individuals. J Clin Psychol 33:1049–1054, 1977

Goldberger ME: Recovery of movement after CNS lesions in monkeys, in Plasticity and Recovery of Function in the Central Nervous System. Edited by Stein D, Rosen J, Butters N. New York, Academic Press, 1974, pp 220–256

Goldstein KH, Scheerer M: Abstract and concrete behavior: an experimental study with special tests. Psychol Monogr 2:53, 1941

Gordon WA, Hibbard MR, Kreutzer JS: Cognitive remediation: issues in research and practice. Journal of Head Trauma Rehabilitation 4:76–84, 1989

Gorham DR: A proverbs test for clinical and experimental use. Psychol Rep 2:1–12, 1956

Gunderson JG, Mosher LR: The cost of schizophrenia. Am J Psychiatry 132:1257–1264, 1975

Halstead WC: Brain and Intelligence. Chicago, IL, University of Chicago Press, 1947

Halstead WC, Wepman JM: The Halstead-Wepman aphasia screening test. Journal of Speech and Hearing Disorders 14:9–15, 1959

Harding CM: Course types in schizophrenia: an analysis of European and American studies. Schizophr Bull 14:633–643, 1988

Harding CM, Brooks GW, Ashikaga T, et al: The Vermont longitudinal study of persons with severe mental illness, I: methodology, study sample, and overall status 32 years later. Am J Psychiatry 144:718–726, 1987

Heaton RK: Wisconsin Card Sorting Test Manual. Odessa, FL, Psychological Assessment Resources, 1981

Hecaen H: Acquired aphasia in children and the ontogenesis of hemispheric functional specialization. Brain Lang 3:114–134, 1976

Horton AM, Miller WG: Brain damage and rehabilitation, in Current Topics in Rehabilitation Psychology. Edited by Golden CJ. New York, Grune & Stratton, 1984, pp 259–277

Horton AM, Sautter SW: Behavioral neuropsychology: behavioral treatment for the brain-injured, in The Neuropsychology Handbook: Behavioral and Clinical Perspective. Edited by Wedding A, Horton AM, Webster J. New York, Springer Publishing Company, 1986, pp 218–251

Horton AM, Wedding D: Clinical and Behavioral Neuropsychology. New York, Praeger, 1984

Jastak S, Wilkinson GS: Wide Range Achievement Test–Revised, Manual. Wilmington, DE, Jastak Associates, 1984

Kennard MA, McCulloch WS: Motor response to stimulation of cerebral cortex in absence of areas 4 and 6 (Macaca mulatta). J Neurophysiol 6:181–190, 1943

Kertesz A: Recovery and treatment, in Clinical Neuropsychology. Edited by Heilman KM, Valenstein E. New York, Oxford University Press, 1985, pp 481–505

Kinsbourne M: The minor cerebral hemisphere as a source of aphasic speech. Arch Neurol 25:302–306, 1971

Kornetsky C: The use of a simple test of attention as a measure of drug effects in schizophrenic patients. Psychopharmacology 24:99–106, 1972

Kraemer S, Sulz KHD, Schmid R, et al: Kognitive therapie bei standard versorgten schizophrenen patienten. Nervenarzt 58:84–90, 1987

Kraepelin E: Dementia praecox (1896), in The Clinical Roots of the Schizophrenia Concept. Edited by Cutting J, Shepherd M. Cambridge, England, Cambridge University Press, 1987, pp 426–441

Lashley KS: Factors limiting recovery after central nervous lesions. J Nerv Ment Dis 88:733–755, 1938

Lewinsohn PM, Danaher BG, Kikel S: Visual imagery as a mnemonic aid for brain-injured persons. J Consult Clin Psychol 45:717–723, 1977

Lezak MD: Neuropsychological Assessment, 2nd Edition. New York, Oxford, 1983

Liu CN, Chambers WW: Intraspinal sprouting of dorsal root axons. Arch Neurol 79:46–61, 1958

Luborsky L, Singer B, Luborsky L: Comparative studies of psychotherapies: is it true that "everyone has won and all must have prizes?" Arch Gen Psychiatry 32:995–1002, 1975

Marengo JT, Harrow M, Lanin-Kettering I, et al: Evaluating bizarre-idiosyncratic thinking: a comprehensive index of positive thought disorder. Schizophr Bull 12:497–511, 1986

May PRA: Treatment of Schizophrenia. New York, Science House, 1968

Meichenbaum DH: The effects of instructions and reinforcement on thinking and language behavior of schizophrenics. Behav Res Ther 7:101–114, 1969

Meichenbaum DH, Cameron R: Training schizophrenics to talk to themselves: a means of developing attentional controls. Behavior Therapy 4:515–534, 1973

Meyer JS, Shinohara Y, Kanda T, et al: Diaschisis resulting from acute unilateral cerebral infarction. Arch Neurol 23:241–247, 1970

Meyer JS, Welch KM, Okamoto S, et al: Disordered neurotransmitter function. Brain 97:654–664, 1974

Nelson HE, O'Connell A: Dementia: the estimation of premorbid intelligence levels using the New Adult Reading Test. Cortex 14:234–244, 1978

Osterreith PA: Le test de copie d'une figure complexe. Archives de Psychologie 30:206–356, 1944

Pribram KH: Languages of the Brain: Experimental Paradoxes and Principles in Neuropsychology. Englewood Cliffs, NJ, Prentice-Hall, 1971

Raven JC: Guide to the Standard Progressive Matrices. London, HK Lewis, 1960

Rey A: L'examen Clinique en Psychologie. Paris, Presses Universitaires de France, 1964

Rosenthal R, Hall JA, DiMatteo MR, et al: Sensitivity to Nonverbal Communication: The PONS Test. Baltimore, MD, Johns Hopkins University Press, 1975

Schneider GE: Early lesions of superior colliculus: factors affecting the formation of abnormal retinal projections. Brain Behav Evol 8:73–109, 1973

Smith A: Speech and other functions after left (dominant) hemispherectomy. J Neurol Neurosurg Psychiatry 29:467–471, 1966

Solovay MR, Shenton ME, Gasperetti C, et al: Scoring manual for the Thought Disorder Index. Schizophr Bull 12:483–496, 1986

Spaulding W, Garbin C, Crinean W: The logical and psychometric prerequisites for cognitive therapy for schizophrenia, in The Role of Mediating Processes in Understanding and Treating Schizophrenia. Edited by Brenner H, Boker W. Zurich, Switzerland, Huber, 1989, pp 116–140

Stavraky GW: Supersensitivity Following Lesions of the Nervous System. Toronto, Canada, University of Toronto Press, 1961

Terman LM, Merrill MA: Stanford-Binet Intelligence Scale. Manual for the Third Revision, Form L-M. Boston, MA, Houghton Mifflin, 1973

Tow PM: Personality Changes Following Frontal Leucotomy. London, Oxford University Press, 1955

Turner WM, Tsuang MT: Impact of substance abuse on the course and outcome of schizophrenia. Schizophr Bull 16:87–95, 1990

Von Monakow C: Die Lokalisation im Grosshirnrinde und der Abbau der Funktion Durch Korticale Herde. Wiesbaden, Germany, JF Bergmann, 1914

Wechsler D: A standardized memory scale for clinical use. J Psychol 19:87–95, 1945

Wechsler D: Wechsler Adult Intelligence Scale–Revised, Manual. New York, Psychological Corporation, 1981

Chapter 3

Psychophysiological Correlates of Cognitive Deficits

Steven L. Schandler, Ph.D., and Michael J. Cohen, Ph.D.

Psychophysiology is a compound science, blending experimental psychology, electrophysiology, and biology into an integrative study of human behavior. The primary tenet is to provide a simultaneous evaluation of human mental behavior and of physiological responses that precede and support behavior. The approach is not general: the behaviors and their physiological substrates are carefully defined and precisely measured. Definition is provided by rigorous research paradigms designed to isolate specific behaviors. Measurement is achieved by the use of sophisticated recording instruments capable of detection, acquisition, and storage of activity simultaneously from diverse biological systems of the body. When psychophysiological studies use both psychological and physiological measures, they provide an exceptionally detailed, yet coherent view of human cognitive function. As such, psychophysiological measures provide essential service in determining the presence and location of cognitive deficits.

A Model of Cognitive Function and Deficit in Clinical Populations

The selection of psychophysiological measures of cognition is guided principally by the cognitive model in which the measures will be applied. For purposes of this discussion, *cognitive function* refers to the psychological operations that occur within the central nervous system (CNS) during the processing of information. In contrast to more spontaneous *thinking*, information processing refers to operations contingent on a particular stimulus. The stimulus is

This chapter describes research supported by a Department of Veterans Affairs Medical Research Grant and Chapman University Faculty Research Grants awarded to Steven Schandler.

externally presented, and its psychophysical dynamics (i.e., duration and intensity) are known or controlled. It is assumed that the psychological properties of the stimulus (i.e., meaningfulness) are sufficiently known to allow discussions of the probability that it would elicit a particular response. Thus, at stimulus presentation, a cognitive deficit is assessed as 1) no response when a response was expected, 2) an incomplete response, or 3) occurrence of a less probable response than that typically expected.

Cognitive operations and their psychophysiological assessment must be considered within a general model of information processing. In their comprehensive review of cognitive clinical psychology, Ingram and Kendall (1986) suggested that cognitive operations occur within a *cognitive taxonomic system.* This model is useful because it relates cognitive mechanisms and processes to the clinical status of the individual. A diagram of this system is displayed in Table 3–1. The architecture of this system is reflected by the *cognitive structure,* which represents both the physical components and the psychological mechanisms involved in information storage. The actual information stored or stored representations of the information content form *cognitive propositions.* Information processing is reflected in *cognitive operations,* and *cognitive products* are the result of interactions between acquired information and cognitive structure, operations, and propositions. Beginning with the input of an informational stimulus, these interactions are multidirectional. Figure 3–1 provides a diagram of these interactions. Note that output behavior is affected by cognitive structure and products, by biochemical and emotional factors, and by influences in the external environment. Traditional psychophysiological measures have been directed at assessments of peripheral activity, such as affective changes and sensory data processing. Later in this chapter, it will be seen that the use of new psychophysiological measures and multiple measures recorded simultaneously allows assessments of cognitive propositions and products.

This system is not intended as the only or most accurate model of cognition. The system does not allow determination of the nature of the cognitive deficit. Rather, Ingram and Kendall (1986) proposed that the system "can be employed to conceptually organize and empirically examine both the unique and shared cognitive features of various forms of psychopathology and psychological dysfunction" (p. 13). For example, if two disorders associated with cognitive dysfunction, such as depression and anxiety, are characterized by intact cognitive structures and similar cognitive operations, then the cognitive deficits that distinguish these disorders must reside in the cognitive propositions area of the taxonomic system.

The cognitive taxonomic system provides a helpful schematic for visualizing the cognitive system and potential locations of cognitive deficits. However, the system does not convey the dynamics of information processing that occur

Table 3–1. Representative constructs with each category of components of the cognitive taxonomic system for integration with clinically relevant theory and research

Schema			
Structure	**Propositions**	**Operations**	**Products**
Short-term memory	Episodic knowledge	Spreading activation	Attributions
		Attention	Decisions
Long-term memory	Semantic knowledge	Cognitive elaboration	Images
Iconic/sensory storage	Internally generated information	Encoding	Thoughts
Cognitive networks/ associative linkages	Beliefs (stored)	Retrieval	Beliefs (accessed)
		Information transfer speed	
Memory nodes			Stimulus detection and recognition

Source. Reprinted from Ingram RE, Kendall PC: "Cognitive Clinical Psychology: Implications of an Information Processing Perspective," in *Information Processing Approaches to Clinical Psychology.* Edited by Ingram RE. Orlando, FL, Academic Press, 1986, pp. 3–21. Used with permission.

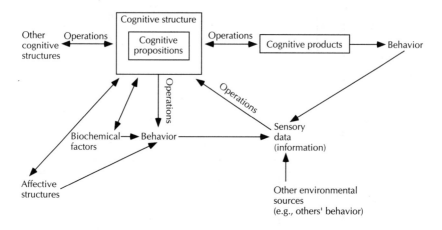

Figure 3–1.   Schematic diagram suggesting the pattern of interrelationships among the various components of the cognitive taxonomic system. *Source.*   Reprinted from Ingram RE, Kendall PC: "Cognitive Clinical Psychology: Implications of an Information Processing Perspective," in *Information Processing Approaches to Clinical Psychology.* Edited by Ingram RE. Orlando, FL, Academic Press, 1986, pp. 3–21. Used with permission.

within the cognitive system and are used to evaluate the presence of cognitive deficits. Information processing begins with the reception of environmental information (stimulus) and its conversion to neuroelectric energy. This energy is conveyed to the CNS. If the information is of sufficient physiological power or of sufficient meaningfulness, then the information will be encoded within short-term memory. Depending on environmental and psychological demands, the information may either remain and decay in short-term memory or be transferred to more permanent long-term memory. Within long-term memory, internal operations may be initiated to act on the information. These operations can include associations and linkages with previously stored information or with information received via other reception channels, or both. Whether the information was stored in long-term memory and, if stored, how the presented information was transformed are shown by what is retrieved. Within this model, retrieval is the only operation that can be measured by behavior. As such, it is critical to clinical evaluations of cognitive deficits. Behavioral evidence of a cognitive deficit is demonstrated by 1) inability to retrieve information, 2) difficulty in retrieving information, or 3) differences between the retrieved information and the information presented for encoding.

The information-processing model is helpful for visualizing the dynamics of cognitive operations. However, behavioral measures of cognition cannot show the operation of individual components of the information-processing model;

therefore, the source(s) of a cognitive deficit cannot be isolated within the model. A cognitive deficit may reflect disruptions in encoding, short-term and long-term memory storage, retrieval from storage, motor systems underlying a response, or any combination of these processes. A disruption in any of these processes can result in the same output behavior.

Fortunately, the cognitive operations of the information-processing model produce concomitant neuroelectric activity. This activity can occur in any area of the CNS and in physiological systems innervated by the CNS. To be psychophysiologically relevant, the operations of information processing must produce physiological changes that can be both reliably measured during information processing and reliably distinguished from routine physical adjustments related to homeostasis. The physiological measures also must conform to and increase the definition of behaviors associated with information processing. It will be seen that these conditions can be met. Psychophysiological paradigms not only help corroborate behavioral measures of cognitive deficit, but also locate the source(s) of the deficit within the information-processing model.

Psychophysiological Measurement and Instrumentation

Interest in the psychophysiology of cognitive activity extends back at least two millennia (see Caccioppo and Petty 1983 for a review). Despite a growing belief in the interaction of mind and body and an increased sophistication in the understanding of the physiological substrates of each, the technology for measuring these substrates and permanently storing the information was unavailable in the 19th century. Precision instrumentation with acceptable reliability and cost was not available until the 1940s. The foundations for the necessary technologies and their applications had roots in the development of bioelectric recording systems pioneered by Matteucci, Lippmann, and Einthoven in the 19th century and by Forbes and Thatcher and Erlanger and Gasser in the 1920s (see Basmajian 1967 and Grings 1954 for reviews). The early 20th century saw the application of this developing technology to psychophysiological studies of cognitive activity. Table 3–2 provides a synopsis of the most prominent psychophysiological measures of cognition and their methods and units of measurement.

One early approach was to measure the electrical activity of the skin associated with activity of the eccrine sweat glands. Originally termed the galvanic skin response or psychogalvanic skin response, the measure is now termed *electrodermal activity* (EDA) or the *electrodermal response* (EDR). Early investigators used EDA to probe mental and emotional states of both psychiatrically normal populations (Jones 1928; Prideaux 1920; Syz 1926; Waller 1918; Wells

Table 3–2. Summary of common psychophysiological measures, response systems, units of measurement, and recording technique

Response system	Primary organ	Unit of measurement	Typical recording technique
Electrodermal	Sweat glands	Microseimens	Electrical voltage or current applied across electrodes on skin area with sweat glands (usually the palm or fingertips)
Heart rate	Heart	Beats per minute	Electrodes placed on opposite sides of the body across the heart (e.g., the wrists)
Blood pressure	Heart, blood vessels	Millimeters of mercury	Sphygmomanometer with a pressure cuff wrapped around the upper arm
Peripheral blood flow Finger pulse volume Blood volume pulse	Blood vessels	Relative change in millimeters	Pressure, photoelectric, or densitometer plethysmography
Neuromuscular activity Electromyogram Muscle action potential	Skeletal muscles	Micro- or millivolts	Electrodes placed on surface of skin above muscle
Brain wave Electroencephalogram Evoked potential	Brain	Microvolts	Electrodes placed on scalp above locations sensitive to the processing of different kinds of environmental information

and Forbes 1911) and populations with severe psychopathology (Peterson and Jung 1907). Because of its direct relationship with autonomic activity, EDA remains a widely used measure of general cognitive status by psychophysiologists. However, increased interest in specific cognitive operations and the limited sensitivity of EDA to such operations have resulted in reduced applications of this measure in recent psychophysiological literature.

In their study of insane patients, Peterson and Jung (1907) also measured limb *blood flow* with a displacement plethysmograph. This instrument operated on the principal that cognitively mediated changes in blood flow to a limb resulted in alterations in limb size. If the limb was sealed in a container of air or fluid, variations in limb size resulted in movement of air (pneumoplethysmograph) or water (hydroplethysmograph) into or out of the container. This device was first used successfully by Glisson and Swammerdam in the late 1600s (see Hyman and Winsor 1961 for a review). In 1881, Mosso used the displacement plethysmograph to measure cognitive activity (Angell and Thompson 1899). He showed that mental activity increased blood flow to the cranium (brain) and decreased blood flow to the periphery. Angell and Thompson (1899) used a displacement plethysmograph to measure limb blood flow in response to sensations and emotions associated with "agreeable" and "disagreeable" stimuli. Although their stimuli were not sufficiently powerful to produce differential responses, the presentation of each stimulus did result in general vasoconstriction. Blood flow measures remain in use by today's psychophysiologists. However, the displacement plethysmograph has been superseded by a variety of more sensitive electronic detectors. The reflectance plethysmograph detects changes in reflected light produced by blood flowing in and out of a small body area, such as a finger or an ear.

Blood flowing into a physical structure produces a darkening of the skin and less reflection of light. The capacitance plethysmograph senses changes in electrical conductivity between two electrodes placed on opposite sides of a physical structure, such as a finger, an arm, or even the body trunk. As blood flows through the structure, the area becomes more dense, and less electrical activity passes between the electrodes. More recently, infrared detectors and optical densitometers have been used for blood flow measurements. Blood carries heat, and an infrared detector can measure minute heat changes associated with blood flow in any body area. Similarly, optical densitometers respond to changes in energy absorption produced by blood flow in any body area. Because of their sensitivity and suitability to any body area, infrared and densitometric plethysmographs offer the ability to obtain localized blood flow assessments, such as measures from individual cranial arteries.

Perhaps to Edmund Jacobson goes credit for the first series of intensive evaluations of the relationship between cognitive activity and physiology.

Jacobson proposed that neuromuscular activity was directly related to cognitive activation and awareness. Neuromuscular measurements require equipment sufficiently sensitive for measuring 10^{-4} volts (microvolts). Equipment capable of multichannel microvolt recordings became available in the late 1920s. Using both ink-writing (polygraph) and electron-beam (oscilloscope) oscillographs, Jacobson (1930a, 1930b, 1930c, 1930d, 1931a, 1931b, 1931c, 1932) reported a series of precision studies of elicited mental events and *electromyographic* (EMG) activity. These studies focused on the psychophysiology of imagination, abstract thinking, and memory. Although the success of these studies was somewhat limited, interest in the EMG as a cognitive index has been renewed by social psychophysiologists in their recent studies of facial EMG activity during emotional expression and thinking.

Jacobson demonstrated the ability to measure very low level neuromuscular electrical signals from electrodes placed on the skin surface over the muscle. As with measures from other peripheral systems, substantial inference was necessary to relate the data to cognitive events. Early psychophysiologists sought more direct measures. In 1929, Karl Lashley published the famous text *Brain Mechanisms and Intelligence.* The book's publication stimulated increased efforts to probe in vivo operations of what John Watson called the "mystery box," the human brain. Newly developed, reliable, and accurate low-level physiological recording instruments were joined with electrodes placed on the scalp surface over different cortical areas. Berger (1929) first used *electroencephalography* (EEG) to discover two distinct electrical rhythms, alpha and beta. He and his colleagues (Gibbs et al. 1935) also reported abnormalities in the brain rhythms of epileptic patients. This finding suggested the applicability of EEG for the clinical diagnosis of CNS disorders. Further support for this application was provided by Walter (1936), who found slow-wave (delta) activity to be localized in tissue surrounding brain tumors.

By the late 1930s, the technologies and research methodologies were available to support reliable psychophysiological evaluations of cognitive function. World War II greatly expedited technological development and increased the use of psychophysiological measures to evaluate cognitive function and dysfunction. This increase occurred for two reasons. First, strong relationships were being discovered between cortical arousal, peripheral arousal, and behavior. These changes could be reliably measured with a variety of psychophysiological indices (Darrow 1936; Davis and Davis 1939; Lindsley 1944; Murray 1938). Second, advancements in medical treatment and neurosurgical techniques resulted in a large number of hospitalized patients surviving the war with traumatic damage to the CNS. These individuals required accurate evaluations of cognitive deficits immediately after injury and during rehabilitation.

Luria and his colleagues developed very effective neuropsychological assessment techniques using behavioral measures to assess cognitive deficits (see Luria 1963 for a review). However, it was quickly recognized that the incorporation of psychophysiological measures during neuropsychological evaluations increased validity and precision for diagnosing the nature of the cognitive deficit, the location of the injury producing the deficit, and the prognosis for rehabilitation. Initially, the limb movement kymograph was incorporated. Later evaluations employed more sensitive psychophysiological measures such as EMG, EEG, EDR, and heart rate.

Today, the EEG is arguably the most widely used psychophysiological measure of cognitive operations. Initially, the EEG was applied as a useful clinical tool to assess brain damage after injury. Within the past two decades, this orientation has broadened to encompass functional assessments. Preeminent within the assessment of functional brain processes has been the use of the event-related potential (ERP). The ERP represents shifting EEG bioelectric levels occurring 50–1,000 milliseconds after brief sensory stimulation. These shifts are best viewed as electrical waves on which faster, asynchronous EEG signals occur. The time of occurrence, size, and shape of the ERP waves relate to different epochs in the information-processing cycle. Relative to information processing, ERP components are differentiated as exogenous and endogenous (see Donchin et al. 1986 for a review). Exogenous components occur early after stimulus onset (<100 milliseconds) and reflect the physical properties of the stimulus. Exogenous components are automatic and are sometimes referred to as evoked potentials. Typically measured at sensory cortical sites, exogenous components are useful in evaluating the functional status of sensory pathways. Endogenous components of the ERP are not automatic; if they occur, they will be found 100–1,000 milliseconds after stimulus onset. Endogenous ERP components are elicited by the demands and significance of the information processing associated with the stimulus. Thus, the occurrence and size of the ERP depends on the informational meaningfulness of the stimulus, the participant's past experience with the stimulus, and perceived contingencies between the stimulus and other environmental influences (see Donchin et al. 1986 and Hillyard and Hansen 1986 for reviews). As such, the ERP is especially sensitive to the status of the human cognitive system; it is being increasingly used as a noninvasive measure for diagnosis and prognosis of cognitive alterations associated with head injury (Greenberg et al. 1976, 1982; Ommaya and Gennarelli 1976). This increased sensitivity is obtained at a substantial price: ERP measurement is very difficult. Because of distraction or momentary changes in cognitive status, or both, the electrical waveform shifts may not occur or may occur differently across each stimulus presentation. The typical approach is to present the same stimulus 80 or more times, record an EEG during each stimulus presentation, and use a computer algorithm to derive an ERP waveform from the average of all EEGs measured.

The ERP is not simply a mirror of cognitive performance but offers unique insight into information processing. Some researchers have suggested that the ERP provides a measure of cognitive deficit that can be recorded free from the necessity of a behavioral response or neuropsychological test (Porjesz and Begleiter 1981, 1985). However, this is asking too much of a single measure. More recent approaches have used the ERP together with other physiological responses to examine psychophysiological patterning during complex problem solving. The objective is to determine the presence of a cognitive deficit, localize it within the information-processing model, and assess its magnitude. The psychophysiological responses are selected to reflect both CNS and autonomic nervous system activity during each stage of information processing. The problem-solving tasks delineate and probe different operations of information processing. The emphasis is on multiple physiological response measures occurring in synchrony with behaviors reflective of different information-processing operations.

This review has focused on the most prominent of what are a large number of physiological systems capable of being tapped by the psychophysiologist. It appears that virtually any physiological system within the body can be measured, often with noninvasive methods such as surface electrodes. However, it would be erroneous to conclude that if a physiological event can be measured, then it is psychophysiologically useful. Rather, the elicitation of a physiological response by a psychological event depends both on the strength of the relation between the response and the event and on the significance of the psychological event. Some measures such as electrodermal activity, heart rate, and blood pulse volume reflect variations in metabolic demands that are neurologically controlled by the autonomic nervous system. As such, these measures are sensitive to the allocation of body resources and general body state, making them particularly useful for assessing resting body activity levels and the presence of stimuli sufficiently powerful to alter these levels. Because of the robustness of their neuroelectric signals, these measures are easier to measure and relatively resilient to noise contamination from other biological systems. EEG activity and its ERP derivatives are CNS controlled. The ERP is most responsive to small, subtle alterations in the neuroelectric activity of brain operations, as would occur during thinking and cognition. However, its very sensitivity makes the ERP highly variable across stimulus presentations and individuals and very susceptible to artifact and noise interference from brain and body operations unrelated to cognition.

Therefore, today's psychophysiologists use multiple measures chosen to assess both general physiological status and specific neuroelectric operations associated with cognitive activity. Consider the evaluation of the orienting response (OR). The OR represents a general somatomotor and autonomic response whose magnitude is directly related to the perception, novelty, and meaningfulness of an external stimulus. Because orienting occurs in virtually all areas of the central and peripheral nervous systems, the measure can be obtained across a variety of physiological systems and species. The OR is highly stimulus selective, reflecting the formation of a CNS "neuronal model" to which subsequent presentations of the stimulus are compared (Sokolov 1963). Generally, the OR is associated with the early components of cognition, such as attention and information reception and encoding. However, during learning, OR formation reflects not only stimulus discrimination but also detection and evaluation of specific contingencies between a stimulus and the surrounding environment. These properties make the OR well suited to evaluations of cognitive operations in persons with severe cognitive dysfunction. For example, Grings et al. (1962) used the OR to index basic information processing in severely retarded patients.

Figure 3–2 presents an example of the type of recordings that might be obtained during the measurement of orienting. Note that the right and left electrooculargrams (R-EOG and L-EOG) are recorded only to determine the presence of eye-movement artifact in the EEG during stimulus presentation. The vertical lines indicate tone stimulus onset. Although each measure shows an initial OR to the stimulus, the size, speed, and time to return to prestimulus level vary for each measure. Differences appear even in measures obtained from the same response system, such as the EEG and the electrodermal measures of skin potential and skin response. It is hoped that by using measures with different dynamics both from the same and different physiological systems, a coherent picture of autonomic nervous system and CNS functional or dysfunctional orienting can be obtained. However, in the absence of behavioral data such as motor responses or verbal reports, the physiological data alone would not provide a valid explanation of orienting.

Öhman and Bohlin (1987) termed this problem the "psycho-physiologist's predicament." Using the OR as an example, they proposed that during orienting, psychological factors play a very limited role in accounting for variation in physiological functions. Öhman and Bohlin in fact found that the best correlations that can be expected between psychological factors and physiological function are .20–.30. The psychophysiologist faces the predicament of deciding whether to jettison the physiological measures, with all their complexity and limited power to explain psychological events, or to adopt the measures for the

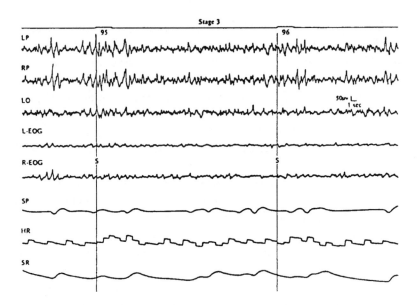

Figure 3–2.   An example of the type of psychophysiological recordings that might be obtained during the measurement of orienting to a specific stimulus. Legend: S = tone stimulus. LP = left parietal (P3). RP = right parietal (P4). LO = left occipital. L-EOG = left oculogram. R-EOG = right oculogram. SP = skin potential. HR = heart rate. SR = skin resistance. *Source.*   Reprinted from Johnson LC, Lubin A: "The Orienting Response During Waking and Sleeping." *Electroencephalography and Clinical Neurophysiology* 22:11–21, 1967. Used with permission.

small but more complete view of cognition that they provide. Psychological and physiological measures in combination provide a view of cognitive function that is unavailable if these factors are measured separately.

Psychophysiology of Cognitive Status and Function

The general status of cognitive function may be conceived in terms of physiological energy. Both a *steady-state energy,* available to support general cognitive operations such as awareness, and a *preparatory energy,* available for release in support of responses to cognitive demands, exist before cognitive demands. Preparatory energy is often referred to as activation.

In her comprehensive review of activation, Elizabeth Duffy (1972) distinguished activation from overt behavior: Activation represents the release of energy into and from physiological systems before an observable response. Critical to this proposition is that cognitive status represents tonic and phasic interactions between cognitive operations and all physiological systems sensitive to CNS operations. There is substantial evidence of the close interaction between cortically mediated activity (e.g., language), cortical operations, and activity in peripheral systems directly controlled both by the CNS and by the autonomic nervous system (Duffy 1962; Lacey et al. 1963; Lindsley 1970). However, considerations of cortical function separate from autonomic function results in a distorted view of the organism's behavior (Duffy 1962, 1972).

Because of their high level of interrelatedness, a cognitive event will be related to changes in several different response systems. However, activation should not be viewed as synchronous increases in activity or arousal in all physiological systems during a cognitive event. For example, under states of low cortical alertness shown by EEG, Lacey (1967) and Sternbach (1960) independently found high autonomic activation in some systems. Activation is more appropriately conceived as physiological systems changing from their steady state in support of event-contingent cognitive operations. These changes can reflect increases or decreases in activity. The most coherent relationships between cognitive and physiological operations are derived from evaluation of patterns across multiple psychophysiological measures.

Evaluations of activation patterns occur at both idiographic and nomothetic levels. During the initiation of a cognitive event, the psychophysiologist views each physiological system in terms of both the normal range of response and the subject's steady-state level of physiological activity before the response; this phenomenon may be explained by the law of initial values (LIV; Wilder 1957, 1958). The LIV postulates an inverse relationship between the steady-state level of physiological activity before stimulus onset and the magnitude of the activation response elicited by the stimulus. Thus, in the highly activated individual, the magnitude and, in extreme cases, the probability of a measurable response would be reduced. This is often referred to as a *ceiling effect*. A converse *basement effect* would be found during lowered activation. Superimposed on LIV is the individual's lability. Lability refers to the variation in an individual's response either to different stimuli or to the same stimulus presented at different times.

Considerations of LIV and lability are critical in psychophysiological studies of cognitive deficit. Because cognitive dysfunction is often associated with or produced by CNS alterations, cognitive deficits are often associated more with general homeostatic and neurophysiological changes than with disruptions in cognitive operations. These conditions can make psychophysiological evaluations of cognitive deficit problematic. Consider the hyperarousal theory of schizophrenia. It has been consistently reported that schizophrenic patients show chronically heightened neurophysiological activity (Bowers 1976; Maaser and Farley 1988; Whatmore and Ellis 1962; Zahn 1988). Psychophysiologically, this is evidenced by elevated EMG, EDA, and heart rate and desynchronized

EEG. Behaviorally, schizophrenic patients will report having stimulus flooding and an inability to focus attention. The condition is sufficiently reliable for some investigators to propose that stimulus overload produces psychophysiological disorganization directly resulting in thought disturbance (Epstein and Coleman 1970). However, controlled studies of activation patterns in psychiatrically normal and clinical populations have shown that the psychophysiological disorganization and hyperarousal of schizophrenic patients are secondary responses to the primary symptom of heightened anxiety (Tucker et al. 1969, 1974).

The importance of psychophysiological pattern analysis in assessing cognitive function has led to the development of several psychophysiological approaches that explicitly consider the interrelatedness of LIV, lability, and homeostasis. One approach presented by Lacey (1956) is the calculation of an autonomic lability score. The autonomic lability score incorporates a mathematical transformation yielding a range-corrected evaluation of the amount of physiological response independent of the preresponse physiological level. Subsequent research on the autonomic lability score showed it to be most valid only if the LIV is in operation (Clifton and Graham 1968; Hord et al. 1964). For example, Hare (1968) found uncorrected heart rate and electrodermal response scores to be most effective in distinguishing attention behaviors in psychopathological and nonpsychopathological populations.

Another approach is to derive a single composite score from the simultaneous responses of several physiological systems during perceptual and cognitive tasks. The clearest example of this approach is Wenger's index of autonomic balance ($\bar{A}$; Wenger 1947; Wenger and Cullen 1972). Wenger extensively studied the interactions between sympathetic nervous system and parasympathetic nervous system functions by observing psychophysiological response patterns during behavioral tasks. High $\bar{A}$ scores are associated with parasympathetic dominance, whereas low $\bar{A}$ scores are associated with sympathetic dominance. The psychophysiological measures included persistence of red dermographia, salivary output, heartbeat period between heartbeats, standing (postural) palmar skin conductance, volar forearm skin conductance, period between respiration cycles, and pulse pressure. Each measure is obtained under very specific conditions, including time of day (between 9 A.M. and 12 noon), room temperature (74–76°F), and room humidity (40%). The cognitive state of the individual is controlled with specified behaviors and postures.

The $\bar{A}$ score was reported to be a sensitive discriminator of chemical, physiological, and psychological conditions affecting individuals. Wenger and Cullen (1972) reported $\bar{A}$ scores that differentiated children on systemic and psychological dimensions. Children with higher $\bar{A}$ scores had lower basal metabolism, had faster physical development, were less emotional, were more patient and neat, and were less distractible. $\bar{A}$ score magnitudes correlated directly with level of adjustment at home and at school. McKelligott (1959) found $\bar{A}$ scores to discriminate between clinically complete cervical, thoracic, and lumbar spinal lesions. Wenger et al. (1960) reported on the sensitivity of autonomic balance scores to chemical ingestion. Specifically, these investigators found that amphetamine, atropine, and epinephrine lowered $\bar{A}$ scores, whereas the injection of Prostigmin resulted in increased scores.

The latter findings conform with Wenger's theory that anxiety is characterized by lowered autonomic balance scores (increased sympathetic nervous system dominance). In fact, Wenger et al. (1956) found significantly lowered $\bar{A}$ scores for graduate students on the day of a test versus 1 month after the test. A number of investigators reported relatively reduced $\bar{A}$ scores in individuals with anxiety-related or anxiety-produced disorders such as peptic ulcers, asthma, and certain forms of carcinoma (Clemens 1954; Little 1955; Wenger 1948).

Autonomic balance has been assessed in patients with cognitive and psychopathological disorders (Darrow 1943). Gunderson (1953) and Sherry (1959) found chemical and psychophysiological evidence of sympathetic nervous system dominance in schizophrenic patients, which was further characterized by lower than normal A scores. Wenger and Cullen (1972) corroborated these results, reporting that their schizophrenic subject population had the lowest $\bar{A}$ scores obtained from any previously examined patient group.

A second approach to psychophysiological patterning is to use experimental procedures and statistical analyses to "lock" physiological responses to cognitive operations. An example of this approach was presented by Germana (1968). He proposed a psychophysiologically indexed activational response process, termed activation peaking (AP), which tracks information processing during learning. As a neutral stimulus takes on a learned significance, psychophysiological activation increases systematically until the point of learning. Additional exposure to the learning situation results in successive decrements in activation. According to Germana, AP reflects processes associated with the orienting response.

Several characteristics of AP make it particularly useful for studies of cognitive activity and cognitive deficits. First, AP is related to the attachment of information to a previously neutral stimulus. The level of activation increases as information is acquired to support learning. Consequently, AP is applicable to complex learning paradigms, which gradually tap several different stages of information processing. Together with behavioral measures of learning, AP allows reliable evaluations of attention and storage. We have successfully applied AP to delineate the area of cognitive deficits within the information processing of detoxified alcoholic persons and persons at risk for alcoholism (Schandler et al. 1988b, 1992). This research is discussed in the next section.

Second, AP appears resistant to alterations in physiological levels (i.e., ceiling and floor effects) produced by pharmacological substances or neurophysiopathy. In a series of studies of the effects of marijuana on learning in persons with and without a heavy history of use, Cohen and his colleagues (Cohen et al. 1975; Rickles et al. 1978) found the physiological floor to lower during intoxication, while AP response patterns remained stable across conditions. Schandler et al. (1984, 1988a) found a similar outcome during psychophysiological studies of information processing in intoxicated alcoholic persons and nonalcoholic persons. Despite the substantial alterations in physiological baselines produced by acute alcohol intoxication and chronic alcohol abuse, AP reliably differentiated between groups of alcohol users and their state of intoxication. In conjunction with behavioral measures of learning, AP showed alcohol ingestion to be associated with the same disruption of information processing regardless of drinking history and physical status.

Finally, AP does not require production of a complex response during learning. As long as the CNS and some autonomic connections exist, the progression of learning can be charted. Thus, AP is applicable to populations with severe cognitive limitations. For example, Uno and Gargiulo (1977) found differential AP patterns of electrodermal responding in trainable mentally retarded participants during different problem-solving tasks. Though the behavioral repertoire was limited and homogenous in these persons, AP magnitude reliably distinguished tasks of varying difficulty.

For these reasons, the AP paradigm used in conjunction with behavioral measures has been useful for evaluating cognitive operations both in special populations and in psychiatrically normal populations under special conditions. Across conditions and populations, AP yields relatively consistent results that provide coherent assessment of cognitive activity.

Psychophysiology Applied to the Evaluation of Cognitive Deficits

Our research with chronic alcoholic persons typifies current applications of psychophysiology to assessing cognitive deficits. We have spent the past decade investigating the effects of alcohol abuse and alcoholism on cognitive function. The overarching objective of this research is to examine the role that cognitive dysfunction plays in the etiology and epidemiology of alcoholism. However, a practical objective is to improve the design and efficiency of alcoholism prevention and treatment programs. Wilkinson and Sanchez-Craig (1981) stressed that a major component of the treatment of alcoholism involves the learning of both simple and complex cognitive coping strategies. Cognitive-based therapies have been particularly effective in comparison to traditional supportive therapies (McCourt and Glantz 1980; Oei and Jackson 1982; Parsons 1980; Sanchez-Craig et al. 1984). The effectiveness of these treatments will ultimately reflect the clarity of understanding concerning cognitive functions of alcoholic persons.

Early in our research, we discarded the view that alcoholic persons display a permanent deficit in global cognitive function after chronic alcohol abuse. As early as 1941, Wechsler noted that alcohol-related mental deficits were selective, reflecting performance alterations on specific cognitive tasks. One very consistent finding is that chronic alcohol abuse reduces visuospatial information processing (Parsons 1986; Ryan and Butters 1983; Wilson 1987). Unlike alcohol-related verbal deficits, visuospatial deficits may not recover after detoxification and abstinence. Alcohol-related deficits in visuospatial-information processing reflect neither a general decrement in intellectual activity nor disruptions of motor activity associated with a response (Glosser et al. 1977; Yohman et al. 1985). Rather, alcohol appears to disrupt one or more cognitive operations during the processing of visuospatial information.

Only recently have attempts been made to define the nature and magnitude of an alcohol-related visuospatial deficit and its location within information-processing structures of the CNS. One persistent problem is that studies of visuospatial deficits in alcoholic persons can be confounded by two factors. First, if alcoholic persons regain verbal but not visuospatial operations, then the cognitive probe task must explicitly be free of verbal content. Unless the verbal content of a task can be removed or controlled, alcoholic persons may display visuospatial deficits that actually represent verbal disruptions.

A second problem is that chronic alcoholic persons are afflicted with substantial peripheral neuropathy. Behavioral measures of cognitive deficit may reflect peripheral rather than central disruptions. Simultaneous measures of central concomitants enhance resolution while coincidentally allowing assessment of the presence and degree of peripheral disruption.

In consideration of these problems, we used a new visuospatial task together with behavioral, autonomic, and ERP-dependent measures. A synopsis of several of our studies illustrates the approach (Cohen et al. 1983, 1989; Schandler et al. 1988a, 1988b, 1991, 1992). Under conditions of intoxication and detoxification, alcoholic persons performed a visuospatial task that required them to learn the spatial position of nonsense shapes that were unlikely to produce verbal associations. During learning, the EDR, heart rate, and ERP were recorded and analyzed.

The learning performance and psychophysiological data indicated three clear effects. The first effect was unexpected; while intoxicated, alcoholic persons' visuospatial learning performance was superior to their performance after detoxification. The superiority was reflected not only in relatively greater speed of learning, but also in terms of relatively fewer errors and nonresponses by these persons. Second, the pattern of physiological activation clearly tracked the learning performance in the intoxicated and detoxified conditions. The superior performance of the intoxicated alcoholic persons was associated with a distinctive physiological pattern that accurately represented their learning performance. The relatively inferior learning performance of the detoxified alcoholic persons was characterized by an undifferentiated activational pattern. Third, compared with their ERPs when detoxified, the intoxicated alcoholic persons showed significantly enhanced ERP components occurring between 50 and 300 milliseconds after stimulus onset.

The finding of superior visuospatial learning in alcoholic persons when intoxicated versus detoxified has not been reported elsewhere in the literature. Any attempt to proceed with a psychophysiological interpretation of the data depended on evaluation of whether the behavioral data were acceptable or aberrant. Several investigators reported that alcohol facilitates affective states related to information processing (Docter and Bernal 1964; Docter and Perkins 1961; Docter et al. 1966; Mendelson 1964). An alcohol-related autonomic balancing theory would have particular significance relative to information processing in alcoholic persons. Using a pharmacological stress test (Funkenstein mecholyl test), Kissin and Hankoff (1959) and Kissin and Platz (1968) concluded that alcohol reduces tension and autonomic imbalance in alcoholic persons. If alcohol causes a pharmacological balancing effect in alcoholic persons, then their attention to and subsequent learning of environmental relationships could be enhanced while intoxicated but depressed while sober. We followed this theoretical route in our subsequent analyses of the studies.

Our behavioral data were consistent with the theory. In addition to achieving the learning criterion more quickly, the intoxicated alcoholic persons had fewer nonresponses and errors relative to when they were detoxified. The higher number of nonresponses by the detoxified alcoholic persons may show that, without alcohol, the alcoholic persons were pharmacologically imbalanced and less able to obtain enough information to support a response. This would locate alcohol's balance and imbalance effects on attention and encoding operations during information processing.

An evaluation of learning performance patterns helped to identify the cognitive operations that are affected by alcohol. By themselves, the learning performance data could only suggest that alcohol's effects may be most disruptive to attentional operations during visuospatial processing. We proceeded to overlay psychophysiological measures on the behavioral data using analyses of AP and of brain waves. The increased resolution that was achieved from these approaches illustrates the value of applying psychophysiological measures to achieve an understanding of cognitive deficits.

The autonomic measures of AP obtained from alcoholic persons during visuospatial learning supported the premise that alcohol affects attention mechanisms. Figures 3–3 and 3–4 present EDR and heart rate data aligned for AP from intoxicated and detoxified alcoholic persons. The intoxicated alcoholic persons displayed a very clear pattern of electrodermal and heart rate AP that correctly tracked their learning performance. Recalling the connection between AP and orienting behavior, these data indicated that, when intoxicated, the alcoholic persons were more effective at scanning and selecting cues from the environment. When detoxified, the alcoholic persons achieved the learning criterion, but their AP pattern was less clear. Orienting appeared reduced. The inferior visuospatial learning displayed by detoxified alcoholic persons may have resulted from reduced scanning and encoding.

The ERP data confirmed this premise. The states of intoxication and detoxification were best delineated by the ERP components associated with attention

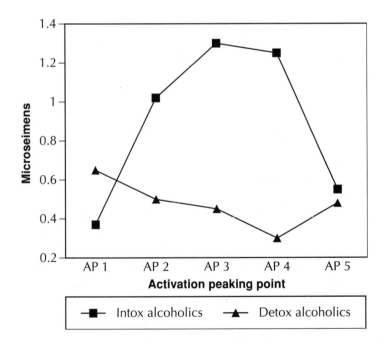

Figure 3–3.   Mean skin conductance (microseimens) levels for intoxicated alcoholic persons and detoxified alcoholic persons during each activation peaking (AP) point.

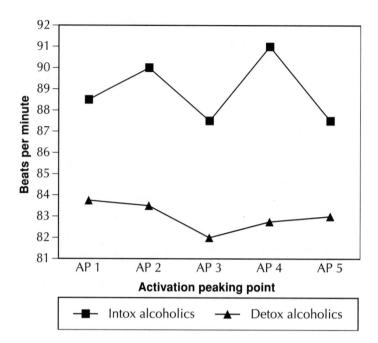

Figure 3–4.   Mean heart rate (beats per minute) levels for intoxicated alcoholic persons and detoxified alcoholic persons during each activation peaking (AP) point.

and information encoding. Support for this proposition was first derived, albeit indirectly, from the finding that both groups maintained an operational memory storage process. This was evidenced by the presence of a clear and consistent P300 component with greater amplitudes regardless of intoxication condition. The P300 is a positive shifting waveform component occurring approximately 300 milliseconds after stimulus onset. It is probably the most investigated of the ERP components and is considered to reflect psychological rather than physical characteristics of an information stimulus. P300 presence and amplitude are most associated with orientation to task-relevant information and with the updating and modifying of information stored in working memory (Fabiani et al. 1986; Johnson and Donchin 1978; Karis et al. 1984).

Chronic alcohol use is consistently associated with reductions in P300 amplitude and increased P300 onset latencies. However, these effects were gleaned from comparisons of detoxified or abstinent alcoholic persons with nonalcoholic persons. The unquestionable central neuropathy produced by prolonged ethanol ingestion would make it very difficult to determine to what degree the P300 aberrations displayed by alcoholic persons represent disruptions in cognitive processes or a general disruption of the cerebral neurostructure. The subjects in our studies possessed similar histories of chronic alcohol abuse, allowing an assumption of equivalent neuropathy. The data indicated a clear and equivalent P300 presence regardless of the intoxicated state of the alcoholic persons, although the P300 presence was lower in magnitude than that displayed by nonalcoholic persons. The finding of similar P300 amplitudes in both conditions indicated essentially similar operational memory processes related to the storage of task-relevant information. Thus, the visuospatial deficit displayed by the alcoholic persons was not due to a disruption in memory storage.

Absence of a memory storage effect does not ipso facto mean that visuospatial deficits of alcoholic persons are the result of differences in attentional information encoding processes. Direct support for such an effect was evident in evaluations of the early components of the ERP. Specifically affected were P2, N1, and N2-P3, reflecting positive and negative brain-wave shifts occurring between 50 and 250 milliseconds after stimulus onset. These ERP components are considered to represent information-processing operations associated with comparisons between the physical characteristics of the stimulus and information contained in working memory obtained from previous experience with the stimulus. Our intoxicated and detoxified alcoholic subjects displayed these components, but the amplitudes were reduced relative to amplitudes displayed by nonalcoholic persons. However, compared with the subjects' state after detoxification, the P2, N1, and N2-P3 amplitudes were significantly greater during intoxication. Previous findings suggest that this effect represents an amplitude depression of components within the detoxified group rather than enhanced amplitudes in intoxicated persons.

Overlaying these ERP findings on the AP and learning performance data began to provide a coherent picture of visuospatial deficits in alcoholic persons. A substantive body of data suggests that the N1 and P2 components represent sensation and attentional processes related to the formation of an OR (Näätänen and Gaillard 1983). Our AP data were consistent with the N1 and P2 findings. Porjesz and Begleiter (1979, 1980, 1981) reported that the amplitudes of the N1-P2 components both are significantly depressed in detoxified alcoholic persons and are the components most sensitive to attentional manipulations of information presented to abstinent alcoholic persons. Based on these data, the investigators have proposed that "sensory-filtering" mechanisms are impaired in abstinent chronic alcoholic persons.

There are data that also indicate that the sensory-filtering and encoding processes are more normal in intoxicated alcoholic persons than in detoxified alcoholic persons, resulting in the intoxicated persons' relatively superior learning performance. It is interesting to note the observation of Porjesz and Begleiter

(1985), who stated that the findings of reduced N1-P2 components in abstinent alcoholic persons corroborated the findings of several other investigators who administered acute doses of alcohol to nonalcoholic persons. They proposed that "brain dysfunction in chronic [abstinent] alcoholics resembles aberrations detected in normal persons under the influence of alcohol" (Porjesz and Begleiter 1981, p 311).

Although the application of psychophysiological measures assists in the framing and addressing of questions, the measures do not—by themselves—answer questions. One might conclude from our data that the brain functions and information-processing behavior of intoxicated alcoholic persons resemble operations present in sober nonalcoholic persons. Such a statement cannot be correct because these groups are so different: All neuroanatomical data show that chronic alcoholic persons possess moderate, alcohol-related structural damage of the CNS. Furthermore, the damage tends to be idiopathic in its relation to alcohol ingestion. For example, the CNS damage displayed by chronic alcoholic persons is not similar to that of normal degenerative processes such as aging. What the behavioral and the psychophysiological data do suggest is that certain chronic alcoholic persons process information more normally when they are intoxicated than when they are detoxified and abstinent. This emphasizes Naitoh's call (1972) for more studies that evaluate what alcohol does *for* rather than *to* the alcoholic person.

Summary

We have attempted to present the process by which modern psychophysiology is applied to the study of cognitive deficit. The research and its interpretations emphasize two principal characteristics of applied psychophysiology.

First, the use of behavioral and physiological measures does not automatically result in useful explanations of cognitive deficit. The effective use of psychophysiology depends on the development of appropriate research designs applied to populations with established and verified cognitive function and dysfunction. The development of proper cognitive probe tasks and the determination of population characteristics must occur before the application of psychophysiological methods. Psychophysiology is expensive; it demands advanced technology and considerable analytical effort. More important, it involves the application of recording devices to the patient. Poorly conceived, superficial psychophysiological studies would be viewed as capricious, potentially violating accepted logistical and ethical cost-benefit ratios. The assessment of cognitive deficit demands the utmost care and sensitivity to the patient's status. That psychophysiology demands the same may explain its special suitability to evaluations of cognitive deficits.

The second principle of psychophysiology is that human cognition represents a dynamic process involving multiple internal and external variables. We also must see cognitive deficits the same way. The application of psychophysiology literally compels the investigator to consider any cognitive deficit as multivariate. As a result, interpretations of psychophysiological data are quite difficult. However, when the interpretations produce coherence, they result in explanations of cognitive deficits that are clearer and more complete than those provided by behavioral measures alone. This increases the therapeutic relevance of these data.

References

Angell JR, Thompson HB: A study of the relations between certain organic processes and the consciousness. Psychol Rev 6:32–69, 1899

Basmajian JV: Control of individual motor units. American Journal of Physical Medicine 46:480–486, 1967

Berger H: Uber das elektrenkephalogramm des menschen. Archiv für Psychiatrie und Nervenkrankheiten 87:527–570, 1929

Bowers MB Jr: Pathogenesis of acute schizophrenic psychosis, in Dimensions in Abnormal Psychology, 2nd Edition. Edited by Shean G. Chicago, IL, Rand McNally, 1976, pp 146–190

Caccioppo JT, Petty RE: Foundations of social psychophysiology, in Social Psychophysiology: A Sourcebook. Edited by Caccioppo JT, Petty RE. New York, Guilford, 1983, pp 3–32

Clemens TL: A preliminary report on autonomic functions in neoplastic diseases, in The Psychological Variables in Human Cancer. Edited by Gengerelli JA, Kirkner FJ. Berkeley, University of California Press, 1954, pp 95–127

Clifton RK, Graham FK: Stability of individual differences in heart rate activity during the newborn period. Psychophysiology 5:37–50, 1968

Cohen MJ, Rickles WH, Naliboff BD: Marijuana influenced changes in GSR activation peaking during paired-associate learning. Pharmacol Biochem Behav 3:195–200, 1975

Cohen MJ, Schandler SL, Naliboff BD: Psychophysiological measures from intoxicated and detoxified alcoholics. J Stud Alcohol 44:271–282, 1983

Cohen MJ, Schandler SL, McArthur DL: Spatial learning of visual "nonsense syllables" during ethanol intoxication. Percept Mot Skills 68:599–606, 1989

Darrow CW: The galvanic skin reflex (sweating) and blood pressure and a preparatory and facilitative functions. Psychol Bull 33:73–94, 1936

Darrow CW: Physiological and clinical tests of autonomic function and autonomic balance. Physiol Rev 23:1–36, 1943

Davis H, Davis PA: Action potentials of the brain: its relation to physiological states and to states of impaired consciousness. Res Publ Assoc Res Nerv Ment Dis 19:50–80, 1939

Docter RF, Bernal ME: Immediate and prolonged psychophysiological effects of sustained alcohol intake in alcoholics. Quarterly Journal of Studies on Alcohol 25:438–450, 1964

Docter RF, Perkins RB: The effects of ethyl alcohol on autonomic and muscular responses in humans. Quarterly Journal of Studies on Alcohol 22: 374–380, 1961

Docter RF, Naitoh P, Smith JC: Electromyographic changes and vigilance behavior during experimentally induced intoxication with alcoholic subjects. Psychosom Med 28:605–615, 1966

Donchin E, Karis D, Bashore TR, et al: Cognitive psychophysiology and human information processing, in Psychophysiology: Systems, Processes, and Applications. Edited by Coles MGH, Donchin E, Porges SW. New York, Guilford, 1986, pp 244–267

Duffy E: Activation and Behavior. New York, Wiley, 1962

Duffy E: Activation, in Handbook of Psychophysiology. Edited by Greenfield NS, Sternbach RA. New York, Holt, Rinehart and Winston, 1972, pp 577–622

Epstein S, Coleman M: Drive theories of schizophrenia. Psychosom Med 32:113, 1970

Fabiani M, Karis D, Donchin E: P300 and recall in an incidental memory paradigm. Psychophysiology 23:298–308, 1986

Germana J: Psychophysiological correlates of conditioned response formation. Psychol Bull 70:105–114, 1968

Gibbs FA, Davis H, Lennox WG: The electroencephalogram in epilepsy and in conditions of impaired consciousness. Archives of Neurology and Psychiatry 3:1133–1148, 1935

Glosser G, Butters N, Kaplan E: Visuoperceptual processes in brain-damaged patients on the digit symbol substitution test. Int J Neurosci 7:59–66, 1977

Greenberg RP, Mayer DJ, Becker DP: The prognostic value of evoked potentials in human mechanical head injury, in Head Injuries: Proceedings of the Second Chicago Symposium on Neural Trauma. Edited by McLaurin RL. New York, Grune & Stratton, 1976, pp 81–88

Greenberg RP, Newlon PG, Becker DP: The somatosensory evoked potential inpatients with severe head injury: outcome prediction and monitoring of brain function. Ann N Y Acad Sci 388:683–688, 1982

Grings WW: Laboratory Instrumentation in Psychology. Palo Alto, CA, National Press, 1954

Grings WW, Lockhart RA, Dameron LE: Conditioning autonomic responses of mentally subnormal individuals. Psychological Monographs 76:1–35, 1962

Gunderson EK: Autonomic balance in schizophrenia (unpublished doctoral dissertation). Los Angeles, University of California, 1953

Hare RD: Psychopathy, autonomic functioning, and the orienting response. J Abnorm Psychol 73: (suppl 3, part 2) 1–24, 1968

Hillyard SA, Hansen JC: Attention: electrophysiological approaches, in Psychophysiology: Systems, Processes, and Applications. Edited by Coles MGH, Donchin E, Porges SW. New York, Guilford, 1986, pp 227–243

Hord DJ, Johnson LC, Lubin A: Differential effect of the law of initial value (LIV) on autonomic variables. Psychophysiology 1:79–87, 1964

Hyman C, Winsor T: History of plethysmography. J Cardiovasc Surg (Torino) 2:506–518, 1961

Ingram RE, Kendall PC: Cognitive clinical psychology: implications of an information processing perspective, in Information Processing Approaches to Clinical Psychology. Edited by Ingram RE. Orlando, FL, Academic Press, 1986, pp 3–21

Jacobson E: Electrical measurements of neuromuscular states during mental activities, I: imagination and movement involving skeletal muscle. Am J Physiol 91:567–608, 1930a

Jacobson E: Electrical measurements of neuromuscular states during mental activities, II: imagination and recollection of various muscular acts. Am J Physiol 94:23–34, 1930b

Jacobson E: Electrical measurements of neuromuscular states during mental activities, III: visual imagination and recollection. Am J Physiol 95: 694–702, 1930c

Jacobson E: Electrical measurements of neuromuscular states during mental activities, IV: evidence of contraction of specific muscles during imagination. Am J Physiol 95:703–712, 1930d

Jacobson E: Electrical measurements of neuromuscular states during mental activities, V: variation of specific muscles contracting during imagination. Am J Physiol 96:115–121, 1931a

Jacobson E: Electrical measurements of neuromuscular states during mental activities, VI: note on mental activities concerning an amputated limb. Am J Physiol 96:122–125, 1931b

Jacobson E: Electrical measurements of neuromuscular states during mental activities, VII: imagination, recollection, and abstract thinking involving the speech musculature. Am J Physiol 97:200–209, 1931c

Jacobson E: Electrophysiology of mental activities. Am J Psychol 44:677–694, 1932

Johnson R, Donchin E: On how P300 amplitude varies with the utility of the eliciting stimuli. Electroencephalogr Clin Neurophysiol 44:424–437, 1978

Jones HE: The galvanic skin reflex in infancy. Child Dev 1:106–110, 1928

Karis D, Fabiani M, Donchin E: P300 and memory: individual differences in the von Restorff effect. Cognitive Psychology 16:177–216, 1984

Kissin B, Hankoff L: The acute effects of ethyl alcohol on the Funkenstein mecholyl response in male alcoholics. Quarterly Journal of Studies on Alcohol 20:696–703, 1959

Kissin B, Platz A: The use of drugs in the long term rehabilitation of chronic alcoholics, in Psychopharmacology: A Review of Progress 1957–1967 (PHS Publ No 1836). Edited by Efron DH. Washington, DC, U.S. Government Printing Office, 1968, pp 835–851

Lacey JI: The evaluation of an autonomic response: toward a general solution. Ann N Y Acad Sci 67:123–164, 1956

Lacey JI: Somatic response patterning and stress: some revisions of activation theory, in Psychological Stress: Issues in Research. Edited by Appley MH, Trumbull R. New York, Appleton-Century-Crofts, 1967, pp 79–95

Lacey JI, Kagan J, Lacey BC, et al: The visceral level: situational determinants and behavioral correlates of autonomic response patterns, in Expression of the Emotions in Man. Edited by Knapp PH. New York, International Universities Press, 1963, pp 161–196

Lashley KS: Brain Mechanisms and Intelligence. Chicago, IL, University of Chicago Press, 1929

Lindsley DB: Electroencephalography, in Personality and the Behavior Disorders. Edited by Hunt JMcV. New York, Ronald, 1944, pp 1033–1103

Lindsley DB: The role of nonspecific reticulo-thalamo-cortical systems in emotion, in Physiological Correlates of Emotions. Edited by Black P. New York, Academic Press, 1970, pp 147–188

Little KB: Effects of vagotomy on autonomic balance. Psychsom Med 17: 227–233, 1955

Luria AR: Restoration of Function After Brain Injury. New York, Macmillan, 1963, pp 78–116

Maaser BW, Farley FH: A review of left hemisphere dysfunction and hyperarousal and the effects of chlorpromazine in schizophrenia. Research Communications in Psychology, Psychiatry and Behavior 13:177–192, 1988

McCourt W, Glantz M: Cognitive behavior therapy in groups for alcoholics: a preliminary report. J Stud Alcohol 41:388–346, 1980

McKelligott JW: Autonomic functions and effective states in spinal cord injury (unpublished doctoral dissertation). Los Angeles, University of California, 1959

Mendelson JH, LaDou J, Solomon P: Experimentally induced chronic intoxication and withdrawal in alcoholics. Quarterly Journal of Studies on Alcohol, pt 3, Psychiatric Findings (suppl 2), 40–52, 1964

Murray HA: Explorations in Personality. New York, Oxford, 1938

Näätänen R, Gaillard AWK: The orienting reflex and the N2 deflection of the event-related potential (ERP), in Tutorials in ERP Research: Endogenous Components. Edited by Gaillard AWK, Ritter W. Amsterdam, The Netherlands, North-Holland, 1983, pp 119–141

Naitoh P: The effect of alcohol on the autonomic nervous system of humans: psychophysiological approach, in Biology of Alcoholism, Vol 2: Physiology and Behavior. Edited by Kissin B, Begleiter H. New York, Plenum, 1972, pp 357–433

Oei TPS, Jackson PR: Social skills and cognitive behavioral approaches to the treatment of problem drinking. J Stud Alcohol 43:532–547, 1982

Öhman A, Bohlin G: Barry's unification of matter, mind, and body: one mental process for each polygraph channel, in Advances in Psychophysiology: A Research Annual, Vol 2. Edited by Ackles P, Jennings JR, Coles MGH. Greenwich, CT, JAB Press, 1987, pp 259–270

Ommaya AK, Gennarelli TA: A physiologic basis for noninvasive diagnosis and prognosis of head injury severity, in Head Injuries: Proceedings of the Second Chicago Symposium on Neural Trauma. Edited by McLaurin RL. New York, Grune & Stratton, 1976, pp 49–75

Parsons OA: Cognitive dysfunction in alcoholics and social drinkers: problems in assessment and remediation. J Stud Alcohol 41:105–106, 1980

Parsons OA: Alcoholics' neuropsychological impairment: current findings and conclusions. Annals of Behavioral Medicine 8:13–19, 1986

Peterson F, Jung CG: Psychophysical investigations with the galvanometer and plethysmograph in normal and insane individuals. Brain 30:153–218, 1907

Porjesz B, Begleiter H: Visual evoked potentials and brain dysfunction in chronic alcoholics, in Evoked Brain Potentials and Behavior. Edited by Begleiter H. New York, Plenum, 1979, pp 277–302

Porjesz B, Begleiter H: Brain dysfunction and alcohol, in Biological Effects of Alcohol. Edited by Begleiter H. New York, Plenum, 1980, pp 415–483

Porjesz B, Begleiter H: Human evoked brain potentials and alcohol. Alcohol Clin Exp Res 5:304–317, 1981

Porjesz B, Begleiter H: Human brain electrophysiology and alcoholism, in Alcohol and the Brain. Edited by Tarter RE, Van Thiel DH. New York, Plenum, 1985, pp 139–182

Porjesz B, Begleiter H, Garozzo R: Visual evoked potential correlates of information processing deficits in chronic alcoholics, in Biological Effects of Alcohol. Edited by Begleiter H. New York, Plenum, 1980, pp 603–623

Prideaux E: The psychogalvanic reflex: a review. Brain 43:50–71, 1920

Rickles WH Jr, Cohen MJ, Naliboff BD, et al: Measures of heart rate and skin conductance to orienting stimuli during repetitive administration of marijuana. Br J Addict 73:69–74, 1978

Ryan C, Butters N: Cognitive deficits in alcoholics, in The Biology of Alcoholism, Vol 7: The Pathogenesis of Alcoholism: Biological Factors. Edited by Kissin B, Begleiter H. New York, Plenum, 1983, pp 485–538

Sanchez-Craig M, Annis HM, Bornet AR, et al: Random assignment to abstinence and controlled drinking: evaluation of a cognitive-behavioral program for problem drinkers. J Consult Clin Psychol 52:390–403, 1984

Schandler SL, Cohen MJ, Naliboff BD: Alcohol influenced changes in activation speaking during paired-associate verbal learning. J Stud Alcohol 45:493–499, 1984

Schandler SL, Cohen MJ, McArthur DL, et al: Activation peaking in intoxicated and detoxified alcoholics during visuospatial learning. J Stud Alcohol 49:126–130, 1988a

Schandler SL, Cohen MJ, McArthur DL: Event-related potentials in intoxicated alcoholics during visuospatial learning. Psychopharmacology 94:275–283, 1988b

Schandler SL, Cohen MJ, McArthur DL, et al: Spatial learning deficits in adult children of alcoholic parents. J Consult Clin Psychol 59:312–317, 1991

Schandler SL, Cohen MJ, Antick JR: Activation, attention and visuospatial learning in adults with and without a family history of alcoholism. Alcohol Clin Exp Res 16:566–571, 1992

Sherry LU: Some effects of chlorpromazine on the physiological and psychological functioning of a group of chronic schizophrenics (unpublished doctoral dissertation). Los Angeles, University of California, 1959

Sokolov EN: Perception and the Conditioned Reflex. New York, Pergamon, 1963

Sternbach RA: Two independent indices of activation. Electroencephalogr Clin Neurophysiol 12:609–611, 1960

Syz HC: Observations on the unreliability of subjective reports of emotional reactions. Br J Psychol 17:119–126, 1926

Tucker GJ, Harrow M, Detre T, et al: Perceptual experiences in schizophrenic and nonschizophrenic patients. Arch Gen Psychiatry 20:159–166, 1969

Tucker GJ, Campion EW, Kelleher PA, et al: The relationship of subtle neurological impairments to disturbances of thinking. Psychother Psychosom 24:165–169, 1974

Uno R, Gargiulo RM: Activational peaking in educable and trainable mentally retarded persons (abstract). Percept Mot Skills 44:1186, 1977

Waller AD: The emotive response to ordinary stimulation, real and imaginary. Lancet 96:380–381, 1918

Walter WG: The location of cerebral tumors by electroencephalography. Lancet 2:305–308, 1936

Wechsler D: The effect of alcohol on mental activity. Quarterly Journal of Studies on Alcohol 2:479–485, 1941

Wells FL, Forbes A: On certain electrical processes in the human body and their relation to emotional reactions. Archives of Psychology 2:1–39, 1911

Wenger MA: Preliminary study of the significance of measures of autonomic balance. Psychosom Med 9:301–309, 1947

Wenger MA: Studies of autonomic balance in Army Air Forces personnel. Comparative Psychology Monographs 19, 1948

Wenger MA, Cullen TD: Studies of autonomic balance in children and adults, in Handbook of Psychophysiology. Edited by Greenfield NS, Sternbach RA. New York, Holt, Rinehart and Winston, 1972, pp 535–576

Wenger MA, Jones FN, Jones MH: Physiological Psychology. New York, Holt, Rinehart and Winston, 1956

Wenger MA, Clemens TL, Darsie ML, et al: Autonomic response patterns during intravenous infusion of epinephrine and norepinephrine. Psychosom Med 22:294–307, 1960

Whatmore GB, Ellis RM: Further neurophysiologic aspects of depressed states. Arch Gen Psychiatry 6:243–253, 1962

Wilder J: The law of initial values in neurology and psychiatry: facts and problems. J Nerv Ment Dis 125:73–86, 1957

Wilder J: Modern psychophysiology and the law of initial value. Am J Psychother 12:199–221, 1958

Wilkinson DA, Sanchez-Craig M: Relevance of brain dysfunction to treatment objectives: should alcohol-related cognitive deficits influence the way we think about treatment? Addict Behav 6:253–260, 1981

Wilson GT: Cognitive studies in alcoholism. J Consult Clin Psychol 55: 325–331, 1987

Yohman JR, Parson OA, Leber WR: Lack of recovery in male alcoholics' neuropsychological performance one year after treatment. Alcoholism: Clinical and Experimental Research 9:114–117, 1985

Zahn TP: Studies of autonomic psychophysiology and attention in schizophrenia. Schizophr Bull 14:205–208, 1988

Chapter 4

Cognitive Deficits in Depression

Shirley Hartlage, Ph.D., and Caroline Clements, Ph.D.

T he past 30 years have shown a proliferation of cognitive models of depression (e.g., Abramson et al. 1989; Alloy et al. 1988a; Beck 1967, 1991; Ingram 1984; Lewinsohn et al. 1985; Rehm 1988). The majority of these models postulate that certain ways of thinking cause, exacerbate, or maintain specific symptoms of depression. Some of the models focus on cognitive *deficits* (i.e., quantitative shortcomings) among depressed and depression-prone individuals. For example, Rehm (1977) postulated that deficits in self-control mechanisms cause depression, and other authors (e.g., Hartlage et al. 1993; Hasher and Zacks 1979) suggested that depressed persons are deficient in effortful processes such as problem solving. However, most cognitive models of depression focus on *qualitative* differences between the thinking of depressed and depression-prone individuals and the thinking of psychiatrically normal persons. For example, Beck (1967, 1991) emphasized that depression develops when depressed persons selectively process negative information (rather than process less information overall), and Blaney (1986) indicated that depressed persons recall more information that is congruent rather than incongruent with their depressed moods.

Ingram and his colleagues (Ingram and Kendall 1986; Ingram and Wisnicki 1991) proposed a taxonomy for categorizing cognitive variables that is adopted in this chapter. They distinguished between cognitive operations and schemata. Specifically, cognitive *operations* refer to the processes by which the information system operates. Examples of operations include encoding, retrieval, and recall. Cognitive *schema* are organized information structures in memory. Cognitive deficits and biases among depressed persons may occur in the way depressed persons process information or in the nature of depressed persons' schemata (e.g., Alloy et al. 1985).

In this chapter, we present a theoretical overview and methodological issues relevant to evaluating the cognitive models of depression. Specific models of depression and depressive cognition that focus on operations and schemata follow. We summarize evidence for and against aspects of each model in turn. Several of the cognitive models of depression have been reformulated or have progressively developed since they were originally presented. Thus, Seligman's original learned helplessness model (1975) became the reformulated learned helplessness model of Abramson et al. (1978) and then the hopelessness model (Abramson et al. 1989; Alloy et al. 1988a). Further, Beck (1991) clarified some earlier misconceptions regarding his model (Beck 1967). Finally, Lewinsohn et al. (1985) developed their earlier reinforcement model (e.g., Lewinsohn et al. 1969) to become what is now termed an integrated model of depression.

Theoretical Overview and Methodological Issues

Several methodological issues are relevant to evaluating studies of cognitive deficits in depression (Alloy et al. 1988b): making correct predictions from the models, recognizing the heterogeneity of depressive disorders, assessing stress, using longitudinal versus cross-sectional research strategies, and using optimal measurement techniques. We discuss each of these in turn.

Most cognitive theorists view depression as a heterogeneous disorder (Abramson et al. 1988; Lewinsohn et al. 1985). That is, although a variety of specific etiologies or causal pathways leading to depression have been proposed, each theorist also states that other conditions, including a genetic predisposition or a biochemical imbalance, may result in depression. Expressed in another way, most cognitive models of depression are *sufficiency* models versus *necessity* models. Each proposes a particular causal mechanism that is sufficient for producing depression, but not necessary (i.e., not the only causal mechanism) for producing depression. Further, models of depression such as the hopelessness model (Abramson et al. 1989) are *diathesis-stress models.* A diathesis is a predisposition to disease. The diathesis in these models is a specified cognitive style, for example, a tendency to attribute negative outcomes to stable factors (Abramson et al. 1989). The models hypothesize that when people who have the cognitive diatheses are confronted with stress in the form of negative life events, they are more likely to become depressed. Each model proposes a different cognitive diathesis leading to depression. Thus, each model presents a etiological account of a particular *cognitive subtype* of depression.

Studies testing cognitive models of depression often compared groups of currently depressed and nondepressed individuals using cross-sectional designs (see Abramson et al. 1988, for review). Investigators predicted that depressed subjects would exhibit the hypothetical diathesis, whereas nondepressed subjects would not (Alloy et al. 1988a). In these experiments, the cognitive diathesis was usually measured by self-report instruments such as the Attributional Style Questionnaire (Seligman et al. 1979). However, if depression is a heterogeneous disorder, then results of such studies would depend on the proportion of subjects in each group who were depressed primarily because of the stress diathesis versus those who were depressed for other reasons (e.g., Abramson 1982; Abramson et al. 1988). For example (see Figure 4–1, which contains imaginary data), if the majority of individuals in the depressed groups (groups B and D) are depressed due to a biochemical

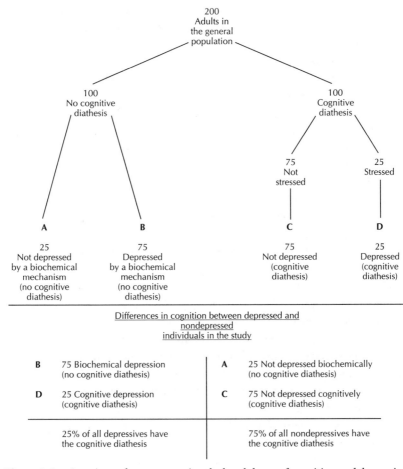

Figure 4–1. Imaginary data representing the breakdown of cognition and depression in the general population. *Source.* Adapted from Abramson LY: "The Cognitive Theories of Depression: Current Status and Future Directions." Paper presented at the Cognitive Theories of Depression Conference, Iowa City, IA, 1982. Used with permission.

mechanism (group B), then these biochemically depressed individuals may not exhibit the hypothetical diathesis. Thus, in our example, only 25 (group D) of 100 depressed persons (groups B and D) exhibit the diathesis. This might lead investigators to conclude that the cognitive models are wrong, even though all of the individuals who had the hypothetical diatheses and were stressed (group D) became depressed.

Additionally, diathesis-stress models imply that individuals who have the hypothetical diathesis must be stressed to become depressed (Abramson et al. 1989; Alloy et al. 1988a). To continue with our hypothetical example, people in the nondepressed groups (groups A and C) may have the diathesis, but may not have been stressed (group C) and therefore may not have become depressed. In our example, 75 (group C) of 100 nondepressed persons (groups A and C) had the diatheses but still did not become depressed because they were not stressed. Again, researchers might erroneously conclude that the cognitive models are incorrect, even though all of the individuals who had the diatheses *and* were stressed (group D) became depressed. The model specifies that both the diatheses and the stress must be present. Further, cross-sectional studies comparing currently depressed and nondepressed subjects, even without methodological problems, can only evaluate the concomitants of depression and not whether certain cognitive characteristics are antecedents to future depression (e.g., Lewinsohn et al. 1985). It may be that the thinking characteristics of persons cognitively prone to future depression are different from the thinking characteristics of persons with current depression (see "Lewinsohn's Integrative Model" below).

Finally, it may be that the cognitive patterns or diatheses, which are characteristic of the depressed state, exist in a latent state but are not apparent unless the individual is currently depressed (e.g., Ingram 1984; Persons and Miranda 1992; Segal and Ingram 1994). The difference between persons who are cognitively prone to depression and those who are not cognitively prone to depression could be that negative cognitions and accompanying sad affect are more easily activated by stress in depression-prone individuals. Thus, studies of diathesis-stress models may need to use methods for activating or uncovering the diathesis in nondepressed subjects. Recently, attempts have been made to activate depressogenic cognitions in nondepressed subjects, in view of suggestions that such cognitions are dormant in nondepressed people (Alloy and Clements 1992; Beck 1991).

Models Focusing on Cognitive Operations

Some theorists developed relatively comprehensive models of depression that focus on cognitive operations. These theorists include Lewinsohn et al. (1985), who emphasized self-focused attention; Ingram (1984), who targeted information processing; and Rehm (1977), who discussed self-control. Other theorists addressed specific aspects of depressed persons' cognitive processing, for example, automatic and effortful processing (Hartlage et al. 1993; Hasher and Zacks 1979; Weingartner 1986); resource allocation during encoding (Ellis and Ashbrook 1988); retrieval (e.g., Clark and Teasdale 1982); and mood congruent recall (e.g., Blaney 1986).

Lewinsohn's Integrative Model

In contrast to most cognitive models of depression, which view depressed mood as arising out of the individual's cognitions, Lewinsohn's theory emphasizes that dysphoria is the central phenomenon in depression. Cognitions (e.g., "I'm inadequate") are viewed as ways people explain to themselves why they are depressed. Lewinsohn suggested that depression is the result of too little positive reinforcement or too much punishment. Positive reinforcement is defined as presentation of a stimulus after a behavior that increases the probability that the behavior will occur again, and punishment is presentation or withdrawal of a stimulus after a behavior that decreases the probability that the behavior will occur again (Skinner 1938). However, Lewinsohn's definition of positive reinforcement generally refers to pleasant experiences. Further, depression may be maintained when attention and other social reinforcement given to the depressed person by significant others increase depressive behaviors. Subsequently, other people in the depressed person's environment may find these behaviors unpleasant and avoid the depressed person.

Social skills deficits among depressed persons were a focus of the original model proposed by Lewinsohn et al. (1969). It was found, for example, that depressed subjects were more uncomfortable in social activities (Youngren and Lewinsohn 1980); were less socially skilled, especially in group situations (Youngren and Lewinsohn 1980), than nondepressed control subjects (e.g., Libet and Lewinsohn 1973); elicited greater feelings of rejection from others (Coyne 1976); and had facial expressions that were difficult to judge, suggesting deficits in nonverbal communication (Prkachin et al. 1977). These findings are generally consistent with the hypothesis that depressed individuals are socially deficient and obtain less positive reinforcement than their nondepressed counterparts in social interactions (Lewinsohn and Hoberman 1982).

Studies also indicated that increased stress or unpleasant life experiences lead to depression (e.g., Brown and Harris 1978). However, in a longitudinal, prospective study, Lewinsohn and Hoberman (1982) found that the frequency of pleasant events did not predict the occurrence of later depression. Hence, Lewinsohn and his colleagues (1985) reformulated their original model and developed what they termed an integrative model of depression. This model purportedly integrates both cognitive and reinforcement theories of depression. It emphasizes self-focus as a mediator between stress or aversive circumstances and negative affect.

According to the integrative theory of depression (Lewinsohn et al. 1985; see Figure 4–2), the chain of events leading to depression begins with the occurrence of a stressful event (variable A). This event disrupts the individual's behavior patterns, which are referred to as "scripted behavior" or automatic behavior (e.g., personal relationships, job tasks; variable B). The disruptions are related to future depression if they result in reduced positive reinforcement or increased aversive experiences (variable C). Initially, people attempt to reduce the impact of stressful events. These attempts will be successful depending on environmental circumstances and on the individual's dispositional characteristics, vulnerabilities (e.g., having poor coping skills), and immunities (e.g., having high self-perceived social competence; variable G) (Lewinsohn et al. 1980). However, if positive reinforcement is not increased or negative circumstances reduced, increased self-awareness will result.

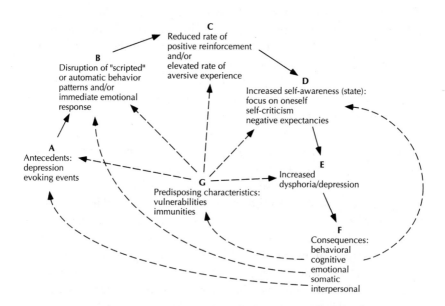

Figure 4–2.   Schematic representation of variables involved in the occurrence of unipolar depression. *Source.*   Reprinted from Lewinsohn PM, Hoberman H, Teri L, et al: "An Integrative Theory of Depression," in *Theoretical Issues in Behavior Therapy.* Edited by Reiss S, Bootzin R. San Diego, CA, Academic Press, 1985, p. 343. Used with permission.

Increased self-awareness (variable D) leads to increased self-criticism (Duval and Wicklund 1972), increased discrepancy between ratings of the ideal self and the real self (Ickes et al. 1973), increased negative expectancies (Carver et al. 1979b), behavioral withdrawal (Carver et al. 1979a), and social difficulties (Fenigstein 1979). Negative expectancies may in turn lead to reductions in effort and persistence (e.g., Carver et al. 1979a; Scheier and Carver 1977). Finally, heightened self-awareness appears to intensify dysphoria (Scheier and Carver 1977). Increased self-awareness and sad mood (variable E) are in turn hypothesized to disrupt the individual's self-protective and self-enhancing self-perceptions (e.g., Alloy and Abramson 1979) and lead to the cognitive, behavioral, and emotional changes (variable F) that are associated with depression.

As indicated, certain aspects of Lewinsohn's integrative theory have been empirically validated. There is fairly strong evidence that stress is related to the onset of depression (e.g., Brown and Harris 1978), particularly first episodes. Further, there is some evidence to support the existence of specific vulnerabilities and immunities (e.g., Lewinsohn et al. 1980, 1995), which play a role in the ability to ward off a potential depressive episode. An increase in self-focused attention does appear to accompany depression (Musson and Alloy 1988). Pyszczynski and Greenberg (1987) argued that increased self-focus leads to depression, whereas Ingram (1990) suggested that self-focused attention is characteristic of psychopathology in general and that the specific content of self-focus determines the nosological category. Finally, depressive realism (e.g., Alloy and Abramson 1979) has been observed among depressed individuals, but it is unclear whether this leads to the changes associated with depression.

Ingram's Information-Processing Model

Ingram's information-processing model of depression (1984) is based on Bower's concept of network theory (1981). Network theory proposes that each emotion, such as depression, has a node in memory (see Figure 4–3). These emotional nodes are linked to associated autonomic reactions, behaviors that express the emotion, and descriptions of situations that lead to the emotion. When an emotional node is activated above a certain threshold, this activation spreads to associatively linked recollections, which makes it easier to remember events associated with the emotion.

According to Ingram's information-processing model (1984), depression occurs when the depression-emotion node is activated. Losses (e.g., of relationships, serious illness) are most consistently and uniquely associated with activation of the depression node and with the onset of depression (Brown 1979; Finlay-Jones and Brown 1981). Although most significant losses are

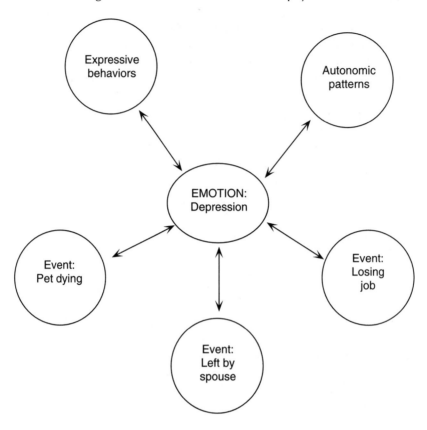

Figure 4–3.   Small portion of the connections surrounding the depression-emotion node. The arrows indicate activation spreading between nodes.

followed by normal grief reactions, such reactions are time limited and lack the self-esteem deficits of typical depression.

Activation of the depression node depends on the *appraisal* (Arnold 1960; Lazarus 1982) or subjective meaning of life events experienced by the individual. Activation subsequently spreads to memories associated with depression. These memories in turn reactivate depressive affective structures and maintain the depression. Further, available thinking capacity is occupied by this recycling of depressive cognitions.

As an example, suppose someone has just been left by a spouse. Presumably, the depression-emotion node will be activated. This activation spreads to associated memories of other losses and rejections. The individual will think about other depressing experiences, which, in turn, further activate the depression-emotion node. Selective recall of negative material will influence the depressed individual's self-evaluation (e.g., "I am unlovable."). Expectations for the future will be negatively affected.

Research is consistent with Ingram's hypotheses that the onset of depression is most closely associated with the experience of loss and depends on the individual's appraisal of life events. Although portions of Ingram's model (1984) are difficult to test directly, predictions based on the model can be evaluated. Specifically, if the spreading-activation hypothesis is correct, then we would expect activation to spread from the depression node to events associated with depression, making depression-relevant information easier to recall. Evidence consistent with Ingram's model suggests that depressed persons recall predominantly information congruent with a negative mood (Blaney 1986; Bradley et al. 1995).

Rehm's Self-Control Model

According to Rehm's model (1977), symptoms of depression occur as the result of deficits in self-control, including self-monitoring, self-evaluation, and self-reinforcement. Self-monitoring entails observing one's own behavior, its antecedents and consequences. Rehm hypothesized that depressed persons primarily attend to negative events resulting in pessimism and negative views of the self, the world, and the future. Depressed persons also may attend to immediate versus delayed outcomes of their behavior, resulting in decreased motivation and hopelessness.

Self-evaluation is defined as comparing one's performance with an internal standard. Rehm (1977) postulated that depressed individuals may apply stringent self-evaluation criteria. Further, depressed persons may develop helplessness (Seligman 1975) in two ways. First, they may make excessive external attributions (i.e., attribute outcomes to factors other than themselves). This leads to passivity even in the face of aversive circumstances. Alternatively, depressed persons may make internal attributions (i.e., attributions to the self) for outcomes, but believe that they are unable to obtain positive results.

Finally, Rehm (1977) proposed that depressed persons are characterized by low rates of overt or covert self-reinforcement and high rates of self-punishment. This perspective of self-control assumes that individuals control their own behavior in the same ways that one person controls another. Low rates of self-reward may be associated with slow rates of behavior, which are typical in depression.

Studies provide scattered evidence that depressed mood affects time spent attending to negative information about the self, but the effect appears to be transitory and may depend on experimental conditions (Rehm 1988).

However, there is fairly consistent evidence that depressed persons set higher standards for themselves, resulting in negative self-evaluations, but not in negative evaluations of others. Results of several studies generally indicate that depressed persons use self-reinforcement less and self-punishment more than nondepressed persons (Nelson and Craighead 1977; Rozensky et al. 1977).

Interference in Effortful Versus Automatic Processing

One way of conceptualizing cognitive deficits in depression is from an automatic-processing versus effortful-processing perspective (e.g., Hartlage et al. 1993; Hasher and Zacks 1979; Weingartner 1986). According to this view, people are limited in the amount of information they can pay attention to at one time. Automatic processes may require less attentional capacity than effortful processes. Examples of processes requiring less attention include driving a car over a familiar route and encoding the frequency of events. A substantial body of evidence suggests that clinical depression interferes with effortful processes such as problem solving (e.g., Price et al. 1978; Stanton et al. 1981), general learning (e.g., Breslow et al. 1980; Cohen et al. 1982), organization (e.g., Weingartner 1986), semantic encoding (e.g., learning material based on its meaning versus its sound; Weingartner et al. 1981), reading comprehension (e.g., Henderson 1987), and performance on motor speed tasks (e.g., Miller 1975; Weckowicz et al. 1978). The reason that depression interferes in effortful processing has not yet been determined. However, extant studies tend to support the hypothesis that available cognitive capacity is reduced when depressed persons use their attentional resources to focus on depression-relevant thoughts (Hartlage et al. 1993).

Although evidence is sparse, depression does not seem to interfere with automatic processes (e.g., Hasher and Zacks 1979). Further, depressive self-relevant content is activated automatically among depressed individuals (Bargh and Tota 1988; Ingram et al. 1994; Segal et al. 1988; Wenzlaff et al. 1988). In other words, even when they are not intending to do so, depressed people appear to readily generate depression-relevant thoughts (e.g., "I am miserable"), which are difficult to suppress.

The automatic-processing versus effortful-processing perspective of depressive cognition has several conceptual and treatment implications (Hartlage et al. 1993). When effortful processes are decreased by depression, individuals may be less able to counteract their negative thoughts through conscious effortful strategies (Barber and DeRubeis 1989), such as counting their blessings and looking for the silver lining (Fiske and Taylor 1984; Taylor et al. 1984). Further, some depression-prone people appear to automatically attribute positive outcomes to the circumstances and negative outcomes to themselves (Hartlage 1990; S. Hartlage, L. B. Alloy, and K. Arduino, unpublished data 1996). Thus, they may be unable to get an ego boost by taking credit for any good things that happen to them. Finally, impaired problem solving among depressed persons may contribute to a continuation of stressful negative life events and, thus, to a perpetuation of depression.

Resource Allocation During Encoding

The resource allocation model (Ellis 1991; Ellis and Ashbrook 1988) was developed in an effort to account for the disruptive effects of depressed mood on memory. It is based on theories of attentional capacity. According to Ellis and Ashbrook, at least two possibilities can occur when depressed-mood subjects (i.e., subjects in a depressed mood who may not have the full syndrome of depression) perform memory tasks. First, at least some portion of the depressed individuals' cognitive capacities can be taken up by one or more of the following: 1) thinking about their sad state, 2) cognitive activities that are directed toward events other than the criterion task (i.e., extra-task processing), and 3) processing features of the task that are not related to the outcome measures set by the examiner (i.e., irrelevant-task processing). Second, sad or depressed mood can quantitatively reduce cognitive capacity. Ellis and Ashbrook made several predictions based on their model. For example, depressive deficits should be greater when encoding demands are more difficult (e.g., when material to be encoded seems to lack meaning or organization). Further, because personally relevant information is thought to be highly integrated and familiar, memory for personally relevant material should demand less effort and thus be less impaired among depressed persons.

Retrieval and Encoding

Retrieval and encoding studies aid in identifying the types of information depressed persons learn and remember. In retrieval studies, investigators ask depressed subjects to remember information learned before the experiment (e.g., recall personal experiences). In studies of encoding, experimenters present subjects with information to be learned or encoded during the course of the experiment. Subjects are then asked to recall or recognize the material. Depressive deficits or distortions in encoding are inferred from the depressed subjects' performances at recall. Further, information to be encoded can be *semantic* (about knowledge or meaning; e.g., positive, neutral, and negative words) or *episodic* (about events in the individual's experience; e.g., positive and negative feedback given to the subject during the experiment). Excellent reviews of depressed persons' performance on encoding and retrieval tasks were compiled by Blaney (1986), Williams et al. (1988), and Ingram and Reed (1986). The findings are summarized below.

Depressed individuals appear to overrecall negative life experiences and underrecall positive life experiences (Ingram and Reed 1986; Williams et al. 1988). Further, these findings do not seem to be solely attributable to depressed persons having experienced more negative events (e.g., Clark and Teasdale 1982).

In general, studies of semantic encoding indicate that depressed individuals underrecall positive as opposed to negative information. Ingram and Reed (1986) suggested that differences among depressed and nondepressed individuals in semantic encoding are primarily attributable to depressed persons' enhanced processing of negative information (e.g., they make more associations to negative information). In contrast, findings are mixed regarding depressive deficits in processing positive information (Ingram et al. 1983; Kuiper and Derry 1982). Blaney (1986) and others (Williams et al. 1988) suggested that selective processing of negative material by depressed persons may only occur when subjects are asked to encode the material in reference to themselves (i.e., to focus during learning on how the words apply to themselves) or when information is evaluated by the subject. One study that used a signal detection paradigm indicated that results of semantic-encoding experiments may actually be measuring response biases (e.g., a tendency for depressed persons to guess more often) rather than a true tendency for depressed persons to overrecall negative material (Zuroff et al. 1983).

Whereas studies of semantic encoding consistently indicate that depressed persons overrecall negative information, studies of episodic encoding indicate that depressed persons underrecall success experiences and positive feedback (see Blaney 1986 and Ingram and Reed 1986 for reviews). This tendency may be particularly true for women (Buchwald 1977) and when the overall content of the feedback is positive (e.g., Craighead et al. 1979).

Case Example

Dr. S. was a tenured university professor who had been depressed for several years. During the initial diagnostic interview, Dr. S. reported low self-esteem, especially in relation to her low writing productivity; believed that her colleagues thought poorly of her; and described an unsatisfactory relationship with her boyfriend. Dr. S. was already on antidepressant medication and had been in psychodynamic psychotherapy for years when she came for cognitive and behavior therapy. She had some insight into the childhood events that had predisposed her to depression, but it had not helped much to change her present experience.

Models of depression based on cognitive operations seem particularly suited to conceptualizing Dr. S.'s case and beginning treatment. From Lewinsohn's perspective, Dr. S.'s depression began when she was divorced (a stressful event). This event disrupted her regular pattern of writing and her relationships with colleagues (scripted behavior), which resulted in receiving fewer accolades from peers (reduced positive reinforcement). Initially Dr. S. tried to force herself to write but was unable to keep working for more than a brief period. Dr. S.'s thinking became increasingly self-focused. She was very critical of herself and did not live up to her own image of who she should be (increased discrepancy between the ideal and the real self). She blamed only herself for not writing but thought it would be virtually impossible to start writing again (negative expectations; she made an internal attribution but thought she was unable to obtain positive results). Dr. S. withdrew from other work-related activities and from colleagues (behavioral withdrawal). She developed difficulties in her relationships with friends and family (social difficulties).

Rehm's model can explain some of Dr. S.'s initial responses to behavior therapy. By the time Dr. S. entered treatment, she had worked through issues directly related to her divorce. Her current depression was more closely associated with her inability to write. Dr. S. was started on a program for increasing her writing behavior. She was instructed to set realistic standards for herself, especially while relearning the writing habit. When Dr. S. met with limited success, she would come into sessions and report, "I failed terribly" (primarily self-monitoring negative events). When she was able to write for 1 or 2 hours, she admitted that after the first 10 minutes she got some satisfaction from performing well (attention to delayed versus immediate outcomes).

In treatment, Dr. S. generated a list of possible reinforcers for use after completing writing tasks. Dr. S. listed romantic evenings with her boyfriend among the alternatives. With his cooperation, Dr. S. found that this reinforcer led to a substantial increase in her writing. Dr. S. was also taught to give herself positive verbal praise (increased self-reinforcement). Learning to take credit for positive outcomes may help Dr. S. ward off future depression when she recovers. Dr. S. reported decreased depression and the positive side effect of an improved relationship with her boyfriend.

The therapist helped Dr. S. to understand why it was so difficult for her to generate positive thoughts. Depressed people appear to generate depression-relevant thoughts automatically and underrecall positive experiences. Dr. S. learned that it is important to practice taking credit for positive outcomes so that some day this will become automatic.

Models Focusing on Cognitive Schemata

Schematic models of depression include the hopelessness model (Abramson et al. 1989), Beck's model (1967, 1991), and the self-worth contingency model of Kuiper et al. (1982, 1988), which is an extension of Beck's model. Each schematic model hypothesizes a cognitive structure or schema that guides interpretation of incoming information in characteristically depressive ways.

The Hopelessness Model

The original learned-helplessness model of depression was based on animal studies. Seligman (1975) observed that dogs exposed to uncontrollable shock exhibited many symptoms characteristic of depression, including passivity, interference with subsequent instrumental learning, lack of aggressiveness and competitiveness, undereating, and weight loss. The key factor in producing the helplessness phenomenon was proposed to be lack of control; with repeated exposure to uncontrollable experiences, the organism apparently learns that reinforcement is not contingent on responding. This belief creates the *expectation* that responses and outcomes are independent, which results in the characteristic manifestations of learned helplessness. Seligman further hypothesized that if the symptoms of learned helplessness and depression are similar, then depression and learned helplessness should have similar causes and cures.

In 1978 Abramson et al. pointed out that the original learned-helplessness model (Seligman 1975) failed to distinguish between cases in which outcomes are uncontrollable for all people (universal) and cases in which outcomes are uncontrollable only for some people (personal). Further, the model did not explain when helplessness is general (global) versus specific, or when it is chronic versus acute. When helplessness is general rather than specific, deficits occur in a broad rather than a narrow range of situations. For example, a teacher who was fired from his job fails to look for another job, cannot get started on his income tax, neglects household chores, and avoids his wife (global helplessness) versus failing only to look for another job and to prepare his income tax (specific helplessness). When helplessness is chronic, deficits are long-lived and recurrent; when helplessness is acute or transient, deficits are short-lived and nonrecurrent. Abramson and her colleagues reformulated Seligman's model and subsequently developed the hopelessness model of depression (Abramson et al. 1989; see Figure 4–4).

According to the hopelessness model, the expectation that highly aversive events are likely—or highly desired events are unlikely—is a proximal (i.e., operating close to the occurrence of symptoms) and sufficient cause of depression. For example, an undergraduate student who has always wanted to become a physician concludes, "I'm sure I did terribly on the MCAT [Medical College Admission Test]" or "I'll never be able to get into med school," and becomes depressed. These expectations are captured by the term *hopelessness*. The hopelessness model also addresses more distal contributory causes of depression. Specifically, the types of attributions that people make for negative life events may increase the likelihood of developing hopelessness. Making stable attributions (e.g., "I failed because they always ask tricky questions on the MCAT") and global attributions (likely to affect many outcomes; e.g., "I failed because I'm stupid") for negative events increases the likelihood of the development of hopelessness. Making internal attributions (caused by something about oneself; e.g., "He didn't ask me out because I'm unattractive") results in depression accompanied by decreased self-esteem. Finally, the hopelessness

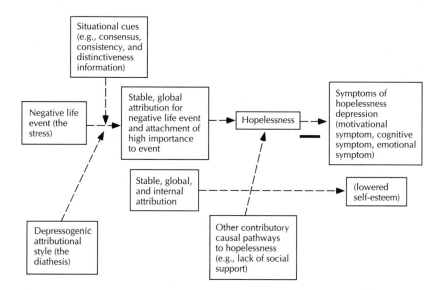

Figure 4–4.   Causal chain specified in the hopelessness theory of depression. The arrow with a solid line indicates a sufficient cause. Arrows with broken lines indicate contributory causes. *Source.*   Reprinted from Abramson LY, Alloy LB, Metalsky GI: "The Cognitive Diathesis-Stress Theories of Depression: Toward an Adequate Evaluation of the Theories' Validities," in *Cognitive Processes in Depression*. Edited by Alloy LB. New York, Guilford, 1988, p. 8. Used with permission.

theory hypothesizes that some people may have a generalized tendency to attribute negative events to internal, stable, and global causes—in other words, a depressogenic attributional style. Such an attributional style makes it more likely that an individual will attribute a specific negative life event to stable and global causes, thus making it more likely that the individual will develop hopelessness depression.

In an extension of the hopelessness theory, Alloy and others (Alloy and Clements 1992; Alloy et al. 1990) suggest that some perception-of-control styles, such as the illusion of control (i.e., persons judge that they have control over outcomes that are, in fact, uncontrollable), make it *less* likely that an individual will develop depression by decreasing the chances that a person will become hopeless when he or she confronts stress. For example, a salesman may fail many times before making a sale. If he believes that his failure is due to something about his sales technique, which he can control, rather than something about his company's product line, which he cannot control, he may be less likely to become hopeless and depressed between sales.

Numerous studies attempted to validate the reformulated learned-helplessness theory of depression (Alloy et al. 1994). Studies of attributional styles of depressed and nondepressed individuals at one point generally supported an association between particular negative attributional styles and depressive symptoms (see Abramson et al. 1989 and Coyne and Gotlib 1983 for reviews). More recently, researchers have begun to use longitudinal-prospective designs to examine the causality issue (e.g., Cutrona 1983; Lewinsohn et al. 1981; Metalsky et al. 1982, 1987). Results of a few studies suggested that negative attributional styles occur before onset of depression (Golin et al. 1981; Seligman et al. 1984) and predict mood change during the course of a therapy session (Peterson et al. 1983). However, other prospective studies were unable to predict future depression from cognitive patterns (Lewinsohn et al. 1981; Peterson et al. 1981). The authors concluded that cognitions are a consequence rather than an antecedent of depression.

Studies of people who have recovered from depression also examine the causality issue. Recovered depressed persons are presumably prone to future depression, so they should have depressogenic attributional styles. The majority of these studies found no differences in cognitive styles between formerly depressed patients and control subjects (Hamilton and Abramson 1983), although in a few studies attributional style was more negative among persons with remitted depression (e.g., Eaves and Rush 1984).

Unfortunately, many of these longitudinal-prospective studies have significant conceptual and methodological limitations, including failure to assess stress, failure to take into account the heterogeneity of depression, derivation of incorrect predictions from the model, and inadequate or less-than-optimal measurement techniques. Therefore, they do not adequately test the causal hypotheses of the theory (see Alloy et al. 1988a, 1988b). Interestingly, some prospective studies that measured stress as well as attributional style supported the model (e.g., Alloy and Clements 1992; Metalsky et al. 1982).

Beck's Model

In 1991 Beck clarified that his model of depression (Beck 1967) primarily addresses the cognitive characteristics of the depressed state and how depression progresses, rather than how depression is caused. According to Beck, depression is characterized by thoughts that arise quickly and automatically. These automatic thoughts consist of negative views of the self, the world, and the future. Even when the depressed person is not aware of having the thoughts, they frequently lead to sad affect.

Additionally, people who are not in the depressed state hold beliefs (e.g., "If I don't succeed, I am nothing") that lie dormant and are inactive (Beck 1967, 1991). These beliefs are generally conditional and are part of a schematic network. The beliefs are elicited by symbolic situations (i.e., situations symbolizing earlier experiences that were responsible for forming the beliefs) to produce the automatic thoughts. For example, a person who holds the belief, "I am worthless unless everyone likes me," and is disliked by someone has the automatic thought, "I am worthless." Finally, in some cases a congruence between personality and stressor may cause depression. For example, an individual who is sensitive to withdrawal of affection may experience rejection and become depressed.

A large body of research evaluated Beck's hypotheses (see Beck 1991 for review). Unfortunately, many of the studies are correlational and have the same methodological flaws as studies testing the reformulated learned-helplessness model (Alloy et al. 1988a; Haaga et al. 1991). The pervasiveness of negative thinking among currently depressed individuals has been the most consistently supported of Beck's hypotheses. This phenomenon is universal and exists among unipolar and bipolar depressed persons, clinically depressed persons, and individuals in a depressed mood state (Hollon et al. 1986). Further, a specific cognitive content (loss, defeat, deprivation) appears to be uniquely associated with depression (e.g., "Nothing good ever happens to me") as opposed to anxiety (e.g., "If I forget my lines in the play, I'll never make it as a professional actress") (Greenberg and Beck 1989; Steer et al. 1995). This association is referred to as the content-specificity hypothesis. Finally, a number of retrospective studies (e.g., Hammen et al. 1989) provide mixed support for the hypothesis that congruence between a personality and stressor may cause depression.

Kuiper's Model

According to the contingency self-worth model of Kuiper et al. (1988), individuals who hold a large number of dysfunctional attitudes (e.g., "If someone disagrees with me, he probably doesn't like me," Kuiper et al. 1988, p. 296) are cognitively prone to depression. These attitudes establish contingencies used by individuals to determine self-worth (e.g., "My value as a person depends upon what others think of me," Kuiper et al. 1988, p. 296). When stressors result in an inability to fulfill self-worth contingencies, the individual first attempts to eliminate the stress. If this attempt fails, diminished self-worth and depression result. Further, clinically depressed and nondepressed individuals are characterized by well-consolidated self-schemata that are negative and positive, respectively. Mildly depressed persons are hypothesized to have self-schemata that are not well consolidated and contain both negative and positive content.

Kuiper and his colleagues (1982, 1988) and others (Prieto et al. 1992) have conducted research that generally provided good support for the self-schema aspect of his model. However, persons with remitted depression, who are presumably depression prone, do not always score higher than control subjects on measures of dysfunctional attitudes (Hamilton and Abramson 1983; Silverman et al. 1984) calling into question whether dysfunctional attitudes play a causal role in depression. Longitudinal studies of the self-worth component of Kuiper's model are needed.

Depressive Realism

Beck (1967) postulated that the thinking of depressed persons is negatively biased. Examples of the errors that he observed in depressive thinking are selective abstraction, overgeneralization, dichotomous thinking, and exaggeration of the negative aspects of experiences. A frequent interpretation of Beck's hypothesis is that depressed persons are characteristically unrealistic relative to nondepressed persons. However, results of a number of studies (e.g., Alloy and Abramson 1979) suggest that the thinking of depressed persons is characteristically accurate, whereas the thinking of nondepressed persons is characteristically positively biased. This apparent phenomenon is known as *depressive realism*. The depressive-realism phenomenon was demonstrated in studies of contingency judgment, predicting outcome, and self-other social comparison, among others (Alloy and Abramson 1979, 1988; Alloy and Ahrens 1987). Depressive realism seems to be particularly accurate with regard to the depressed individuals' perceptions and judgments about themselves, but not about others (Alloy and Abramson 1988), as well as when self-perceptions are assessed immediately after performance (Alloy and Abramson 1988). What causes the depressive-realism phenomenon? Dykman and his colleagues (1989) suggested that both depressed and nondepressed individuals interpret information so as to be consistent with their schemata. However, depressed persons have more negative content (e.g., negative views of the self, the world, and the future) than nondepressed persons in their schemata.

Case Example

Mr. J. was a good-looking young man who had graduated from a top business school and was recently promoted to a high-visibility position in his company. Nonetheless, when anything bad happened to him, he had negative thoughts and became depressed. When he lost at racquetball, he thought, "I'm a complete failure," became depressed, recalled his other imperfections, and became more depressed. When he broke up with his girlfriend, he thought, "She broke up with me because I have a lousy personality," and then, "I'll never be married." He again became depressed.

Each of the schematic models explains different aspects of Mr. J.'s depression. The hopelessness model best delineates a clear causal pathway from Mr. J.'s breakup with his girlfriend (the stressor) to his depression. Mr. J. attributes the breakup to his personality (a stable, global attribution) and concludes that he will never be married (an expectation that a highly desired event is unlikely). Mr. J.'s attribution is also internal, suggesting that his depression in this instance will be accompanied by decreased self-esteem. Although the hopelessness model best explains Mr. J.'s depression after breaking up with his girlfriend, the contingency self-worth model best explains the cause of Mr. J.'s depression after losing at racquetball. In this case, Mr. J. concludes that he is a complete failure. Mr. J. appears to hold the attitude, "If I fail at anything, I am a complete failure" (a self-worth contingency). His depression is more about his lack of self-worth than about an expected outcome, as in Abramson et al.'s (1989) model.

Beck's model (1991) has less to say about how Mr. J.'s depression is caused than about how it develops. Thus, once he is depressed after losing at racquetball, Mr. J. automatically recalls his other imperfections (negative views of the self). With regard to depressive realism, at first glance it appears that Mr. J.'s thinking is negatively biased, as Beck postulated. However, Mr. J. may be somewhat awkward socially compared with others because of his negative self-view.

Summary

The most consistent finding from research on cognitive models of depression is that negative thinking, including negative views of the self, the world, and the future, is more prevalent among depressed than nondepressed individuals. Compared with nondepression, current depression has been associated with negative self-schemata (e.g., Kuiper et al. 1982, 1988); cognitive content involving loss, defeat, and deprivation (e.g., Beck et al. 1987); and negative attributional styles (e.g., Abramson et al. 1989). Further, depressed persons appear to process information in ways that are consistent with their schemata (e.g., Alloy and Abramson 1979; Dykman et al. 1989).

Compared with nondepressed individuals, depressed individuals also seem to recall more negative personal experiences and fewer positive personal experiences (Clark and Teasdale 1982), successes, and positive feedback (Blaney 1986). In fact, the thinking capacity of depressed persons may be occupied by the recycling of negative thoughts (Ingram 1984), leaving few attentional resources for performing tasks that demand thinking capacity (Ellis and Ashbrook 1988; Hartlage et al. 1993). Specifically, clinically depressed persons appear to be deficient in problem solving, organization, semantic encoding, reading comprehension, and performance on motor speed tasks.

Additionally, depression seems to be accompanied by increased self-focus (e.g., Carver and Scheier 1981). Research suggests that depressed individuals set high standards for themselves, but not for others (Rehm 1988). Depressed persons may be less apt to reinforce themselves and more apt to be self-punitive (Rehm 1988). They also exhibit social skills deficits (Youngren and Lewinsohn 1980) and may elicit more feelings of rejection from others (Coyne 1976).

Research on cognitive models of depression yielded less definitive results regarding the cause of depression. It does appear that stress or negative life experiences are associated with the onset of depression (Brown and Harris 1978). Further, the effect of negative events may depend on the individual's appraisal of those events (Lazarus 1982). Results of a few studies that adequately tested the cognitive diathesis-stress models of depression tend to support those models (Alloy et al. 1988a). For example, a negative attributional style may be a distal cause of depression (e.g., Metalsky et al. 1982). However, in general, adequate tests of the models remain to be conducted (Alloy et al. 1988b).

Therapeutic interventions based on cognitive models of depression emphasize changing behavior or altering cognitions from negative to positive. In a later chapter (Roberts and Hartlage, Chapter 14), implications of the theories for treating depression are discussed.

References

Abramson LY: The cognitive theories of depression: current status and future directions. Paper presented at the Cognitive Theories of Depression conference, Iowa City, IA, 1982

Abramson LY, Seligman MEP, Teasdale J: Learned helplessness in humans: critique and reformulation. J Abnorm Psychol 87:49–74, 1978

Abramson LY, Alloy LB, Metalsky GI: The cognitive diathesis-stress theories of depression: toward an adequate evaluation of the theories' validities, in Cognitive Processes in Depression. Edited by Alloy LB. New York, Guilford, 1988, pp 3–30

Abramson LY, Metalsky GI, Alloy LB: Hopelessness depression: a theory based subtype of depression. Psychol Rev 96:358–372, 1989

Alloy LB, Abramson LY: Judgment of contingency in depressed and nondepressed students: sadder but wiser? J Exp Psychol Gen 108:441–485, 1979

Alloy LB, Abramson LY: Depressive realism: four theoretical perspectives, in Cognitive Processes in Depression. Edited by Alloy LB. New York, Guilford, 1988, pp 223–265

Alloy LB, Ahrens AH: Depression and pessimism for the future: biased use of statistically relevant information in predictions for self versus others. J Pers Soc Psychol 52:366–378, 1987

Alloy LB, Clements CM: Illusion of control: invulnerability to negative affect and depressive symptoms after laboratory and natural stressors. J Abnorm Psychol 101:234–245, 1992

Alloy LB, Clements C, Kolden G: The cognitive diathesis-stress theories of depression: therapeutic implications, in Theoretical Issues in Behavior Therapy. Edited by Reiss S, Bootzin R. San Diego, CA, Academic Press, 1985, pp 379–410

Alloy LB, Abramson LY, Metalsky GI, et al: The hopelessness theory of depression: attributional aspects. Br J Clin Psychol 27:5–21, 1988a

Alloy LB, Hartlage S, Abramson LY: Testing the cognitive diathesis-stress theories of depression: issues of research design, conceptualization, and assessment, in Cognitive Processes in Depression. Edited by Alloy LB. New York, Guilford Press, 1988b, pp 31–73

Alloy LB, Kelly KA, Mineka S, et al: Comorbidity of anxiety and depressive disorders: a helplessness-hopelessness perspective, in Comorbidity of Mood and Anxiety Disorders. Edited by Maser JD, Cloninger CR. Washington, DC, American Psychiatric Press, 1990, pp 499–543

Alloy LB, Lipman AJ, Abramson LY: Attributional style as a vulnerability factor for depression: validation by past history of mood disorders. Special issue: cognitive vulnerability to psychological dysfunction. Cognitive Therapy and Research 16:391–407, 1994

Arnold MB: Emotion and Personality. New York, Columbia University Press, 1960

Barber JP, DeRubeis RJ: On second thought: where the action is in cognitive therapy for depression. Cognitive Therapy and Research 13:441–457, 1989

Bargh JA, Tota ME: Context-dependent automatic processing in depression: accessibility of negative constructs with regard to self but not others. J Pers Soc Psychol 54:925–939, 1988

Beck AT: Depression: Causes and Treatment. Philadelphia, PA, University of Pennsylvania Press, 1967

Beck AT: Cognitive therapy: a 30-year retrospective. Am Psychol 46:368–375, 1991

Beck AT, Brown G, Steer RA, et al: Differentiating anxiety and depression: a test of the cognitive content-specificity hypothesis. J Abnorm Psychol 96:179–183, 1987

Blaney PH: Affect and memory: a review. Psychol Bull 99:229–246, 1986

Bower GH: Mood and memory. Am Psychol 36:129–148, 1981

Bradley BP, Mogg K, Williams R: Implicit and explicit memory for emotion-congruent information in clinical depression and anxiety. Behav Res Ther 33:755–770, 1995

Breslow R, Kocsis J, Belkin B: Memory deficits in depression: evidence utilizing the Wechsler Memory Scale. Percept Mot Skills 51:541–542, 1980

Brown GW: The social etiology of depression—London studies, in The Psychobiology of the Depressive Disorders: Implications for the Effects of Stress. Edited by Depue RA. San Diego, CA, Academic Press, 1979, pp 263–290

Brown GW, Harris T: Social Origins of Depression. New York, The Free Press, 1978

Buchwald AM: Depressive mood and estimates of reinforcement frequency. J Abnorm Psychol 86:443–446, 1977

Carver CS, Scheier MF: Attention and Self-Regulation: A Control-Theory Approach to Human Behavior. New York, Springer-Verlag, 1981

Carver CS, Blaney PH, Scheier MF: Focus of attention, chronic expectancy, and responses to a feared stimulus. J Pers Soc Psychol 37:1186–1195, 1979a

Carver CS, Blaney PH, Scheier MF: Reassertion and giving up: the interactive role of self-directed attention and outcome expectancy. J Pers Soc Psychol 37:1859–1870, 1979b

Clark DM, Teasdale JD: Diurnal variation in clinical depression and accessibility of memories of positive and negative experiences. J Abnorm Psychol 91:87–95, 1982

Cohen RM, Weingartner H, Smallberg SA, et al: Effort and cognition in depression. Arch Gen Psychiatry 39:593–597, 1982

Coyne JC: Depression and the response of others. J Abnorm Psychol 85:186–193, 1976

Coyne JC, Gotlib IH: The role of cognition in depression: a critical appraisal. Psychol Bull 94:472–505, 1983

Craighead WE, Hickey KS, DeMonbreun BG: Distortion of perception and recall of neutral feedback in depression. Cognitive Therapy and Research 3:291–298, 1979

Cutrona CE: Causal attributions and perinatal depression. J Abnorm Psychol 92:161–172, 1983

Duval S, Wicklund A: A Theory of Objective Self-Awareness. San Diego, CA, Academic Press, 1972

Dykman BM, Abramson LY, Alloy LB, et al: Processing of ambiguous and unambiguous feedback by depressed and nondepressed college students: schematic biases and their implications for depressive realism. J Pers Soc Psychol 56:431–445, 1989

Eaves G, Rush AJ: Cognitive patterns in symptomatic and remitted unipolar major depression. J Abnorm Psychol 93:31–40, 1984

Ellis HC: Focused attention and depressive deficits in memory. J Exp Psychol Gen 120:310–312, 1991

Ellis HC, Ashbrook PW: Resource allocation model of the effects of depressed mood states on memory, in Affect, Cognition and Social Behavior. Edited by Fiedler K, Forgas J. Gottingen, Federal Republic of Germany, Hogrefe, 1988, pp 25–43

Fenigstein A: Self-consciousness, self-attention, and social interaction. J Pers Soc Psychol 37:75–86, 1979

Finlay-Jones R, Brown GW: Types of stressful life event and the onset of anxiety and depressive disorders. Psychol Med 11:803–815, 1981

Fiske ST, Taylor SE: Social Cognition. Reading, MA, Addison-Wesley, 1984

Golin S, Sweeney, PD, Shaeffer DE: The causality of causal attributions in depression: a cross-lagged panel correlational analysis. J Abnorm Psychol 90:14–22, 1981

Greenberg MS, Beck AT: Depression versus anxiety: a test of the content-specificity hypothesis. J Abnorm Psychol 98:9–13, 1989

Haaga DAF, Dyck MJ, Ernst D: Empirical status of cognitive theory of depression. Psychol Bull 110:215–236, 1991

Hamilton EW, Abramson LY: Cognitive patterns and major depressive disorder: a longitudinal study in a hospital setting. J Abnorm Psychol 92:173–184, 1983

Hammen C, Ellicott A, Gitlin M, et al: Sociotropy/autonomy and vulnerability to specific life events in patients with unipolar depression and bipolar disorders. J Abnorm Psychol 98:154–160, 1989

Hartlage S: Automatic processing of attributional inferences in depressed and cognitively depression-prone individuals (unpublished doctoral dissertation). Evanston, IL, Northwestern University, 1990

Hartlage S, Alloy LB, Vazquez C, et al: Automatic and effortful processing in depression. Psychol Bull 113:247–278, 1993

Hasher L, Zacks RT: Automatic and effortful processes in memory. J Exp Psychol Gen 108:356–389, 1979

Henderson JG: Effects of depression upon reading: a case for distinguishing effortful from automatic processes. Percept Mot Skills 64:191–200, 1987

Hollon SD, Kendall PC, Lumry A: Specificity of depressotypic cognitions in clinical depression. J Abnorm Psychol 95:52–59, 1986

Ickes WJ, Wicklund RA, Ferris CB: Objective self-awareness and self-esteem. J Exp Soc Psychol 9:202–219, 1973

Ingram RE: Toward an information-processing analysis of depression. Cognitive Therapy and Research 8:443–477, 1984

Ingram RE: Self-focused attention in clinical disorders: review and a conceptual model. Psychol Bull 107:156–176, 1990

Ingram RE, Kendall PC: Cognitive clinical psychology: implications of an information processing perspective, in Information Processing Approaches to Clinical Psychology. Edited by Ingram RE. San Diego, CA, Academic Press, 1986, pp 3–21

Ingram RE, Reed MR: Information encoding and retrieval processes in depression: findings, issues, and future directions, in Information Processing Approaches to Clinical Psychology. Edited by Ingram RE. San Diego, CA, Academic Press, 1986, pp 131–150

Ingram RE, Wisnicki K: Cognition in depression, in Cognitive Bases of Mental Disorders. Annual Review of Psychopathology, Vol 1. Edited by Magaro PA. Newbury Park, CA, Sage, 1991, pp 187–230

Ingram RE, Smith TW, Brehm SS: Depression and information processing: self-schemata and the encoding of self-referent information. J Pers Soc Psychol 45:412–420, 1983

Ingram RE, Partridge S, Scott W, et al: Schema specficity in subclinical syndrome depression: distinctions between automatically versus effortfully encoded state and trait depressive information. Cognitive Therapy and Research 18:195–209, 1994

Kuiper NA, Derry PA: Depressed and nondepressed content self-reference in mild depressives. J Pers 50:67–80, 1982

Kuiper NA, Derry PA, MacDonald MR: Self-reference and person perception in depression, in Integrations of Clinical and Social Psychology. Edited by Weary G, Mirels H. London, Oxford University Press, 1982, pp 79–103

Kuiper NA, Olinger LJ, MacDonald MR: Vulnerability and episodic cognitions in a self-worth contingency model of depression, in Cognitive Processes in Depression. Edited by Alloy LB. New York, Guilford, 1988, pp 289–309

Lazarus RS: Thoughts on the relations between emotion and cognition. Am Psychol 37:1019–1024, 1982

Lewinsohn PM, Hoberman H: Depression, in International Handbook of Behavior Modification and Therapy. Edited by Bellack AS, Hersen M, Kazdin AE. New York, Plenum, 1982, pp 397–431

Lewinsohn PM, Weinstein M, Shaw D: Depression: a clinical-research approach, in Advances in Behavior Therapy. Edited by Rubin RD, Frank CM. San Diego, CA, Academic Press, 1969, pp 231–240

Lewinsohn PM, Mischel W, Chaplin W, et al: Social competence and depression: the role of illusory self-perceptions. J Abnorm Psychol 89:203–212, 1980

Lewinsohn PM, Steinmetz JL, Larson DW, et al: Depression-related cognitions: antecedent or consequence? J Abnorm Psychol 90:213–219, 1981

Lewinsohn PM, Hoberman H, Teri L, et al: An integrative theory of depression, in Theoretical Issues in Behavior Therapy. Edited by Reiss S, Bootzin R. San Diego, CA, Academic Press, 1985, pp 331–359

Lewinsohn PM, Gotlib IH, Seeley JR: Adolescent psychopathology, IV: specificity of psychosocial risk factors for depression and substance abuse in older adolescents. J Am Acad Child Adolesc Psychiatry 34:1221–1229, 1995

Libet, JM, Lewinsohn PM: The concept of social skill with special reference to the behavior of depressed persons. J Consult Clin Psychol 40:304–312, 1973

Metalsky GI, Abramson LY, Seligman MEP, et al: Attributional styles and life events in the classroom: vulnerability and invulnerability to depressive mood reactions. J Pers Soc Psychol 43:612–617, 1982

Metalsky GI, Halberstadt LJ, Abramson LY: Vulnerability to depressive mood reactions: toward a more powerful test of the diathesis-stress and causal mediation components of the reformulated theory of depression. J Pers Soc Psychol 52:386–393, 1987

Miller WR: Psychological deficit in depression. Psychol Bull 82:238–260, 1975

Musson RF, Alloy LB: Depression and self-directed attention, in Cognitive Processes in Depression. Edited by Alloy LB. New York, Guilford, 1988, pp 193–220

Nelson RE, Craighead WE: Selective recall of positive and negative feedback, self-control behaviors, and depression. J Abnorm Psychol 86:379–388, 1977

Persons JB, Miranda J: Cognitive theories of vulnerability to depression: reconciling negative evidence. Special issue: Cognitive vulnerability to psychological dysfunction. Cognitive Therapy and Research 16:485–502, 1992

Peterson C, Schwartz SM, Seligman MEP: Self-blame and depressive symptoms. J Pers Soc Psychol 41:253–259, 1981

Peterson C, Luborsky L, Seligman MEP: Attributions and depressive mood shifts: a case study using the symptom-context method. J Abnorm Psychol 92:96–103, 1983

Prieto SL, Cole DA, Tageson CW: Depressive self-schemas in clinic and nonclinic children. Cognitive Therapy and Research 16:521–534, 1992

Price KP, Tryon WW, Raps CS: Learned helplessness and depression in a clinical population: test of two behavioral hypotheses. J Abnorm Psychol 87:113–121, 1978

Prkachin K, Craig K, Papageorgis D, et al: Nonverbal communication deficits and response to performance feedback in depression. J Abnorm Psychol 86:224–234, 1977

Pyszczynski T, Greenberg J: Self-regulatory perseveration and the depressive self-focusing style: a self-awareness theory of reactive depression. Psychol Bull 102:122–138, 1987

Rehm LP: A self-control model of depression. Behavior Therapy 8:787–804, 1977

Rehm LP: Self-management and cognitive processes in depression, in Cognitive Processes in Depression. Edited by Alloy LB. New York, Guilford, 1988, pp 143–176

Rozensky RA, Rehm LP, Pry G, et al: Depression and self-reinforcement behavior in hospitalized patients. J Behav Ther Exp Psychiatry 8:35–38, 1977

Scheier MF, Carver CS: Learned Helplessness or Egotism: Do Expectancies Matter? Pittsburgh, PA, Carnegie-Mellon University, 1977

Segal ZV, Hood JE, Shaw BF, et al: A structural analysis of the self-schema construct in major depression. Cognitive Therapy and Research 12:471–485, 1988

Segal ZV, Ingram RE: Mood priming and construct activation in tests of cognitive vulnerability to unipolar depression. Clinical Psychology Review 14:663–695, 1994

Seligman MEP: Helplessness: On Depression, Development, and Death. San Francisco, CA, WH Freeman, 1975

Seligman MEP, Abramson LY, Semmel A, et al: Depressive attributional style. J Abnorm Psychol 88:242–247, 1979

Seligman MEP, Peterson C, Kaslow NJ, et al: Attributional style and depressive symptoms among children. J Abnorm Psychol 93:235–238, 1984

Silverman JS, Silverman JA, Eardley DA: Do maladaptive attitudes cause depression? Arch Gen Psychiatry 41:28–30, 1984

Skinner BF: The Behavior of Organisms. New York, Appleton-Century-Crofts, 1938

Stanton RD, Wilson H, Brumback RA: Cognitive improvement associated with tricyclic antidepressant treatment of childhood major depressive illness. Percept Mot Skills 53:219–234, 1981

Steer RA, Clark DA, Beck AT, et al: Common and specific dimensions of self-reported anxiety and depression: a replication. J Abnorm Psychol 104:542–545, 1995

Taylor SE, Lichtman RR, Wood JV: Attributions, beliefs about control, and adjustment to breast cancer. J Pers Soc Psychol 46:489–502, 1984

Weckowicz TE, Tam CI, Mason J, et al: Speed in test performance in depressed patients. J Abnorm Psychol 87:578–582, 1978

Weingartner H: Automatic and effort-demanding cognitive processes in depression, in Handbook for Clinical Memory Assessment of Older Adults. Edited by Poon LW, Crook T, Davis KL. Washington, DC, American Psychological Association, 1986, pp 218–225

Weingartner H, Cohen RM, Murphy DL, et al: Cognitive processes in depression. Arch Gen Psychiatry 38:42–47, 1981

Wenzlaff RM, Wegner DM, Roper DW: Depression and mental control: the resurgence of unwanted negative thoughts. J Pers Soc Psychol 55:882–892, 1988

Williams JMG, Watts FN, MacLeod C, et al: Cognitive Psychology and Emotional Disorders. Chichester, England, John Wiley, 1988

Youngren MA, Lewinsohn PM: The functional relation between depression and problematic interpersonal behavior. J Abnorm Psychol 89:333–341, 1980

Zuroff DC, Colussy SA, Wielgus MS: Selective memory and depression: A cautionary note concerning response bias. Cognitive Therapy and Research 7:223–232, 1983

Chapter 5

Cognitive Deficits in Psychotic Disorders

William D. Spaulding, Ph.D., Dorie Reed, Ph.D.,
Jeffrey Poland, Ph.D., and Daniel M. Storzbach, Ph.D.

In this chapter, we review theories, paradigms, and constructs of cognitive psychology to account for the etiology, development, and expression of psychotic disorders. Normally, the term psychotic disorders connotes a number of specific diagnoses whose symptoms include prominent and protracted psychosis. The exact definition of psychosis has changed over the years, but its core meaning has remained fairly constant, reflecting the colloquial concept of insanity. In current clinical parlance and in the official nosology of DSM-IV (American Psychiatric Association 1994), psychosis refers to syndromes of specific perceptual experiences, thought patterns, and behaviors that suggest that the patient is in an altered state, phenomenologically separated from consensual social reality. Symptoms include disorientation, hallucinations, bizarre ideas and beliefs, unintelligible or meaningless speech, impoverishment of verbal or affective expression, anomalous affective expression, and bizarre motor behavior.

Psychosis is distinguished from other altered states when the syndrome is associated with significant failures in the patient's adaptive abilities. Psychotic disorders include pervasive developmental disorders (childhood schizophrenia and autism), schizophrenia, schizoaffective disorder, depression with psychotic features, bipolar disorder with psychotic features, and a variety of organic and toxic neuropathological conditions.

Despite the variety of diagnoses that qualify as psychotic disorders, cognitive accounts of adult-onset psychotic disorders have focused almost entirely on schizophrenia. Relatively little attention has been directed to other adult-onset psychotic disorders. There is a distinct and extensive cognitive literature on pervasive developmental disorders, which have a childhood onset; that literature is beyond the scope of this chapter.

The emphasis on schizophrenia derives partly from the fact that for many years, schizophrenia was defined more inclusively than it is today. By diagnostic standards of the time, earlier researchers thought they were studying schizophrenia; in fact, however, they were studying heterogeneous populations that included a number of different psychotic disorders. As specific disorders were separated from schizophrenia, explanatory cognitive constructs sometimes accompanied them. However, these constructs usually were borrowed from the original schizophrenia work rather than developed anew for different disorders.

Another reason for the focus on schizophrenia has been that—in contrast to other psychotic disorders—the clinical characteristics of schizophrenia suggest hypotheses about the etiological primacy of cognitive abnormalities. In affective disorders, for example, cognitive abnormalities appear to be secondary effects of the affective abnormality: The grandiose beliefs (a cognitive abnormality) of a manic patient appear to the clinical observer to be driven by psychophysiological arousal and euphoria. Similarly, the cognitive expressions of organic and toxic conditions appear to be caused by neurophysiological conditions. Theories of schizophrenia, on the other hand, have credibly hypothesized the reverse order of causality—with primary cognitive abnormalities driving other symptom expressions. For this reason, schizophrenia has been more interesting to cognitive theorists than other psychotic disorders.

On the other hand, cognitive study of schizophrenia has not been a monolithic enterprise. Despite more exclusive modern diagnostic criteria, no single, unified model can account definitively for all of the cognitive characteristics of schizophrenia or other psychotic disorders. Similarly, schizophrenic cognition is not always clearly different from cognitive abnormalities in other disorders because even the rigorously defined psychotic syndromes of DSM-IV do not necessarily represent the best possible categorization. Current taxonomy is a "best guess" about which symptom syndromes reflect common etiological factors or other important relationships.

There is no compelling reason to conclude that any two subtypes of schizophrenia have more in common than one subtype of schizophrenia and another psychotic disorder. Contemporary research studies often attempt to make key diagnostic distinctions and qualify conclusions accordingly, but teasing out all the similarities and differences, even between subtypes of schizophrenia, will take a long time. This is as true in the cognitive domain as in the genetic, neurophysiological, and developmental domains. Therefore, researchers potentially could apply what they learn about cognitive factors in schizophrenia to other disorders.

Current research that illuminates the psychobiological origins of schizophrenia and related disorders undermines some of the old reasons for the cognitive study of psychosis. For example, it now appears very unlikely that there is a single etiological factor within the cognitive domain that can account for all types of schizophrenia. Nevertheless, cognitive research on schizophrenia is more intense today than ever. The context of such research has changed, however, from a search for cognitive origins to a search for cognitive clues about neurobiological origins and development, cognitive mechanisms by which neurobiological abnormalities are expressed in behavior, cognitive measures that yield clinically useful information about patients' biopsychosocial status, and cognitive targets for treatment.

A complete appreciation of current cognitive research on psychotic disorders is not possible without an understanding of the historical evolution of cognitive paradigms as applied to schizophrenia. Therefore, we will briefly review that history, leading to the integrated cognitive neuroscience paradigms that recently have converged from different lines of research.

Evolution of Cognitive Models of Schizophrenia

Emil Kraepelin's descriptive and nosological accounts of schizophrenia—which he called *dementia praecox* (early-onset dementia)—mark the beginning of modern scientific study of the disorder (see Boyle 1990). Chief among Kraepelin's (1896) observations was long-term deterioration of mental functioning, which was the characteristic that led him to include dementia in the diagnostic label.

Mental functioning was a familiar term in Kraepelin's era. Before Binet's pioneering work on intelligence testing (Pollock and Brenner 1969) elevated the concept to a level of definition suitable for scientific study, however, mental functioning was a protoscientific cognitive construct—cognitive because it referred to mental abilities and the brain functions that support them, protoscientific because those abilities had not yet been objectively, quantitatively measured or subjected to experimental analysis.

When scientific study of intelligence began, researchers immediately recognized that mental functioning was composed of a number of discrete and relatively independent abilities. This realization raised the question of whether Kraepelin's perception of global and pervasive mental deterioration had been unduly influenced by poorly grounded assumptions about the nature of mental functioning.

The next major schizophrenia theorist, Eugen Bleuler (1950), disputed several of Kraepelin's conclusions (see Boyle 1990), partly because Bleuler observed cases that were not characterized by an unremitting deterioration and partly because the concept of mental functioning was by then a more differentiated and measurable construct. However, Bleuler implicitly accepted the Kraepelinian assumption that psychiatric disorders in general can be differentiated into discrete, nonoverlapping disease categories.

The Earliest Cognitive Models

Bleuler introduced modern cognitive concepts into theories of schizophrenia. Among the diagnostic hallmarks of the disorder—autism, affective anomalies, associative anomalies, attentional problems, and ambivalence (Bleuler's familiar "5 A's")—association and attention clearly reflect cognitive constructs that were being actively studied in experimental psychology laboratories of that era. Bleuler used these constructs to explain various behavioral expressions of the disorder. Although he disagreed with Kraepelin about the nature and inevitability of schizophrenic cognitive deterioration, he generally accepted Kraepelin's clinical description and subcategorization of the disorder. Thus, Bleuler superimposed his cognitive view of schizophrenia on Kraepelin's nosologically oriented clinical descriptions.

Bleuler's work set the stage for subsequent lines of theory and research, which endeavored to articulate with increasing specificity the causal relationships between cognitive abnormalities and classic clinical expressions (the "symptoms"). In retrospect, this particular approach embodied a *symptom-linkage* theory.

Symptom-linkage theories use mechanistic explanations of symptomatic behavior, in terms of underlying cognitive causes. Ultimately, however, symptom-linkage theories are limited as etiological explanations because they do not address the causes of cognitive abnormalities. Bleuler, like Kraepelin, vaguely postulated a "metabolic" disorder, probably genetically determined, operating over an unspecified developmental period. In addition, the symptom-linkage approach fails to recognize the possibility of significant relationships between cognitive abnormalities and important behavioral characteristics that are not classic symptoms. For example, although deficits in emotional and behavioral aspects of social functioning are not classic symptoms, they have received much attention in contemporary schizophrenia research, and cognitive abnormalities are strongly suspected to have a role in producing them (Cramer et al. 1989; Cutting 1981; Harrow et al. 1989; Liberman et al. 1982; Wallace and Boone 1984). The cognitive abnormalities that underlie these expressions probably are different from those that produce the classic symptoms.

A Bifurcation of Research Paradigms

In the 1920s and 1930s, the limitations of pure symptom-linkage approaches produced a bifurcation in the evolution of cognitive theories of schizophrenia.

One branch continued to use Kraepelinian description and nosology as its conceptual basis; the other did not.

The non-Kraepelinian branch was dominated by experimental psychology. It focused increasingly on the nature of cognitive abnormalities that could be detected and measured in the laboratory and deemphasized relationships between cognition and classic symptoms. This branch was founded in the work of David Shakow, and over the years it became the cognitive domain of experimental psychopathology (see Shakow 1977a). Until recently, there has been only a modest amount of mutual influence between experimental cognitive psychopathology and Kraepelinian nosology, in large part because the Kraepelinian categories of psychotic disorders seemed to be only slightly related to important cognitive abnormalities.

The Kraepelinian branch became primarily concerned with developing integrative theories of etiology and expression, wherein cognitive constructs play a mediating role between the two. Psychoanalytic etiological models dominated this branch for about three decades.[1] Thereafter, neurophysiological models became dominant, inspired primarily by psychopharmacological findings. The cognitive constructs in this branch changed considerably over the years, although a Kraepelinian view of diagnostic categories and a Bleulerian view of symptom-linkage remained.

In the psychoanalytic era, cognitive constructs of the Kraepelinian branch generally were derived from traditional notions of ego functioning. The origins of schizophrenia were thought to lie in developmental psychodynamics that produced specific pathogenic flaws in ego functions (see, e.g., Arieti 1955). In the neurophysiological era, researchers borrowed cognitive constructs from cybernetics and the nascent cognitive neuroscience of the time or reformulated Kraepelinian descriptive concepts (see, e.g., Klein et al. 1980). In the former case, the constructs provided a heuristic method for understanding how pathological neurophysiological processes might produce more molar brain dysfunction. In the latter case, researchers modernized traditional symptom descriptions by using the terminology of psychology, psycholinguistics, and related disciplines. In both cases, cognitive constructs were considered mechanisms that mediate between neurobiological origins, either specified or unspecified, and their ultimate consequences in adaptive personal and social functioning.

---

[1]Freud himself was unsympathetic to the Kraepelinian and Bleulerian views. When Bleuler suggested that rapproachment may be possible between those views and psychoanalysis, Freud is said to have replied that Bleuler had fallen victim to one of his own A's, ambivalence. Nevertheless, later psychoanalytic theorists did manage to combine Kraepelinian nosology, Bleulerian symptom-linkage, and psychodynamic developmental etiology.

Limitations of Earlier Cognitive Models

The practice of applying new terms to old Kraepelinian concepts created problems for developing cognitive models in both the psychoanalytic and neurophysiological eras. As we noted above, Bleuler, in his era of psychological research, was led to reconsider Kraepelin's notion of mental functioning. Further developments in cognitive psychology required reconsideration of other Kraepelinian notions; failure to recognize this has been costly.

The concept of *thought disorder* is an example. Originally, it seemed clear that the disorganized verbal behavior often observed in schizophrenic patients reflected an underlying disturbance in cognitive mechanisms that organize language. In common parlance, thought was considered to be internal speech, so it seemed a small conceptual step to infer thought disorder from language disorder. Subsequent research endeavored to specify the flaws in thought that could account for schizophrenic language. This work produced some interesting terms and tools for characterizing schizophrenic speech abnormalities (e.g., Andreasen 1986); some, such as *derailment*, are even included in the DSM-IV diagnostic criteria. Arieti's interpretation of schizophrenia (Arieti 1955) elegantly combined psychoanalytic motivational theory with a cognitive model that traces symptom expression to failures in syllogistic logic.

This research failed, however, to clarify the nature of cognitive abnormalities in schizophrenia. By the end of the 1950s, experimental psychologists concluded that language does not have an isomorphic relationship with the cognitive processes that support it. Studying language, therefore, is not necessarily equivalent to studying cognition (see Asarnow and MacCrimmon 1982).

Another example is the collection of explicit and implicit assumptions associated with the Kraepelinian concept of *delusion*. A delusion is understood to be a kind of belief or attribution. The processes associated with belief and attribution have been studied extensively with experimental methods. Many of the chapters in this volume draw heavily from that experimental literature for theory and clinical application. The literature is convoluted. Belief and attribution processes are themselves complex, interacting systems of cognitive, affective, behavioral, and social phenomena (see, e.g., Jones et al. 1971; Lipe 1991). Nevertheless, Kraepelin's protoscientific understanding of belief and attribution, as preserved in his nosology, serves today as the diagnostic basis for understanding abnormalities in these complex systems. As a result, researchers have learned very little about the relevance of delusions to scientifically understood belief and attribution processes (see Oltmanns and Maher 1988).

Problems such as these illustrate the importance of considering basic principles of experimental cognitive psychology as well as descriptive nosology when constructing models of cognitive psychopathology. Naive protoscientific concepts such as thought disorder and delusions survived—and are in common professional and scientific use today—because they were formalized in Kraepelinian nosology despite an inadequate psychological perspective.

Even constructs that have been through the experimental sieve become suspect as cognitive paradigms evolve. For example, constructs associated with familiar phenomena such as attention and memory undergo continuous reconstruction in contemporary cognitive science. Researchers and clinicians cannot assume that colloquial concepts of mental functioning are applicable to psychopathology.

Reformulations of Schizophrenia

By the mid-1960s, genetic and pharmacological research had accumulated considerable evidence for biological origins of schizophrenia, but this evidence was not advancing a cognitive understanding of schizophrenia or its behavioral expression. Experimental psychopathology had articulated and quantified key cognitive characteristics of schizophrenia but had done little to clarify the role of these characteristics in the disorder's etiology or expression. Non-Kraepelinian views of schizophrenia set in motion a much-needed paradigmatic convergence.[2]

The proposition that schizophrenia is a *diathesis-stress disorder*—that is, one in which diathesis or vulnerability interacts with stress (pathogenic environmental factors) to produce the disorder—was a key development. The diathesis-stress concept is implicit in some earlier theories of schizophrenia (such as Arieti's). A model proposed by Meehl (1962, 1989) was the first to lead to a strategy for integrating biological and psychological paradigms. Meehl hypothesized three states in the development of schizophrenia: schizotaxia, schizotypy, and schizophrenia itself. Schizotaxia is the genetic configuration that produces vulnerability, and schizotypy is the biopsychological result of schizotaxia. Pre-

---

[2]Schizophrenia is itself a Kraepelinian concept, so "non-Kraepelinian views of schizophrenia" may seem an oxymoron. However, one may accept the proposition that there is a family of psychotic disorders whose categorical boundaries are unclear, but which for some purposes can be usefully included under the rubric "schizophrenia and related disorders" or "schizophrenia spectrum disorders." Use of the term does not necessarily imply acceptance of the Kraepelinian assumption that it is a unitary disease-like entity with clear categorical boundaries. Within Kraepelinian thinking the precise boundaries between diagnoses are subject to ambiguity. For example, there is continuing controversy about whether schizoaffective disorder should be a subcategory of schizophrenia or a separate category. Related to this is the proposition that continuous dimensions of functioning within a "schizophrenic" population may have more meaning than diagnostic subcategory boundaries.

sumably, schizotypy includes neurological, psychophysiological, cognitive, and behavioral vulnerabilities.

The implications of a cognitive vulnerability to schizophrenia were not lost on experimental psychopathologists. The early concept of symptom-linkage was expanded to accommodate diathesis-stress models by making a distinction between symptom-linked and vulnerability-linked cognitive abnormalities. By the end of the 1970s, several theorists had proposed a number of cognitive abnormalities as possibly linked to vulnerability to schizophrenia (Cromwell and Spaulding 1978; Erlenmeyer-Kimling and Cornblatt 1978; Spring and Zubin 1978; Zubin and Spring 1977). In keeping with the non-Kraepelinian view, researchers generally did not take strong positions on whether such abnormalities are congenital or acquired; biological or psychosocial in origin; actual causative factors or mere markers of other etiological processes; closely linked to classical symptoms or respectful of diagnostic boundaries. Current research is gradually articulating the nature and role of various cognitive abnormalities with respect to vulnerability to schizophrenia and related disorders.

Other developments of the 1960s and 1970s indicated a need for more complex cognitive theories of schizophrenia than had been previously imagined. Researchers increasingly viewed schizophrenia as an *episodic* disorder, wherein episodes of psychotic exacerbations are preceded by vulnerable and prodromal states and followed by residual and remitted states (Zubin and Spring 1977). Currently, cognitive models in schizophrenia research include abnormalities that fall into five course-related categories. *Vulnerability-linked abnormalities* can be detected before any clinical expression of disorder emerges—sometimes in early childhood. Vulnerability-linked abnormalities also may occur in individuals who are genetically at risk for schizophrenia but who never express the disorder. *Episode-linked abnormalities* appear with the onset of a psychotic episode and disappear when the episode ends. *Episode-sensitive vulnerabilities* are vulnerability-linked but also exhibit variations in severity associated with the onset of psychotic episodes. *Symptom-linked abnormalities* directly influence the quality of specific symptoms during psychotic episodes. *Residual abnormalities* appear during psychotic episodes and persist in the residual and remitted states, possibly creating new vulnerabilities to relapse (future episodes) or new deficits in personal and social functioning.

Another important non-Kraepelinian dimension of schizophrenia research in the 1960s and 1970s subdivided schizophrenia into a *process* subtype and a *reactive* subtype. Process schizophrenia is characterized by a family history of schizophrenia, earlier onset (mid-adolescence), poor premorbid functioning with insidious onset of the frank disorder, disorganized and/or undifferentiated symptomatology, little functional difference between psychotic and remitted states, and poorer prognosis despite better short-term symptomatic response to neuroleptic drugs. Reactive schizophrenia is characterized by later onset (early adulthood), normal premorbid functioning, dramatic onset of florid and bizarre symptoms, clear episodes of psychosis interspersed with relatively remitted states, and better prognosis despite more questionable short-term drug response. The presence or absence of a clear paranoid syndrome (delusions of persecution and/or hallucinations of persecutory voices) was another important distinction between the process and reactive subtypes (Cromwell and Pithers 1981). Few process schizophrenic patients exhibit a paranoid syndrome, whereas most reactive patients predominantly show either paranoid or schizoaffective symptoms.

Experimental psychopathology research identified many cognitive differences between process and reactive subjects, as well as between paranoid and nonparanoid subjects. Some theoretical cognitive models relied heavily on these differences. The use of these differences in research decreased precipitously in the 1980s, however—due partly to the introduction of DSM-III (American Psychiatric Association 1980). It was hoped that the new (but still basically Kraepelinian) diagnostic criteria in DSM-III would clear up the confusion created by the previous *Diagnostic and Statistical Manuals*. DSM-III led to a revival of interest in classic Kraepelinian symptomatology. Researchers developed new instruments to identify and quantify symptoms rather than pursue process/reactive or paranoid/nonparanoid differences.

In addition, it became clear that the process/reactive and paranoid/nonparanoid distinctions reflect continuous dimensions rather than discrete subtypes (Cash 1973). Much of the cognitive research had artificially constructed categories based on extreme values on the two dimensions, and the findings from these studies became suspect. Cognitive research on schizophrenia also was drawn away from hypotheses about symptom-linkage because findings on vulnerability-linkage and residual deficits seemed more promising. Ironically—in light of the fact that linkage to classic Kraepelinian symptoms was the original cognitive hypothesis in modern schizophrenia research—hypotheses about specific symptom-linkage remain the most poorly supported in the cognitive domain (see Neale et al. 1985).

Moreover, the Kraepelinian revival was tempered somewhat by lessons of the past. This moderating influence is evident in the creation by neo-Kraepelinians of the positive/negative symptom distinction (Andreasen and Olsen 1987; see also J. Strauss et al. 1974). These symptoms mostly are new categories for classic nosology, but negative symptoms also include non-Kraepelinian concepts such as social competence (Bellack et al. 1990). There is evidence, for example, that low social competence is associated with cognitive abnormalities (Cramer et al. 1989, 1992); by definition, therefore, the positive/negative distinction creates the possibility of symptom-linked cognitive deficits.

The effect on the scientific community of the semantic wordplay embodied in the positive/negative distinction has been to reduce pointless debate, encourage paradigmatic rapprochement, and help broaden the scope of neurobiological, cognitive, and social-behavioral research. The value of the positive/negative distinction, however, appears to depend on viewing the two terms as at least two continuous dimensions, rather than as Kraepelinian subcategories (Andreasen et al. 1990).

The Influence of Neuropsychology

The introduction of clinical neuropsychology into schizophrenia research (Goldstein 1986; Levin et al. 1989; Goldstein 1991) was an important development in cognitive research. Clinical neuropsychology originated in neurosurgery services as an application of the experimental analysis of brain-behavior relationships for the assessment of brain injury. Through tests of cognitive performance, clinical neuropsychologists were remarkably accurate in determining the anatomical locations of brain lesions and, more importantly, their functional implications.

Ironically, when the neuropsychological assessment approach was first applied to schizophrenia, its value was not widely recognized because it failed to discriminate chronic schizophrenia from chronic brain injury. In the early 1980s, however, researchers realized that perhaps, in some sense, chronic schizophrenia *is* chronic brain injury. Using computerized neuroimaging techniques and the traditional paradigms of experimental psychopathology, neuropsychological researchers began to identify not only the cognitive abnormalities of schizophrenia but also the brain structures and functions with which those abnormalities might be associated.

The concept of *cognitive deficit* had appeared in models of schizophrenia at least since the 1930s, but by the 1980s the concept had evolved considerably. Originally, researchers used the term cognitive deficit almost interchangeably with cognitive abnormality. Later models sometimes postulated specific cognitive factors that influence the qualitative expression of schizophrenia, without being abnormal themselves or contributing to the severity of functional impairments. Combined with the perception of schizophrenia as an episodic disorder and the introduction of clinical neuropsychology, this approach designates a cognitive deficit as a particular type of abnormality that directly impairs personal and social functioning—but not necessarily by producing classic Kraepelinian symptoms.

The difference between an abnormality and a deficit may seem trivial, but it has significant implications for basic and clinical research. Theories of the phenomenology, etiology, and development of schizophrenia make extensive use of many kinds of cognitive abnormalities, whereas clinical assessment and treatment models tend to focus on cognitive deficits.

The Era of Cognitive Science

During the 1970s and 1980s, a Kuhnian paradigm shift (Kuhn 1970) occurred in psychology (Baars 1986). Progress in experimental psychology, neuropsychology, cybernetics, and the biological brain sciences converged to the degree that researchers considered cognition in the context of a comprehensive, unifying model of behavior. Theorists labeled this movement cognitive science.

Some researchers in cognitive science have linked their work to biological brain structure. *Connectionist* models, for example, include hypotheses about how cellular architecture supports information processing. Researchers often evaluate such models by constructing computer programs that simulate hypothetical brain processes, including pathological processes. Neuropsychological models of cognition also address brain structure, although their focus tends to be on neurophysiology and interactions of anatomical subsystems. Researchers traditionally have used psychological test data to evaluate these models; increasingly, however, they are relying on analysis of animal behavior in the presence of known brain lesions.

Other cognitive models address the nature of information processing independent of its biological medium. We refer to these as *classical cognitive models* because they reflect the original independence of cognitive psychology from hypotheses about brain structure and function.

The psychopathology of psychotic disorders reflects developments in cognitive science. Researchers have introduced new laboratory paradigms in experimental research and studied those paradigms as possible vulnerability factors, episode markers, symptom-linked abnormalities, or residual deficits— much like traditional cognitive paradigms. Researchers also have applied general theoretical concepts from the new paradigms in models of abnormal cognition. The most important of these models is the notion of *systemic organization* (see Brenner 1987; Engel 1980; E. Goldberg and Bilder 1987; Spaulding 1986). Systems theory, which is rooted in a number of disciplines that contribute to cognitive science, organizes information processing systems into *functional components* and *levels of organization*.

Researchers define the functional components of a system in terms of the information processing operations those components perform. Traditional cognitive concepts such as attention and memory reflect a nascent understanding of the componential or modular nature of systems, although the components included in systemic cognitive models do not necessarily correspond closely to colloquial concepts. Applied to psychopathology, the component concept suggests that cognitive impairments may be associated with failures of the cognitive system within or between specific components. Some models of psychotic cognition developed during the era of cognitive science emphasize the localization of primary impairments within system components (see Cromwell and Spaulding 1978).

Biological systems are organized hierarchically with respect to both structure and function: Elemental or *molecular* subsystems are subsumed within more superordinate or *molar* subsystems. Cognition is the processing of information within and across subsystems. In "upward" processing, raw data is progressively analyzed by increasingly molar components; in "downward" processing, interpretations of raw data modulate and modify the activity of molecular components. In the context of psychopathology, this model suggests that molecular impairments produce molar impairments by passing faulty information upward, and molar impairments produce molecular impairments by failing to properly regulate molecular components. Determining causality, however, may be problematic in such a situation because of the reciprocal regulatory relationships between components. A component process may be "upstream" with respect to the information it processes but "downstream" with respect to the neuroregulatory consequences of some other impairment. Thus, *heterarchical* or modular organization may be a more apt characterization of cognition than hierarchical organization.

In the light of systems theory, the limitations of traditional hypotheses about psychotic cognition become more apparent. In systemic terms, overly simplistic hypotheses about unidirectional causation between cognitive and behavioral impairments imply *cascade models* of causation (Corrigan et al. 1991). In these models, impairments flow from one abnormality to the next in a hierarchical cascade of consequences, eventually expressing themselves in behavioral expression. Kraepelinian views of psychopathology, for example, embody a cascade model of causation in which mutually exclusive categories of disorders imply single, noninteracting causal processes. Cognitive and behavioral abnormalities do not always behave as cascades, however. Although some research still endeavors to identify the most molecular level at which cognitive impairments can be detected, theorists no longer assume that such impairments are necessarily the origin of molar impairments.

The distinction between a linear cascade view and a reciprocally causal systemic view of cognitive psychopathology has important implications for treatment as well as etiological theory. A hierarchical, cascade model suggests that the appropriate target for intervention is the most molecular or "original" deficit. A heterarchical, modular view of cognition suggests that intervention at any number of levels may produce benefits for systemic functioning (see Figure 5–1). Failure to recognize the systemic characteristics of psychiatric disorders leads to an overdependence on the most molecular levels of treatment— in other words, neuropharmacology—and neglect of other potentially useful avenues of intervention.

The unifying concepts of systems theory have led to paradigmatic rapprochement in psychopathology in the era of cognitive science. Classical, connectionist, and neuropsychological models exhibit increasing correspondence. The integration is far from complete, however. A number of classical cognitive constructs still have undetermined correspondence to brain

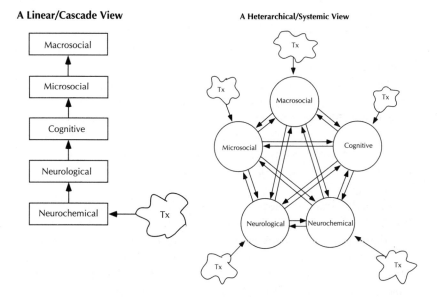

Figure 5–1. Linear/cascade model versus heterarchical/systemic model of causation and treatment. Each box or circle represents a level of organismic functioning; arrows represent causal pathways by which functioning at one level may affect functioning at another level. Linear model implies that most effective treatment must be directed at causal origin of disorder; heterarchical/systemic model implies that changes in any level of functioning may affect performance in other levels. Hence, treatment directed at any impaired level may potentially have broadly distributed effects.

structure or process, although they are empirically linked to vulnerability, psychotic symptoms or episodes, or residual impairments.

Impairments Within the Cognitive System

We turn now to a selective review of paradigms that continue to be useful in understanding cognition in psychotic disorders. Some of these paradigms are specifically associated with classical, connectionist, or neuropsychological models; others incorporate two or more models. In keeping with the notion of heterarchical, modular organization of biological systems, we will proceed from molecular to molar levels of cognitive functioning. The paradigms, the putative cognitive abnormalities they measure, and their probable etiological roles are summarized in Table 5–1.

Preattentional Processes

The most molecular end of the cognitive spectrum consists of processes that rapidly and automatically translate the physical features of stimuli into coded representations for further processing. Researchers have studied visual and auditory modalities most extensively in this regard, both in clinical and in nonclinical populations.

Researchers in experimental psychology have developed and applied a number of approaches to measure the parameters of icon construction and translation. With regard to the visual modality, there appear to be no differences between nonschizophrenic and schizophrenic subjects in the rate and efficiency with which icons are initially constructed or in their persistence (Knight 1984; Spaulding et al. 1980). There are differences in the auditory modality, however.

Researchers have studied these auditory differences primarily with *two-click threshold* paradigms (Freedman et al. 1993). In this approach, brief auditory stimuli ("clicks") are presented to subjects pairwise, at time intervals in the 50-millisecond range. Researchers monitor the subject's response to each click electroencephalographically to determine whether the subject's auditory system detects the two clicks separately or fuses them into a single stimulus. Schizophrenic patients exhibit fused detection at shorter interstimulus intervals than nonschizophrenic subjects (see Spaulding et al. 1980). Researchers believe that this fused detection reflects an abnormality in a neurochemical inhibitory mechanism that normally helps to organize stimulus sequences temporally as the auditory icon is constructed. Researchers have found this abnormality in schizophrenic patients in psychotic and remitted states, as well as in

Table 5–1. Summary of cognitive impairments, examples of measurement paradigms, and probable etiological role of impairments

Level of functioning	Deficit	Laboratory paradigm	Probable etiological role
Preattentional	Auditory icon construction	Two-click threshold	Vulnerability-linked
Preattentional	Visual icon decoding	Backward masking	Episode-sensitive vulnerability
Preattentional	Visual icon decoding	Span of apprehension	Vulnerability-linked
Preattentional	Visual icon decoding	Degraded-image CPT	Vulnerability-linked
Attentional	Continuous attention	Uncomplicated CPT	Episode-linked
Attentional	Distractibility (visual)	CPT with distraction	Episode-linked
Attentional	Distractibility (auditory)	Dichotic listening	Episode-linked
Attentional	Segmental attentional set	"AX" CPT	Vulnerability-linked
Attentional	Segmental attentional set	RT crossover	Vulnerability-linked
Memory organization	Reduced STM capacity	Digit span	Episode-linked
Memory organization	Mnemonic failure	Various learning tasks	Residual
Memory organization	Unstable personal constructs	Repertoire grids	Unknown
Memory organization	Skill and role deficits	Role-playing assessments	Vulnerability-linked, residual
Memory accessing	Node activation anomalies	Negative priming	Unknown
Memory accessing	Classical anamnestic syndrome	Various memory tasks	Residual
Conceptual	Categorization anomalies	Object sorting tasks	Episode-linked, residual
Conceptual	Abstraction deficits	Proverb interpretation	Vulnerability-linked
Executive	Working memory deficit	Spacial memory task	Unknown
Executive	Response bias anomalies	Ambiguous stimulus tasks	Symptom-linked
Executive	Planning and evaluation deficit	Card sorting tasks	Vulnerability-linked, episode-linked, residual

unaffected relatives—suggesting that it is a genetically based, vulnerability-linked impairment. Researchers have not determined whether the impairment is found in disorders other than schizophrenia (see Spaulding et al. 1980).

Researchers also have found numerous differences between nonclinical and clinical subjects in icon decoding processes, which they have studied primarily with *backward masking* (Braff et al. 1991; Green and Walker 1986; Sacuzzo and Braff 1981) and *span of apprehension* paradigms (Asarnow et al. 1991; M. E. Strauss et al. 1984). Theorists believe that both of these approaches measure the processes that translate literal featural information from the icon.

In backward masking, researchers use a tachistoscope to present a visual target stimulus (e.g., alphanumeric characters) followed by another stimulus (the "mask") to the subject. When the interstimulus interval is brief enough, the subject cannot report the target stimulus content. In schizophrenic and schizotypal subjects, the masking effect persists at longer interstimulus intervals, indicating that those subjects require more time to translate a given amount of information from the icon (Braff et al. 1991). There is some evidence that the abnormality is more severe in the psychotic state and is reduced by antipsychotic medication (Braff et al. 1991).

In the span of apprehension approach, a subject briefly views a matrix of several characters and is asked to determine whether a designated character is present. Performance on the task reflects the amount of information the subject can process during the stimulus presentation. Impaired span of apprehension has been demonstrated in psychotic and remitted schizophrenic patients and in children at risk for schizophrenia (Asarnow et al. 1991; M. E. Strauss et al. 1984). Researchers also have found deficits in other psychotic disorders during acute psychosis, but the deficits do not appear in premorbid or remitted states (Asarnow et al. 1991; Strauss et al. 1984).

A related visual processing test is the degraded-image continuous performance task (Nuechterlein 1991; Nuechterlein et al. 1986). Continuous performance tasks (CPTs) usually address performance at the attentional rather than the preattentional level of cognition. In a typical CPT, the subject watches a series of simple alphanumeric stimuli, presented at the rate of about 1 per second, and is instructed to press a button when a specifically designated target stimulus appears. The task thus demands continuous attention, vigilance, and readiness to respond over a period of several minutes. In the degraded-image version, the stimuli are blurred, making it more difficult to decide quickly whether any particular stimulus is the target. Presumably, the degraded stimulus image imposes a higher demand on preattentional feature analytic processes than a sharp image, so the degraded-image CPT represents a measure of preattentional processing. Subjects with schizophrenia show impairment on traditional and degraded-image CPTs (Nuechterlein 1991; Nuechterlein et al. 1986). However, the impairment on traditional CPTs is episode-sensitive and is found in other psychotic disorders, whereas degraded-image CPT performance is independent of episodic changes in clinical status and is more specific to schizophrenia.

Taken together, studies of psychotic disorders using preattentional paradigms provide strong evidence of vulnerability-linked abnormalities at this level. These abnormalities appear to be specific to schizophrenia, but further study of other disorders, especially in nonacute states, is needed. The fact that these abnormalities occur in remitted and unaffected subjects suggests that the impairments are not part of a pathogenic cascade leading directly to subsequent impairments at more molar cognitive levels. Instead, they could simply be vulnerability markers—indicators of structural or neurochemical abnormalities that actually lie upstream in the causal flow. On the other hand, there also is increasing evidence that at least some unaffected relatives and other high-risk subjects show subclinical abnormalities in personal and social functioning, as well as in preattentional processing (Chapman and Chapman 1987). This could mean that preattentional impairments contribute to relatively subtle difficulties in proprioception, social perception, or other molar processes, which in turn create enduring vulnerabilities in the behavioral domain.

Preattentional deficits may be significant for clinical application in several areas. If such deficits are downstream indicators of a pathogenic neurochemical process related to psychosis, they may provide useful information about the current status of that process. Clinicians might use this information to predict onset or relapse in vulnerable individuals or to assess the effects of pharmacological interventions earlier than they can using clinical behavioral criteria. On the other hand, preattentional deficits may be part of a cascade that produces subtle functional impairments in nonacute or nonpsychotic states, which clinicians may need to take into account in the design of skill training and related interventions that are typically implemented in the residual phase of a disorder, or in early detection and prevention techniques. Similarly, assessment of these abnormalities could prove useful in the assessment and treatment of nonpsychotic disorders in the schizophrenia spectrum, especially schizotypal personality disorder.

Attention

As we noted earlier in this chapter, theorists have propounded impairments in attention since the advent of cognitive views of schizophrenia. A century of research in experimental psychology has produced a rich and complex understanding of the various cognitive processes associated with the colloquial concept of attention. Although this approach is beneficial from a scientific point of view, it creates difficulty in discussing the relevance of attentional impairments to psychopathology. Instead, researchers have developed a number of specific paradigms to study specific processes under the "attention" rubric.

Researchers have used CPTs extensively to study vigilance impairments in psychotic disorders (Cornblatt et al. 1988; Nuechterlein 1983, 1991); often, they add extraneous and/or irrelevant stimulation to the CPT in order to assess the effects of distraction.[3] Other researchers have thoroughly studied a similar type of vigilance and distraction in the auditory system with dichotic listening tasks (Berlin and McNeal 1976; Friedes 1977; Gruzelier and Hammond 1980; Naatanen 1986; Spring et al. 1991; Wielgus and Harvey 1988). Subjects listen to spoken messages delivered through earphones, with target messages delivered to one ear and irrelevant messages or other distractions delivered concurrently to the other ear. The task is to verbally repeat the target message as it is delivered (called shadowing) or to press a button upon hearing a designated word or other signal in the target message.

Although CPTs and dichotic listening tasks seem similar with respect to their cognitive demands, researchers do not know whether performance is highly correlated within individuals. Impairments on both are common in patients with psychotic disorders, with little evidence of specificity to any particular disorder. Researchers observe impairments most often in the acute phase. Uncomplicated CPTs with low distraction levels show minimal impairment in remitted patients, although an impairment in children may be associated with vulnerability to schizophrenia (Berlin and McNeal 1976; Friedes 1977; Gruzelier and Hammond 1980; Naatanen 1986; Spring et al. 1991; Wielgus and Harvey 1988). Researchers have not extensively studied the possible vulnerability linkage of dichotic listening impairment.

Another CPT variant is sometimes called the "AX" CPT because the target is an "X" specifically following an "A." As with distraction, this additional

---

[3]It is important to note that distraction so defined refers to stimulus information whose processing is irrelevant to task performance. This is distinct from a situation in which stimulus information must be processed for its informational content to discriminate signal from non-signal. Distraction impairs performance by disrupting sustained attention to a selected channel and all the preattentional processes operating on that channel. for expample, if the signal stimulus is a particular word, the information processed in reading a series of words containing the target is not distraction. A flash of light which interrupts reading the word series (and perhaps shifts attention to investigating the light flash) is distraction. Sustained use of preattentional stimulus-analytic processes such as reading involves cognitive operations quite different than for ignoring extraneous or irrelevant stimulus events.

complexity amplifies the CPT impairments found among psychotic subjects (Cohen and Servan-Schreiber 1992). The interplay of processes that the AX CPT addresses has recently become a focus for connectionist theories of schizophrenic impairment (Cohen and Servan-Schreiber 1992).

A key concept in this work is context: the information that a subject must continuously access during a task to guide performance and accomplish a goal. Instructions stored in working memory (described later) and accessed during performance provide much of the contextual information in CPTs and other tasks. Researchers can incrementally manipulate context processing demands by adding complexities such as the contingent response rule of the AX CPT.

Theorists suggest that schizophrenic subjects have impaired context processing; when the complexity of contextual information exceeds their limited processing ability, they show a performance deficit. Characteristic of the connectionist approach, researchers propose a cellular configuration as part of this model, to explain how the continuous accessing of contextual information during an AX CPT is accomplished and how continuous performance is interrupted when that process fails. Computer programs can model the cellular configuration and mimic the task performance it produces in schizophrenic and nonschizophrenic subjects.

Researchers also have used simple reaction time (RT) tasks to study impaired vigilance in psychotic disorders (Nuechterlein 1977; Rist and Cohen 1991; Rosenbaum et al. 1988). Most psychotic patients show an overall slowing of RT, although separating the contributions of cognitive, motor, and motivational factors makes interpretation difficult.

The effects of various configurations of preparatory intervals (PIs) across many RT trials have been of particular interest to researchers. In nonschizophrenic subjects, RT generally is faster when all PIs in a series are of equal length, compared with series of PIs that vary randomly from 1 to 20 seconds. Paradoxically, in schizophrenic patients, RT is slower when the PIs are of equal length, if the PIs are 7 seconds or longer (although some studies show slower RT at shorter PIs; see Nuechterlein 1977). Graphic comparisons of RT in schizophrenic subjects as a function of PI, under regular (equal length) and irregular (varying length) PI conditions, show RT for regular PI trials overtaking and "crossing over" RT for irregular trials, with the intersection occurring at a PI of about 6 seconds (see Figure 5–2). Hence, researchers have termed the phenomenon *RT crossover*. Researchers have observed RT crossover in a number of clinical and normal subject groups, but it occurs most frequently in process schizophrenic subjects and their first-degree relatives.

Based on his studies of the RT crossover effect, Shakow (1977b) reviewed a theory of schizophrenic attentional impairment that is strikingly complementary to the connectionist view of context processing. Normal performance

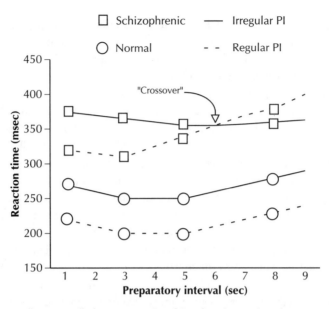

Figure 5–2. "Crossover" phenomenon in schizophrenic reaction time.

on an RT task, Shakow argued, is guided by a *major set*—a state of psychological preparedness that incorporates contextual information about the entire task. As subjects perceive that a PI series is regular, they adopt a particular set that optimizes their speed in responding to a signal having known temporal characteristics. When subjects perceive that the PIs are irregular, they adopt a different set, which optimizes response speed when the temporal characteristics are unpredictable.

Schizophrenic patients exhibit crossover when PIs are 7 seconds or longer because they are unable to use the contextual information of PI regularity to speed up their response. Instead, they construct a *minor set* using limited information about the task, such as the length of the immediately preceding PI. Thus, schizophrenic task performance is guided by sequential use of suboptimal minor sets, which Shakow collectively termed a *segmental set*.

Further studies of RT in schizophrenia identified other peculiarities associated with PI configurations; these results initially cast some doubt on Shakow's original interpretation (Bellissimo and Steffy 1972, 1975; Kaplan 1974; Nuechterlein 1977). Now, however, although there are some vicissitudes in schizophrenic RT performance, segmental set apparently remains a viable explanation of the crossover effect and schizophrenic attentional impairments in general. An integrated model of psychotic attentional impairments—wherein a segmental set makes the patient more prone to distraction because in a minor set any particular stimulus is more likely to be "unexpected" or "out of context" (Cohen et al. 1991)—now appears possible.

Abnormal psychophysiological arousal levels common in psychosis make distractions even more likely to disrupt sustained attention (Gjerede 1983)—which makes creation of a major set more difficult, which augments vulnerability to distraction, ad infinitum. There is some direct experimental evidence that RT crossover is linked to a genetic vulnerability to schizophrenia (DeAmicis and Cromwell 1979).

Studies of uncomplicated vigilance performance generally suggest that impairments in vigilance are common in psychotic disorders but not specific to any particular disorder. Impairments are most evident in the psychotic state, and their severity lessens as clinical status improves. Impairments in this domain do not seem to be vulnerability-linked or residual, except when the task is complicated by high demands for preattentional and contextual processing.

This qualification may be trivial because in the real world almost any natural vigilance task is accompanied by significant demands on preattentional and contextual processing. For example, waiting to speak in a social conversation is a vigilance task that requires extensive preattentional processing of cues (facial expressions, etc.), a complex contextual set (the topic of conversation and the social relationships among the conversants) and a complex motor response (speech). The complexity of natural situations often will be more than enough to produce functional impairment even in a remitted patient who shows no deficits in an uncomplicated laboratory CPT.

The process that produces RT crossover does seem to be vulnerability-linked to schizophrenia (DeAmicis and Cromwell 1979). Impaired AX CPT performance may reflect the same contextual processing deficit, so it also may be vulnerability-linked. In patients with schizophrenia or schizotypal personality disorder, vulnerability-linked impairments in preattentional processing may further amplify the effects of natural complexity on attention, and abnormalities in psychophysiological arousal may amplify the effects of distraction.

Memory Capacity and Organization

Memory is a colloquial concept that generally refers to an individual's ability to store information so that it can be accessed later for further processing. The concept of memory has persisted in cognitive science as a rubric rather than a specific type of process. Many processes share the characteristic of storing information but have little else in common.

Sensory icons are a type of memory, although they persist for only a few hundred milliseconds; we discussed impairments associated with iconic process in the section on preattentional deficits above. *Short-term memory* (STM) refers to processes that store encoded information for periods of several seconds. *Working memory* is similar to short-term memory but is specialized for handling the information necessary to plan and conduct complex behaviors. *Long-term memory* (LTM) is a virtually limitless information bank that contains declarative knowledge of the world acquired during a lifetime.

Contemporary accounts of human memory include several other types, although terminology is not perfectly consistent and some types appear to overlap with others. In this chapter, only a brief review of STM and LTM in psychotic disorders is practical. We discuss working memory under executive processes, for reasons that will become apparent.

Researchers have studied STM functioning in psychotic disorders extensively with the familiar digit span task, wherein the subject repeats a string of digits recited by the examiner. Researchers have had difficulty, however, determining whether subjects' impaired performance on this task is due to actual STM failure or to problems with the preattentional, attentional, psychophysiological, and more molar processes that store and use the information in STM (Oltmanns 1978). Whatever the cause, the STM capacity of people with psychotic disorders appears to be normal under minimally demanding conditions but extremely vulnerable to "shrinkage" in the presence of distraction or other cognitive demands (Oltmanns 1978). Since "minimally demanding conditions" usually prevail only in the laboratory, researchers frequently observe STM failures in psychotic patients in naturalistic situations (see Calev 1990). Moreover, researchers note STM impairments in actively psychotic patients irrespective of diagnosis (Oltmanns 1978), suggesting that the impairments are episode-linked and not etiologically specific. There is insufficient evidence about whether STM impairments also may be vulnerability-linked or residual in some disorders.

People naturally use *mnemonic strategies* to facilitate transfer of information from STM to LTM. Experimental studies suggest that schizophrenic subjects tend not to use simple mnemonics when other subjects would do so automatically (Calev 1990; Koh 1978; Koh and Kayton 1974; Koh et al. 1976). When specifically cued to use mnemonics, however, schizophrenic subjects can use them, and their memory performance improves accordingly (Caler 1990; Koh 1978; Koh and Kayton 1974; Koh et al. 1976). Thus, schizophrenia appears to be associated with a failure to use routine mnemonic strategies, with an attendant impairment in tasks that require rapid transfer of STM information to LTM. This impairment could be because LTM organization is not conducive to the use of mnemonics or because a process that normally identifies mnemonically useful associations is deficient. Researchers know little about this subject, but mnemonic failure seems likely to be a residual impairment in some patients, with obvious implications for skill acquisition. Inasmuch as mnemonic failure appears to involve processes that operate on memory, it may be best understood in terms of executive impairment (discussed below).

LTM usually is divided into *episodic memory* and *declarative memory*. Episodic memory is a record of events and experiences; declarative memory is a comprehensive store of relational knowledge. Researchers have studied the organizational structure of declarative LTM at many levels, though there is no universally accepted nomenclature. For present purposes, declarative LTM organizational levels include *elemental associations, semantic associations, motor programs, personal constructs, scripts, metascripts,* and *social roles. Elemental associations* enable an individual to recognize raw stimulus features as familiar objects. *Semantic associations* connect words, objects, and concepts with related characteristics. *Motor programs* are bodies of procedural information that support the performance of skilled sequential movements, such as walking (less complex) or playing a musical instrument (more complex). *Personal constructs* are organized collections of the various dimensions by which people are understood and categorized, such as friendly/hostile or selfish/generous. *Scripts* are bodies of declarative and procedural information necessary to support the interactive performance of complex activities, such as driving a car or playing a game of tennis. *Metascripts* are collections of scripts related through contextual information, necessary for guiding behavior through complex and varying situations. *Social roles* are bodies of information that provide the overarching context for using scripts and metascripts—organizing complex social behavior over extended periods of time and ultimately giving it "meaning."

Although one of the oldest cognitive hypotheses in psychopathology is that "loosening of associations" is a hallmark of schizophrenia, severe psychiatric disorders probably are not associated with abnormalities in elemental associations, semantic associations, or motor programs. Schizophrenic speech does sometimes suggest abnormal associative relationships between words and concepts, but laboratory analysis of these abnormalities generally suggests that the problem is in attentional, conceptual, and executive functioning, rather than associative structure (Asarnow and Watkins 1982; Grove and Andreasen 1991; Rochester 1978; Wagener et al. 1986). Evidence that schizophrenic subjects have difficulty recognizing facial expressions (Bellack et al. 1992) may indicate that they have abnormal associations involving facial features; the fact that these associations are limited to certain kinds of affective expression (e.g., disapproval, anger), however, suggests that higher-level processing of contextual information (the emotional "meaning" of particular facial expressions) causes the difficulty (see Cramer et al. 1989, 1992).

The *personal constructs* of chronic schizophrenic patients in the residual phase tend to be simplistic, impoverished, and unstable (Dingamans et al. 1983; Klion 1988). Researchers in psychopathology have not extensively studied scripts and metascripts, but the well-known social incompetence of chronic schizophrenic patients probably is due in part to inadequate or incomplete information in these LTM structures (Bellack et al. 1989). This effect also applies to social roles, although researchers have long known that schizophrenic patients do strategically select and perform particular social roles that help maintain their status as "crazy," incapacitated, and dependent people (Braginsky et al. 1969). Given the potential relevance of these higher-level LTM structures to disordered social functioning, further research appears to be needed.

Although episodic memory is impaired in schizophrenia (Calev 1990), the implications of this impairment are unknown. A better understanding awaits more complete models of the relationships between various types of memory, attention, and executive processes.

Accessing Information in Memory

The virtue of a representation in STM or LTM is its ability to make additional information available for processing when called upon. Models of *informational node activation* describe the mechanics of this accessing function; the concept of information processing through heterarchical activation of nodes serves as a building block for a comprehensive view of cognition (Andersen 1990; Anderson and Bower 1974).

Researchers usually measure node activation in the laboratory in terms of the probabilities that information activated through a node will be utilized in a given task. In *priming tasks*, researchers intentionally activate or prime subjects' nodes by manipulating the demands of a preliminary task and then analyzing the effects of the prime on a subsequent task. Research on priming tasks has shown that node activation operates at molar as well as molecular levels of memory organization, affecting the use of entire metascripts and social roles (Bargh and Gollwitzer 1994).

Negative priming involves activation of a node that causes impairment on a subsequent task. Negative priming may occur because the activated nodes are not useful for performing the task, but they occupy capacity in STM that otherwise would be occupied by other nodes that are useful. Alternatively, it may occur because useful nodes are inhibited. Negative priming has the methodological appeal of creating situations in which impaired performance is "normal," and abnormal node activation could cause unimpaired task performance. Thus, failure to show a performance impairment in a negative priming task could indicate impaired node activation. Schizophrenic and schizotypal subjects have shown an absence of negative priming effects in simple conditioning experiments (Beech and Claridge 1987; Gray et al. 1991).

Broadly distributed node activation properties or biases may have significant influence in determining the general quality of behavior in schizophrenia. Magaro (1980, 1984) constructed a model in which paranoid and nonparanoid schizophrenia are distinguished by the degree to which activation of memory (old information channels) predominates over activation of perceptual processing (new information channels). Overactivation of memory processing leads to overuse of old information in executive planning and evaluation operations (described later), which results in behavior that is guided by preconceptions to the exclusion of new information. Underactivation of memory processing eliminates the influence of conceptual information on behavior, causing behavior to become directionless. Memory overactivation is associated with the rigidity and insensitivity to disconfirming information that is characteristic of paranoia, and underactivation is associated with the directionlessness ("low motivation") and conceptual impoverishment of undifferentiated schizophrenia.

The concept of node activation impairments appears to have considerable potential to help researchers understand cognitive deficits. Research in this area is relatively new, however, and more is needed to establish even the basic parameters of priming abnormalities in psychotic disorders. The distinction between node activation that proceeds automatically in the course of memory entry and retrieval, as opposed to controlled and effortful selection of memory information, and programs that occur as part of executive functioning, is especially important in this regard. This distinction ultimately may prove artificial, but it will have to be more fully understood before the meaning of node activation abnormalities in psychotic disorders becomes clear.

Node activation abnormalities may explain the fact that patients with chronic psychotic disorders often have impairments on a diversity of tasks that measure retrieval of information from LTM, especially from episodic memory (Saykin et al. 1991; Tamlyn et al. 1992). The pattern of deficits is similar to that observed in a number of progressive neuropathological conditions and is known as the *general anamnestic syndrome*. The relationship of this syndrome to chronicity in schizophrenia, as well as to other chronic conditions, strongly suggests that it is a residual deficit—possibly the result of a progressive neuropathological process. Researchers do not know, however, to what extent the deficits are due to problems with retrieval from LTM, as opposed to problems with initial encoding of information in LTM.

Conceptual Processing

The dynamic interplay between STM and LTM, as information is stored and activated for further processing, gives rise to conceptualization. Concepts are symbols that guide access to the larger bodies of information that the concepts incorporate. Concepts are stored in LTM and activated for use in situations that require appropriate organization of complex information. *Abstraction* refers to the ability to manipulate conceptual information for the purpose of applying relational rules to complex situations. At a molecular level, this allows people to categorize objects for further processing on the basis of common abstract characteristics (e.g., a banana and an apple can be categorized as "fruit"). At more molar levels, abstraction supports the ability to communicate and learn through metaphor and analogy.

Payne et al. (1972) studied a relatively molecular level of conceptual processing in the laboratory with the object sorting task. In this task, a subject is presented with a tray of miscellaneous objects (a candle, a bicycle bell, a hammer, etc.) and instructed to organize the objects into categories. The number and quality of categories that the subject uses are taken to represent important characteristics of the subject's conceptual processing. Psychotic patients show a number of anomalies on this task. Some use more or fewer categories than normal, sometimes putting each object in its own category or all the objects in a single category. Some use categories that are unusual, bizarre, or incoherent (Payne et al. 1972).

Unfortunately, most of the research with this task was done before researchers understood the importance of phase in psychotic disorders and before contemporary diagnostic conventions were in common use; as a result, interpretation of the data is difficult. Psychophysiological arousal does appear to influence conceptualization as measured in object sorting tasks; therefore, some impairments in this domain probably are episode-linked. Other impairments, especially those found in patients with chronic schizophrenia, persist at moderate levels of arousal and probably are residual deficits.

Harrow and Quinlan (1985) studied a more molar level of conceptual processing with proverb interpretation tasks. Patients with acute psychotic disorders showed impairments in interpreting proverbs, which suggests that they were unable to comprehend or process the abstract concepts that make the proverb applicable to a range of situations—or that they were unable to discriminate the relevant abstraction from irrelevant and incidental concepts. The former impairment produces speech traditionally described as concrete; the latter produces behavior associated with traditional descriptors such as flight of ideas and loosening of associations.

In patients with schizophrenia, proverb interpretation impairments are observed in the residual phase. Impairments in this domain probably contribute heavily to "thought disorder" as it is measured in the laboratory (primarily with measures of speech fluency and coherence). Inasmuch as thought disorder appears in unaffected relatives of schizophrenic patients, concept processing impairments of this type may be vulnerability-linked for schizophrenia.

Executive Processing

As the term implies, executive processing operates at the "highest" (most molar) cognitive level to organize and guide meaningful behavior. Neuropsychologically, this activity is associated primarily with the frontal lobes (E. Goldberg and Bilder 1987). It involves apprehension and continuous use of contextual information that determines the overall purpose and value of behavior—processes traditionally understood in psychology as *motivation*. Executive processing also includes planning: the selection and activation of specific motor programs and scripts to accomplish specific goals. Planning and execution of programs entails ongoing management of cognitive resources, such as the storage capacity available in STM. Thus, executive processing models usually include *working memory*, a specialized type of STM whose function is retention of information that must be accessed continually during executive operations (Goldman-Rakic 1990; Miller et al. 1991).

In familiar situations, executive processing mostly involves the selection of highly organized programs and scripts that, when activated, proceed automatically, without further executive control. (As we noted above, the distinction between automatic node activation in memory and program selection in executive functioning is not yet clear.) Automation of molar programs and scripts is identical in principle to automatic molecular processing of stimulus feature analysis.

In unfamiliar situations, executive processing must involve the use of less organized information, with more frequent reference to contextual information such as verbally encoded instructions or environmental circumstances—which slows down processing and uses working memory less efficiently. Thus, executive processing can be impaired by many of the more molecular deficits we reviewed above—including less efficient automatic (preattentional) processing, failure to recognize familiar elements in situations, inappropriately organized information in LTM, or over/underactivation of memory channels.

In addition, schizophrenia is associated with specific working memory deficits directly related to frontal lobe functioning (Park and Holzman 1992). Because the frontal lobes receive input from so many other brain regions, executive functioning may be disrupted by pathophysiological processes in remote locations, most notably limbic/hippocampal structures (Weinberger and Berman 1988) and the nondominant temporal lobe (Hermann et al. 1988).

Evaluation is an important aspect of executive functioning (Gray et al. 1991). As behavior proceeds, its execution and its impact on the environment must be continuously analyzed. Changes in the environmental situation, whether brought about by the individual's own behavior or other factors, often demand adjustments and changes. Evaluative information becomes part of the contextual information required to guide behavior. The change in preparatory set induced by a regular series of RT trials probably represents a molecular level of this process. At more molar levels, evaluation is more complex, involving comparison of expected sequences of events encoded in scripts with actual sequences in the environment.

Response biasing processes may be related to evaluation processes in executive functioning. Researchers have studied response biasing extensively in the experimental psychology of perception, primarily in a signal detection paradigm. In perception, a response bias is the result of a subject's appraisal of perceptual certainty. In the simplest example, a subject's performance on a vigilance task is influenced by the subject's understanding of the consequences of missing a target stimulus (an error of omission) versus responding when the target was not really present (an error of commission). If the subject appraises the consequences of an omission error as less undesirable than the consequences of a commission error, the subject will adopt a "conservative" response bias: In other words, the subject will require higher certainty that the target is present before responding.

Researchers have long known that chronic schizophrenic subjects use abnormal response criteria—that is, they require a higher or lower than normal level of certainty before responding to a stimulus (see Spaulding et al. 1980). Interestingly, changes in response bias characteristics accompany social behavioral improvements in the long-term course of treatment (Spaulding 1993). This result may mean that in some circumstances, patients have some information about their molecular attentional and preattentional impairments and attempt to compensate for them through response biasing. Even more interestingly, response bias abnormalities may operate in some schizophrenic subjects to influence the formation of beliefs and attributions. Such subjects collect less perceptual information before reaching conclusions about the nature of a stimulus; this effect may be related to the clinical expression of delusions (Cromwell and Spaulding 1978; Garety et al. 1991). If response biasing is an executive function involving selection and control of specific stimulus processing and evaluation programs, hallucinations and delusions may be consequences of the limbic-frontal impairment that researchers suspect is central to schizophrenia.

The Wisconsin Card Sorting Test (WCST) (Heaton 1985) has become a popular tool for studying executive processing in schizophrenic subjects

(Wagman and Wagman 1992). The WCST is popular because the task represents an intermediate level of executive complexity; it requires a combination of conceptual, memory-accessing, contextual, and evaluative operations; and it is associated with neurophysiological activation of frontal cortical areas that researchers think are the primary substrate for executive processing.

In the WCST, a subject is required to sort cards into four bins based on the color, number, or shape of figures on the cards. The instructions do not specify which concept is the sorting criterion; the subject must determine that criterion through trial-wise feedback ("right" or "wrong"). After a number of correct sorts, the criterion unexpectedly changes; the subject must recognize the new criterion from the changing feedback and revise sorting strategy accordingly (see Figure 5–3).

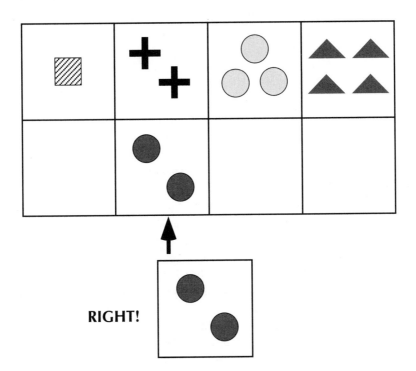

Figure 5–3. Format for computerized card sorting task similar to Wisconsin Card Sorting Test. The computer has dealt a card in the lower box. Subject has responded by moving selection arrow to second sorting bin, indicating subject's choice of "number" as sorting criterion. The computer shows card in selected bin, displays "RIGHT!" message, and plays pleasing beep to indicate selection was correct. Incorrect response results in "WRONG!" message and annoying buzzer.

In general, psychotic subjects have difficulty with this task, although performance returns to normal in nonschizophrenic subjects as the acute phase passes (Penn et al. 1993). Nonpsychotic schizotypal subjects show some impairment on the task (though not as much as psychotic subjects), suggesting that the impairment may be vulnerability-linked for schizophrenia (Spaulding et al. 1989). Residual impairments are fairly common in chronic schizophrenic populations (T. E. Goldberg et al. 1987).

The strength of the WCST—its integration of several executive processes—is a weakness with respect to interpretation. Impairment on the task could be caused by deficits in sustained attention, STM capacity, conceptualization, abstraction, contextual processing, or evaluative processing. The systematic research required to isolate the specific causes of impairment in specific subgroups and individuals has begun only recently. The ubiquity of WCST impairments in chronic schizophrenic populations, however, indicates that sorting performance is an important domain of functioning to consider in psychosocial treatment and rehabilitation approaches, regardless of the molecular origins of the impairments.

Conclusions

Psychotic disorders are associated with abnormalities across the entire range of cognitive functioning, from the most molecular processes to the most molar. These abnormalities generally produce impairments and deficits in information processing, contributing to behavioral ineffectiveness and disorganization. The impairments usually are more numerous, pervasive, and severe in the acute phase of the disorder. Especially in schizophrenia, impairments are present in the vulnerability and residual phases as well.

Not all cognitive abnormalities produce direct detrimental effects on behavior. In some cases, vulnerability and residual impairments may only be markers of other pathogenic processes. In other cases, they may produce relatively subtle deficits in personal and social functioning—or negative symptoms, in the case of schizophrenia.

Researchers have identified a number of preattentional impairments in schizophrenic, schizotypic, and high-risk populations. In nonschizophrenic psychotic disorders, these impairments generally are found only in the acute phase, suggesting that they are vulnerability-linked only for schizophrenia. Researchers have not clearly established vulnerability-linked impairments for other psychotic disorders.

In the psychopathology of schizophrenia, a number of theories are focusing on a crucial impairment in executive processing, wherein contextual information that normally is necessary for optimal task performance is inadequately processed. This impairment has implications for attentional processing at molecular levels of cognition and for performance of complex skills at more molar levels. Cognitive theories of this impairment have begun to converge with neuropsychological, neuroanatomical, and neurophysiological theories of schizophrenia. The cognitive impairment appears to be linked to metabolic underactivation of the frontal lobe and to abnormalities in neural pathways between the frontal lobe, the temporal lobe, and the limbic cortex.

Transient periods of extreme psychophysiological arousal may produce transient cognitive impairments, especially in attention and STM, independent of the phase of the disorder. This effect is an important consideration in clinical assessment because mistaking a transient arousal-linked impairment for a chronic residual impairment could have detrimental effects on treatment selection and outcome. Psychophysiological abnormalities are common in psychotic disorders, and clinicians should always consider their potential role in cognitive dysfunction. Similarly, when clinicians assess the implications of any particular cognitive deficit, they must always consider the phase of the disorder in which it occurs.

Residual deficits in schizophrenia are common, and they cover the entire cognitive spectrum. These deficits probably are significant obstacles to rehabilitation, although researchers are just beginning to verify this hypothesis empirically. Study of residual cognitive deficits promises to have the most direct implications for the cognitive treatment and rehabilitation of schizophrenia. Most of these deficits are quite different from those addressed in cognitive therapeutic approaches to other disorders; therefore, they probably will require different treatment procedures. On the other hand, cognitive abnormalities addressed in the cognitive treatment of anxiety, depression, and personality disorder are not necessarily irrelevant to schizophrenia and other psychotic disorders. They probably are relevant for many patients, but their successful use may require preliminary treatment of the more molecular and pervasive deficits residual to psychosis.

There is no cognitive abnormality unique to any particular psychotic disorder. Within diagnostic categories, patients have unique constellations of impairments and deficits. Traditional diagnostic methods reveal little or nothing about these deficits. Assessment for clinical purposes must use methods borrowed from the research laboratory. Until researchers know more about the implications of specific impairments and deficits, clinicians must undertake assessment and treatment in hypothetico-deductive steps—whereby assessment generates testable hypotheses about the impact of cognitive factors on individual patients' personal and social functioning, and treatment is an experimental intervention that clinicians must evaluate in terms of its effects on patients' personal and social functioning as well as on targeted cognitive impairments.

References

American Psychiatric Association: Diagnostic and Statistical Manual of Mental Disorders, 4th Edition. Washington, DC, American Psychiatric Association, 1994

American Psychiatric Association: Diagnostic and Statistical Manual of Mental Disorders, 3rd Edition. Washington, DC, American Psychiatric Association, 1980

Andersen P: The main features of long-term potentiation: a model for the formation of memory traces, in The Principles of Design and Operation of the Brain. Edited by Eccles JC, Creutzfeldt J. New York, Springer-Verlag, 1990, pp 368–382

Anderson JR, Bower GH: Human Associative Memory, 2nd Edition. Washington, DC, Hemisphere, 1974

Andreasen N: Scale for the assessment of thought, language and communication (TLC). Schizophr Bull 12:473–482, 1986

Andreasen NC, Olsen S: Negative versus positive schizophrenia: Definition and validation. Arch Gen Psychiatry 39:789–794, 1987

Andreasen N, Flaum M, Swayze V, et al: Positive and negative symptoms in schizophrenia: a critical reappraisal. Arch Gen Psychiatry 47:615–621, 1990

Arieti S: Interpretation of Schizophrenia. New York, R Brunner, 1955

Asarnow RF, MacCrimmon DJ: Attention/information processing, neuropsychological functioning, and thought disorder during the acute and partial recovery phases of schizophrenia: a longitudinal study. Psychiatry Res 7:309–319, 1982

Asarnow RF, Watkins JM: Schizophrenic thought disorder: linguistic incompetence or information processing impairment? Behavioral and Brain Sciences 5:589–590, 1982

Asarnow RF, Granholm E, Sherman T: Span of apprehension in schizophrenia, in Handbook of Schizophrenia: Neuropsychology, Psychopathology and Information Processing, Vol 5. Edited by Steinhauer SR, Gruzelier JH, Zubin J. Amsterdam, The Netherlands, Elsevier, 1991, pp 335–370

Baars B: The Cognitive Revolution in Psychology. New York, Guilford, 1986

Bargh J, Gollwitzer P: Environmental control of goal-directed action: automatic and strategic contingencies between situations and behavior, in Nebraska Symposium on Motivation: Integrative Views of Motivation, Cognition and Emotion, Vol 41. Edited by Spaulding W. Lincoln, University of Nebraska Press, 1974, pp 71–124

Beech A, Claridge G: Individual differences in negative priming: relations with schizotypal personality traits. Br J Psychol 8:329–356, 1987

Bellack AS, Morrison RL, Mueser KT: Social problem solving in schizophrenia. Schizophr Bull 15:101–116, 1989

Bellack A, Morrison R, Wixted J, et al: An analysis of social competence in schizophrenia. Br J Psychiatry 156:809–818, 1990

Bellack A, Mueser K, Wade J, et al: The ability of schizophrenics to perceive and cope with negative affect. Br J Psychiatry 168:473–480, 1992

Bellissimo A, Steffy RA: Redundancy-associated deficit in schizophrenic reaction time performance. J Abnorm Psychol 80:299–307, 1972

Bellissimo A, Steffy RA: Contextual influences on crossover in the reaction time performance of schizophrenics. J Abnorm Psychol 84:210–220, 1975

Berlin CI, McNeal MR: Dichotic listening, in Contemporary Issues in Experimental Phonetics. Edited by Lass NJ. New York, Academic Press, 1976

Bleuler E: Dementia Praecox or the Group of Schizophrenias (1911). New York, International Universities Press, 1950

Boyle M: The non-discovery of schizophrenia? in Reconstructing Schizophrenia. Edited by Bentall R. London, Routledge, 1990

Braff DL, Sacuzzo DP, Geyer MA: Information processing dysfunctions in schizophrenia: studies of visual backward masking, sensorimotor gating, and habituation, in Handbook of Schizophrenia: Neuropsychology, Psychopathology and Information Processing, Vol 5. Edited by Steinhauer SR, Gruzelier JH, Zubin J. Amsterdam, The Netherlands, Elsevier, 1991, pp 303–334

Braginsky BM, Braginsky DD, Ring K: Methods of Madness: The Mental Hospital as Last Resort. New York, Holt, Rinehart & Winston, 1969

Brenner H: On the importance of cognitive disorders in treatment and rehabilitation, in Psychosocial Treatment of Schizophrenia. Edited by Strauss J, Baker W, Brenner H. Toronto, Ontario, Canada, Huber, 1987, pp 136–152

Calev A: Memory in schizophrenia, in International Perspectives in Schizophrenia: Biological, Social and Epidemiological Findings. Edited by Weller M. London, John Libbey, 1990, pp 29–41

Cash T: Methodological problems and progress in schizophrenia research. J Consult Clin Psychol 40:278–286, 1973

Chapman LJ, Chapman JP: The search for symptoms predictive of schizophrenia. Schizophr Bull 13:497–503, 1987

Cohen JD, Servan-Schreiber D: Context, cortex, and dopamine: a connectionist approach to behavior and biology in schizophrenia. Psychol Rev 99:45–77, 1992

Cohen JD, Dunbar K, McClelland JL: On the control of automatic processes: a parallel distributed processing account of the Stroop Effect. Psychol Rev 97:332–361, 1991

Cornblatt BA, Risch NJ, Faris G, et al: The Continuous Performance Test, identical pairs version: new findings about sustained attention in normal families. Psychiatry Res 26:223–238, 1988

Corrigan P, Wallace C, Green M, et al: Cognitive dysfunction and psychosocial skill learning in schizophrenia. Paper presented at the annual meeting of the American Psychiatric Association, New Orleans, LA, May 1991

Cramer P, Weegmann T, O'Neil M: How accurately do schizophrenics judge the emotional states of others? Br J Psychiatry 155:229–232, 1989

Cramer P, Bowen J, O'Neill M: Schizophrenics and social judgement. Br J Psychiatry 160:481–487, 1992

Cromwell R, Pithers W: Schizophrenic/paranoid psychoses: determining diagnostic divisions. Schizophr Bull 7:674–688, 1981

Cromwell RL, Spaulding W: How schizophrenics handle information, in The Phenomenology and Treatment of Schizophrenia. Edited by Fann WE, Karacan I, Pokorny AD, et al. New York, Spectrum, 1978, pp 127–162

Cutting J: Judgement of emotional expression in schizophrenics. Br J Psychiatry 139:1–6, 1981

DeAmicis L, Cromwell R: Reaction time crossover in process schizophrenics, their relatives and control subjects. J Nerv Ment Dis 167:593–600, 1979

Dingamans P, Space L, Cromwell R: How general is the inconsistency in schizophrenic behavior? in Applications of Personal Construct Theory. Edited by Adams-Webber J, Mancuso J. New York, Academic Press, 1983

Engel G: The clinical application of the biopsychosocial model. Am J Psychiatry 137:535–544, 1980

Erlenmeyer-Kimling L, Cornblatt B: Attentional measures in a study of children at high risk for schizophrenia, in The Nature of Schizophrenia: New Approaches to Research and Treatment. Edited by Wynne LC, Cromwell RL, Matthysse S. New York, Wiley, 1978, pp 359–365

Freedman R, Waldo M, Adler L, et al: Schizotaxia and sensory gating, in Schizophrenia: Origins, Processes, Treatment and Outcome. Edited by Cromwell R, Snyder R. New York, Oxford University Press, 1993, pp 98–110

Friedes D: Do dichotic listening procedures measure lateralization of information processing or retrieval strategy? Percept Psychophys 21:254–263, 1977

Garety PA, Hemsley DR, Wessely S: Reasoning in deluded schizophrenic and paranoid patients: biases in performance on a probabilistic inference task. J Nerv Ment Dis 179:194–201, 1991

Gjerede PF: Attentional capacity dysfunction and arousal in schizophrenia. Psychol Bull 93:57–72, 1983

Goldberg E, Bilder RM Jr: The frontal lobes and hierarchical organization of cognitive control, in The Frontal Lobes Revisited. Edited by Perecman E. New York, IRBN Press, 1987, pp 159–187

Goldberg TE, Weinberger DR, Berman KF, et al: Further evidence for dementia of the prefrontal type in schizophrenia? A controlled study of teaching the Wisconsin Card Sorting Test. Arch Gen Psychiatry 44:1008–1014, 1987

Goldman-Rakic PS: The prefrontal contribution to working memory and conscious experience, in The Principles of Design and Operation of the Brain. Edited by Eccles JC, Creutzfeldt J. New York, Springer-Verlag, 1990, pp 390–407

Goldstein G: The neuropsychology of schizophrenia, in Neuropsychological Assessment of Neuropsychiatric Disorders. Edited by Grant I, Adams K. New York, Oxford University Press, 1986

Goldstein G: Comprehensive neuropsychological test batteries and research in schizophrenia, in Handbook of Schizophrenia: Neuropsychology, Psychopathology, and Information Processing, Vol 5. Edited by Steinhauer S, Gruzelier J, Zubin J. Amsterdam, The Netherlands, Elsevier, 1991, pp 525–551

Gray JA, Feldon J, Rawlins JNP, et al: The neuropsychology of schizophrenia. Behavioral and Brain Sciences 14:1–84, 1991

Green M, Walker E: Symptom correlates of vulnerability to backward masking in schizophrenia. Am J Psychiatry 143:181–186, 1986

Grove WM, Andreasen NC: Thought disorder in relation to brain function, in Handbook of Schizophrenia: Neuropsychology, Psychopathology and Information Processing, Vol 5. Edited by Steinhauer SR, Gruzelier JH, Zubin J. Amsterdam, The Netherlands, Elsevier, 1991, pp 485–503

Gruzelier J, Hammond V: Lateralized deficits and drug influences on the dichotic listening of schizophrenic patients. Biol Psychiatry 15:759–779, 1980

Harrow M, Quinlan D: Disordered thinking and schizophrenic psychopathology. New York, Gardner Press, 1985

Harrow M, Lanin-Kettering I, Miller JG: Impaired perspective and thought pathology in schizophrenic and psychotic disorders. Schizophr Bull 15: 605–623, 1989

Heaton R: Wisconsin Card Sorting Test. Odessa, TX, Psychological Assessment Resources, 1985

Hermann B, Wyler A, Richey E: Wisconsin Card Sorting Test performance in patients with complex partial seizures of temporal lobe origin. J Clin Exp Neuropsychol 10:467–476, 1988

Jones E, Kanouse D, Kelly H, et al: Attribution: Perceiving the Causes of Behavior. Morristown, NJ, General Learning Press, 1971

Kaplan R: The crossover phenomenon: three studies of the effect of training and information on process schizophrenic reaction time. Unpublished doctoral dissertation, University of Waterloo, Ontario, Canada, 1974

Klein D, Gittelman R, Quitkin F, et al: Diagnosis and Drug Treatment of Psychiatric Disorders: Adults and Children, 2nd Edition. Baltimore, MD, Williams & Wilkins, 1980

Klion K: The construct system organization and schizophrenia: the role of construct integration. Journal of Social and Clinical Psychology 6:439–447, 1988

Knight R: Converging models of cognitive deficit in schizophrenia, in Nebraska Symposium on Motivation: Theories of Schizophrenia and Psychosis, Vol 31. Edited by Spaulding W, Cole J. Lincoln, University of Nebraska Press, 1984, pp 93–156

Koh SD: Remembering in schizophrenia, in Language and Cognition in Schizophrenia. Edited by Schwartz S. Hillsdale, NJ, Lawrence Erlbaum, 1978

Koh SD, Kayton L: Memorization of "unrelated" word strings by young nonpsychotic schizophrenics. J Abnorm Psychol 83:14–22, 1974

Koh SD, Kayton L, Peterson RA: Affective encoding and consequent remembering in schizophrenic young adults. J Abnorm Psychol 85:156–166, 1976

Kraepelin E: Psychiatrie, 5th Ed. Leipzig, Germany, Barth, 1896

Kuhn T: The Structure of Scientific Revolution. Ciicago, IL, University of Chicago Press, 1970

Levin S, Yurgelun-Todd D, Craft S: Contributions of clinical neuropsychology to the study of schizophrenia. J Abnorm Psychol 98:341–356, 1989

Liberman RP, Nuechterlein KH, Wallace CJ: Social skills training and the nature of schizophrenia, in Social Skills Training: A Practical Handbook for Assessment and Treatment. Edited by Curran JP, Monti PM. New York, Guilford, 1982, pp 5–56

Lipe MG: Counterfactual reasoning as a framework for attribution theories. Psychol Bull 109:456–471, 1991

Magaro PA: Cognition in Schizophrenia and Paranoia: The Integration of Cognitive Processes. Hillsdale, NJ, Lawrence Erlbaum, 1980

Magaro PA: Psychosis and schizophrenia, in The Nebraska Symposium on Motivation. Edited by Spaulding W, Cole JK. Lincoln, University of Nebraska Press, 1984, pp 157–230

Meehl PE: Schizotaxia, schizotypy and schizophrenia. Am Psychol 17:827–838, 1962

Meehl PE: Schizotaxia revisited. Arch Gen Psychiatry 46:935–944, 1989

Miller EK, Li L, Desimone R: A neural mechanism for working and recognition memory in inferior temporal cortex. Science 254:1377–1379, 1991

Naatanen R: Processing of the unattended message during selective dichotic listening. Behavioral and Brain Sciences 9:43–44, 1986

Neale J, Oltmanns T, Harvey P: The need to relate cognitive deficits to specific behavioral referents in schizophrenia. Schizophr Bull 11:286–291, 1985

Nuechterlein KH: Reaction time and attention in schizophrenia: a critical evaluation of the data and theories. Schizophr Bull 3:373–382, 1977

Nuechterlein KH: Signal detection in vigilance tasks and behavioral attributes among offspring of schizophrenic mothers and among hyperactive children. J Abnorm Psychol 92:4–28, 1983

Nuechterlein KH: Vigilance in schizophrenia and related disorders, in Handbook of Schizophrenia: Neuropsychology, Psychopathology and Information Processing, Vol 5. Edited by Steinhauer SR, Gruzelier JH, Zubin J. Amsterdam, The Netherlands, Elsevier, 1991, pp 397–433

Nuechterlein KH, Edell WS, Norris M, et al: Attentional vulnerability indicators, thought disorder, and negative symptoms. Schizophr Bull 12:408, 1986

Oltmanns TF: Selective attention in schizophrenia and manic psychoses: the effects of distraction on information processes. J Abnorm Psychol 87:212–225, 1978

Oltmanns TF, Maher B: Delusional Beliefs. New York, Wiley, 1988

Park S, Holzman P: Schizophrenics show spatial working memory deficits. Arch Gen Psychiatry 49:975–982, 1992

Payne R, Hawks D, Friedlander D, et al: The diagnostic significance of overinclusive thinking in an unselected psychiatric population. Br J Psychiatry 120:173–182, 1972

Penn D, Vander Does J, Spaulding W, et al: Information processing and social-cognitive problem solving in schizophrenia. J Nerv Ment Dis 181:13–20, 1993

Pollack RW, Brenner MW: The Experimental Psychology of Alfred Binet: Selected Papers. New York, Springer, 1969

Rist F, Cohen R: Sequential effects in the reaction times of schizophrenics: crossover and modality shift effects, in Handbook of Schizophrenia: Neuropsychology, Psychopathology and Information Processing, Vol 5. Edited by Steinhauer SR, Gruzelier JH, Zubin J. Amsterdam, The Netherlands, Elsevier, 1991, pp 241–271

Rochester S: Are language disorders in acute schizophrenia actually information processing problems? in The Nature of Schizophrenia: New Approaches to Research and Treatment. Edited by Wynne L, Cromwell R, Matthysse S. New York, Wiley, 1978

Rosenbaum G, Shore DL, Chapin K: Attention deficit in schizophrenia and schizotypy: marker versus symptom variables. J Abnorm Psychol 97: 41–47, 1988

Sacuzzo DP, Braff DL: Early information processing deficits in schizophrenia: new findings using schizophrenic subgroups and manic controls. Arch Gen Psychiatry 38:175–179, 1981

Saykin A, Gur RC, Gur RE, et al: Neuropsychological functioning in schizophrenia: selective impairment in memory and learning. Arch Gen Psychiatry 48:618–624, 1991

Shakow D: Schizophrenia: Collected Papers. New York, International Universities Press, 1977a

Shakow D: Segmental set: the adaptive process in schizophrenia. Am Psychol 32:129–139, 1977b

Spaulding W: Assessment of adult-onset pervasive behavior disorders, in Handbook of Behavior Assessment. Edited by Adams H, Calhoun K. New York, Wiley, 1986, pp 631–669

Spaulding W: Spontaneous and induced changes in cognition during psychiatric rehabilitation, in Schizophrenia: Innovations in Theory and Treatment. Edited by Cromwell RL. New York, Oxford University Press, 1993, pp 299–312

Spaulding W, Rosenzweig L, Huntzinger R, et al: Visual pattern integration in psychiatric patients. J Abnorm Psychol 89:635–643, 1980

Spaulding W, Garbin C, Dras S: Cognitive functioning in chronic psychiatric patients and schizotypal college students. J Nerv Ment Dis 177:717–728, 1989

Spring B, Weinstein L, Freeman R, et al: Selective attention in schizophrenia, in Handbook of Schizophrenia: Neuropsychology, Psychopathology and Information Processing, Vol 5. Edited by Steinhauer SR, Gruzelier JH, Zubin J. Amsterdam, The Netherlands, Elsevier, 1991, pp 371–396

Spring BJ, Zubin J: Attention and information processing as indicators of vulnerability to schizophrenic episodes, in The Nature of Schizophrenia: New Approaches to Research and Treatment. Edited by Wynne LC, Cromwell RL, Matthysse S. New York, Wiley, 1978, pp 366–375

Strauss J, Carpenter W, Bartko J: Speculations on the processes that underlie schizophrenic symptoms and signs. Schizophr Bull 11:61–75, 1974

Strauss ME, Bohannon WE, Stephens JH, et al: Perceptual span in schizophrenia and affective disorders. J Nerv Ment Dis 172:431, 1984

Tamlyn D, McKenna P, Mortimer A, et al: Memory impairment in schizophrenia: its extent, affiliations and neuropsychological character. Psychol Med 22:101–115, 1992

Wagener DK, Hogarty GE, Goldstein MJ, et al: Information processing and communication deviance in schizophrenic patients and their mothers. Psychiatry Res 18:365–377, 1986

Wagman A, Wagman W: On the Wisconsin, in Progress in Experimental Personality Research, Vol 15. Edited by Walker E, Dworkin R, Cornblatt B. New York, Springer-Verlag, 1992, pp 162–182

Wallace CJ, Boone SE: Cognitive factors in the social skill of schizophrenic patients: implications for treatment, in Nebraska Symposium on Motivation: Theories of Schizophrenia in Psychosis, Vol 31. Edited by Spaulding WD, Cole JK. Lincoln, University of Nebraska Press, 1984, pp 283–318

Weinberger DR, Berman KF: Speculation on the meaning of cerebral metabolic hypofrontality in schizophrenia. Schizophr Bull 14:157–168, 1988

Wielgus MS, Harvey PD: Dichotic listening and recall in schizophrenia and mania. Schizophr Bull 14:689–700, 1988

Zubin J, Spring B: Vulnerability: a new view of schizophrenia. J Abnorm Psychol 86:103–126, 1977

Chapter 6

Cognitive Assessment and Treatment of Social Phobia

Thomas V. Merluzzi, Ph.D.

Social Anxiety and Social Phobia: Background

Social anxiety and social phobia are characterized by a pervasive fear of most social situations. These disorders commonly are associated with specific situations such as public speaking, walking into a crowded waiting room, meeting someone for the first time, or writing one's name for a clerk at a hotel. Most people are able to manage the mild apprehension they may feel in these situations; that is, the coping capacity of the individual exceeds the debilitating effects of the anxiety. For the socially anxious and particularly the socially phobic individual, however, such situations are debilitating even when the individual can perform the task.

The *Diagnostic and Statistical Manual of Mental Disorders* did not include social phobia as a type of anxiety disorder until DSM-III (American Psychiatric Association 1980); the description changed little in DSM-III-R (American Psychiatric Association 1987). However, the definition of social phobia was refined in DSM-IV: "The essential feature of this disorder is a marked and persistent fear of social or performance situations in which embarrassment may occur" (American Psychiatric Association 1994, p. 411). Table 6–1 lists the DSM-IV criteria for the diagnosis of social phobia.

The DSM-IV criteria reflect empirically based analyses of the DSM-III-R criteria. Turner and Beidel (1989) suggested that certain behaviors listed in the DSM-III-R criteria might not be entirely accurate. They argued, for example, that choking on food is indicative of panic disorder or generalized anxiety disorder rather than social phobia. They further suggested that the more common features of social phobia include "public speaking phobias and generalized social phobia, manifested by the general fear of saying or doing something foolish or the inability to answer questions in social situations" (Turner and Beidel 1989, p. 4). The criteria in DSM-IV are consistent with these research findings. The focus of the diagnosis is on the fear of consequences and intolerable humiliation and embarrassment in social situations.

Table 6–1.   Diagnostic criteria for social phobia

A.   A marked and persistent fear of one or more social or performance situations in which the person is exposed to unfamiliar people or to possible scrutiny by others. The individual fears that he or she will act in a way (or show anxiety symptoms) that will be humiliating or embarrassing.
B.   Exposure to the feared social situation almost invariably provokes anxiety, which may take the form of a situationally bound or situationally predisposed Panic Attack.
C.   The person recognizes that the fear is excessive or unreasonable.
D.   The feared social or performance situations are avoided or else are endured with intense anxiety or distress.
E.   The avoidance, anxious anticipation, or distress in the feared social or performance situation(s) interferes significantly with the person's normal routine, occupational (academic) functioning, or social activities or relationships, or there is marked distress about having the phobia.
F.   In individuals under age 18 years, the duration is at least 6 months.
G.   The fear or avoidance is not due to the direct physiological effects of a substance (e.g., a drug abuse, a medication) or a general medical condition and is not better accounted for by another mental disorder (e.g., Panic Disorder With or Without Agoraphobia, Separation Anxiety Disorder, Body Dysmorphic Disorder, a Pervasive Developmental Disorder, or Schizoid Personality Disorder).
H.   If a general medical condition or another mental disorder is present, the fear in Criterion A is unrelated to it, e.g., the fear of Stuttering, trembling in Parkinson's disease, or exhibiting abnormal eating behavior in Anorexia Nervosa or Bulimia Nervosa.

Specify if:
Generalized: if the fears include most social situations (also consider the additional diagnosis of Avoidant Personality Disorder).

Source.   Reprinted from American Psychiatric Association: *Diagnostic and Statistical Manual of Mental Disorders,* 4th Edition. Washington, DC, American Psychiatric Association, 1994, p. 246. Used with permission.

Prevalence of Social Phobia

Prevalence studies have reported that social phobia occurs in about 2%–3% of the general population and seems to be equally prevalent in men and women (American Psychiatric Association 1994). Pollard and Henderson (1988), however, reported a prevalence rate of 22.6%. They suggested that other studies may underestimate actual prevalence rates because many people reduce their distress by successfully avoiding phobic situations. Excluding low-distress phobic individuals, the prevalence rate in the Pollard and Henderson study is 2%, as in other findings.

Marks (1985) suggested that key symptoms of social phobia may be related to certain specific interpersonal situations; more characterological behavior, however, suggests an Axis II category such as avoidant personality. According to DSM-IV, avoidant personality disorder is characterized by a "pervasive pattern of social inhibition, feelings of inadequacy, and responsivity to negative evaluation, beginning by early adulthood and present in a variety of contexts" (American Psychiatric Association 1994, p. 283). Persons with avoidant personality disorder are extremely sensitive to rejection and are unwilling to engage in relationships unless there is a virtual guarantee of unconditional acceptance. These individuals usually have impoverished social systems because of their inability to attain completely uncritical relationships.

As DSM-IV notes, social phobia and avoidant personality disorder may coexist. At one time, researchers thought the disorders were different: Social phobia was characterized by the fear of some but not all specific situations, whereas persons with avoidant personality disorder actively avoid most social situations and have few or no close relationships. There is growing evidence, however, that persons with generalized social phobia are more likely to be at risk for avoidant personality disorder (Holt et al. 1992). Although generalized social phobia is somewhat less severe than avoidant personality disorder, the differences may be a matter of degree rather than kind (Herbert et al. 1992). In one study, 89% of persons with generalized social phobia exhibited avoidant personality disorder as well, whereas only 21% of those with discrete social phobias demonstrated that comorbidity (Schneier et al. 1991).

DSM-III-R included subtypes of social phobia; subsequent research indicated that the subtypes have very different prevalence rates. Pollard and Henderson (1988) studied the incidence of four types of social phobias listed in DSM-III-R: public speaking/performing, eating in restaurants, writing in public, and using public restrooms. They found that social phobia related to public speaking/performing was by far the most prevalent. They suggested that speaking phobias may need to be classified as separate from the other types. Social phobias related to writing in front of others, eating in public, and using public restrooms were much less prevalent. Individuals with public speaking anxiety only are able to modify their lives so that the phobia does not interfere with day-to-day living; they apparently are not otherwise significantly impaired.

DSM-III-R and DSM-IV describe a generalized subtype of social phobia that may differ from the public speaking type. Based on the Anxiety Disorders Interview Schedule (DiNardo et al. 1983), Heimberg et al. (1990c) identified

35 persons with generalized social phobia and 22 with public speaking phobia and investigated whether these two groups differed with regard to relevant psychological and demographic variables. Although the two groups were similar in some ways—for example, on self-reported social phobic and public speaking anxiety and on self-ratings of performance in a simulated social situation—they differed in other ways. Persons with public speaking phobia exhibited more physiological reactivity and were poorer judges of their performance than those with generalized social phobia. On the other hand, "generalized social phobics were younger, less educated, more likely to be unemployed, more generally anxious and depressed and their phobias were judged more severe by clinical interviewers" (Heimberg et al. 1990c, p. 177). In addition, persons with generalized social phobia reported more general social anxiety and had more negative thoughts about outcomes. Thus, persons with generalized phobia appear to be more debilitated, and that debilitation seems to occur early in their lives. Heimberg et al. could not determine, however, whether the generalized social phobia was the sole cause of the problems or part of a syndrome that included other disorders such as depression.

Etiological Considerations

Buss (1980) and Barlow (1988) offered several theories concerning the etiology of social anxiety and social phobia. Buss suggested that parents may foster sensitivity to social evaluation in a child by isolating the child, preventing the child from gaining experience in a variety of situations, emphasizing the importance of the opinions of others, or overprotecting the child. Buss also suggested that children whose temperament is characterized by high emotionality are likely to respond more intensely to rejection than children who are low in emotionality. The conditions for social phobia are optimal if parenting practices foster isolation and concern about evaluation and the child is predisposed by temperament to respond emotionally. Similarly, Barlow (1988) described a biological vulnerability for persons who develop anxieties. Persons who are vulnerable to anxious apprehension and experience social interactions associated with high arousal may develop social anxiety. Both Buss and Barlow noted that adolescence is a developmental period during which individuals may be especially vulnerable. Adolescents are expected to negotiate social relationships without the family and engage in new social roles such as dating, at a time when they feel most vulnerable to public scrutiny.

Independent research supports these theories. There appears to be a genetic component to shyness that may be an antecedent to social anxiety and social phobia (Bruch 1989). Moreover, socially anxious individuals reported, retrospectively, that their mothers were avoidant and fearful. Socially phobic persons also viewed their parents' child-rearing practices as fostering isolation, promoting sensitivity to evaluation, and not promoting family sociability (Bruch 1989). In addition, socially phobic individuals recalled a high degree of self-consciousness in junior high school and dated minimally (Bruch et al. 1989).

Social Anxiety and Shyness

Zimbardo (1977) reported that 42% of "normal" college students said that they were shy; Lazarus (1982) reported similar rates for a sample of children. Clearly, therefore, not all shy people are socially phobic, given the 2%–3% prevalence rates for the DSM-IV diagnosis of social phobia.

There are some noteworthy differences between social phobia and shyness. First, the severity of avoidance in social phobia is quite different from the apprehension that may be experienced by someone who is shy. In addition, the impact of social phobia on work, school, and social relationships may be quite large relative to the impact of shyness; in particular, a person with generalized social phobia will be more debilitated than a shy person. Finally, psychologists notice shyness—which they consider to be a fairly stable personality trait— much earlier than social phobia, which typically has its onset in early to late adolescence (Turner et al. 1990).

Social Cognitive Conceptualizations of Social Anxiety and Social Phobia

There are several conceptual representations of social anxiety and social phobia that may facilitate an understanding of the cognitive aspects of the disorders. In this section, I present a sample of those characterizations, beginning with the notion that each conceptualization is a form of cognitive vulnerability.

Cognitive Vulnerability

Psychologists have implicated attribution style in the development and maintenance of depression. That is, in the face of major stressors, certain dysfunctional inferential styles may put an individual at risk for depression. An attribution style in which an individual sees negative events as stable, global, and internal is the diathesis that interacts with stress to produce depression.

There are patterns of cognitive processes in social anxiety and social phobia that may lead to greater vulnerability, exacerbating or maintaining a tendency to withdraw from social situations. Hypersensitivity to rejection may result in a faulty interpretation of social cues: For example, a simple question from another person may be interpreted as criticism.

In addition to developing general conceptual models of cognitive vulnerability for psychopathology, Ingram and Kendall (1987) articulated several cognitive features that are unique to anxiety disorders; these features include schema content and functioning, temporal distortion in which the focus is on negative aspects of future events, and task-irrelevant cognitive content. In the following sections, I describe several dominant cognitive conceptual frameworks.

Self-Schema

Individuals with social phobia have a hypersensitivity to social evaluation and perceive threats even in situations that may not be particularly harmful. Thus, they have a schema for processing social information that is vigilant for social rejection and may distort information that is nonthreatening to make it appear threatening. This schema forms a basis for describing and defining the self.

Hope et al. (1990) found that individuals with social phobia had longer color-naming latencies in a Stroop task for social threat words (e.g., embarrassed) but shorter latencies for physical threat words (e.g., illness) than subjects with panic disorder. In addition, the more socially phobic the individual, the greater the latencies to social threat words. Longer latencies represent a defensiveness that is moderated by arousal. This initial processing of information happens relatively quickly and may affect the type of information that eventually will be processed more deeply. This would mean that, in social situations, the individual pays too much attention to the socially threatening information in the environment and therefore is unable to attend to salient information.

Self-Discrepancy

In another line of investigation related to the self, researchers have studied the role of self-comparisons or discrepancies in the development or maintenance of psychopathology. Researchers have shown that two types of self-discrepancies are associated with vulnerability to emotional problems: 1) a discrepancy that pits an individual's perceptions of actual attributes of his or her self against an ideal self (actual/own versus ideal/own), and 2) a discrepancy that pits the individual's actual self against the self that represents what the person feels others want him or her to be (actual/own versus ideal/other). Comparing clinically depressed subjects with socially phobic subjects, Straumen (1989) found that subjects with depression have greater discrepancies between their actual/own and ideal/own selves. On the other hand, subjects with social phobia had greater discrepancies between their actual/own and ideal/other selves. For example, socially anxious individuals typically talk quite a bit about their concern about the expectations and evaluations of significant (and not-so-significant) others. Although anxious persons do not have perfectionistic standards, they believe that they will fall short of others' standards (Wallace and Alden 1991). In fact, socially anxious individuals tend to think that events are controlled by powerful others (Cloitre et al. 1992).

Self-Presentation

According to self-presentation theory, social interaction is a process in which an individual tries to create a certain impression (real or imagined). The impression that the individual is trying to create may be construed as an interaction goal; the individual may assess the degree to which the goal is being achieved during the course of the real or imagined interaction. The process of assessing the attainment of that interaction goal reveals the relationship between the individual's goal and the individual's actual behavior.

In most instances, a socially anxious individual may assess an actual interaction as not approaching the goal (Schlenker and Leary 1982; Schlenker and Weingold 1992). At first, the individual may adopt an acquisitive style that is intended to attain social approval. As the interaction progresses—in real life or in the mind of the socially anxious person—the individual may be hypersensitive to social cues. The individual may misinterpret certain cues as disinterest or rejection and then switch to a protective style that is designed to minimize the loss of approval. This style may be characterized by less talk, less self-revelation, or minimal nonverbal communication in an attempt to avoid rejection or disapproval. The result may be a deficiency in the development of relationships or a decision not to engage in any interaction because the expected outcome is negative. Finally, the self-protective style may result in negative reactions from others that reinforce the anxious individual's expectations (Meleshko and Alden 1993).

Public Self-Consciousness

Socially anxious individuals may be characterized as chronically self-focused; that is, they tend to experience a high degree of self-awareness, in which the individual's attention is focused on the self as a social public object (Buss 1980). This chronic state of self-focused attention may be associated with other cognitive aspects of psychopathology. For example, persons who are chronically self-focused may have more negative affect and anxiety (Ingram 1990).

This theory relates to the self-discrepancy and self-presentation theories because self-focused attention increases the salience of discrepancies between interaction goals and actual behavior or discrepancies between aspects of self. Individuals with severe public self-consciousness are overly concerned about others' opinions of them and are susceptible to pressure to conform; they exaggerate the personal relevance of others' behavior (Buss 1980).

Alden et al. (1992) found that women with low social efficacy were more likely to withdraw from social interaction in a self-focused condition—with a video camera in the room—than when the camera was absent. Heightened self-awareness led to a tendency to withdraw, which indicates that the dominant feelings of anxiety and fear in social situations are more salient when an individual is self-focused. In addition, women with low social efficacy felt that the individuals with whom they were interacting did not like them, and, based on ratings by the other individuals in these interactions, low-efficacy women actually were less liked than high-efficacy women. Women with low social efficacy appeared to engage in a self-preservation strategy and withdrew; as a consequence, others rejected them socially.

Focus of Attention

Socially anxious or phobic persons may appraise social situations as challenging or frightening; the thoughts that accompany such appraisals usually are intrusive and negative in affect valence. The result of such preoccupation with negative thoughts is that attention to the functional aspects of a task is attenuated as a certain amount of that attention is devoted to worry. Because socially anxious individuals devote so much attention to internal processes, they do not encode cues in the environment well, or they distort those cues by exaggerated self-relevance; performance suffers as a result (Sarason et al. 1990).

Thus, socially anxious individuals spend their attention on self-critical and self-deprecating thoughts and do not attend to salient cues. An extremely socially anxious or phobic individual might miss important signals concerning how to take turns in discussion, for example. Moreover, cues that are encoded might be used to provide evidence that is consistent with the negative thoughts that the individual generates. For example, Malone et al. (1993) found that under certain circumstances, attending to one's partner in a social interaction can provide cues that may undermine the socially anxious individual's performance. If a socially phobic person views the other person in the interaction as more socially competent, the socially anxious individual's negative preoccupation may be exacerbated.

States of Mind

According to the states of mind model, deviation from an optimal balance of positive and negative thoughts is associated with psychopathology. This model is empirically derived from research that assessed positive and negative thoughts; it makes differential predictions about psychological functioning based on the relative proportion of positive to negative statements.

The five states of mind are positive dialogue, negative dialogue, internal dialogue of conflict, positive monologue, and negative monologue (Schwartz and Garamoni 1986). According to Schwartz and Garamoni (1986), the optimal state of mind is positive dialogue, which comprises 62% ± 6% positive statements and 38% ± 6% negative statements. Positive dialogue provides a positive coping style, yet includes enough negative statements for an individual to be sensitive to salient and threatening information. The negative dialogue pattern is the opposite of the positive dialogue: 62% negative and 38% positive. Internal dialogue of conflict is represented by 50% positive and 50% negative self-statements. Positive monologue is characterized by a large proportion of positive statements (greater than 62%), and negative monologue is characterized by a large proportion of negative self-statements (greater than 62%).

Schwartz and Garamoni suggested that optimal adjustment is associated with positive dialogue, mild psychopathology with negative dialogue, and more severe psychopathology with the negative monologue state. Heimberg et al. (1990a) found that, on average, a socially phobic individual's state of mind, as assessed by a structured questionnaire, was characterized by negative dialogue; such an individual's state of mind was characterized by negative monologue, however, when it was assessed by a more open-ended approach such as the thought-listing method.

Cognitive Assessment of Social Anxiety and Social Phobia

Many aspects of social anxiety and social phobia are consistent with the conceptual formulations described earlier. In the following sections, I review assessment strategies that clinicians use to measure these formulations.

Thoughts/Self-Statements

Although some of the conceptual frameworks described above refer to cognitive processes that may account for or characterize social anxiety, clinicians rarely incorporate those processes in the cognitive assessment of psychopathology. Instead, as Ingram and Kendall (1987) note, clinicians typically assess the by-products of cognitive processes.

One of the most well-researched products of cognitive processes is the thought or self-statement. Glass and Merluzzi (1981) and Merluzzi (1993) offered a taxonomy of self-statement assessment that included recognition, recall, prompted recall, and expressive and projective methods. Subsequently, Glass (1993) suggested that assessment methods may be categorized according to how they relate to four dimensions: structure, timing, response mode, and nature of stimulus.

Structure refers to the method of obtaining self-statements: The production method requires subjects to generate thoughts, whereas the endorsement method requires subjects to rate how frequently they had a certain thought (Glass 1993). Timing refers to the time frame for reporting thoughts: Retrospective reports require the subject to endorse or produce thoughts from some time in the past (usually the immediate past); concurrent reports ask the subject to report thoughts as they occur. Response mode consists of either written or oral reporting of thoughts. Finally, nature of stimulus refers to the type of social situation about which the subject is asked to provide thought data (e.g., imagined, role-played, or in vivo).

In an overview of cognitive assessment methods for social anxiety and social phobia, Arnkoff and Glass (1989) reviewed several methods of self-statement assessment. In the following sections, I review several approaches to self-statement assessment, using Glass's structure dimension (production vs. endorsement) as a method of labeling the type of assessment method. Arnkoff and Glass (1989), Glass (1993), Martzke et al. (1987), Merluzzi (1993), and Merluzzi and Boltwood (1990) provide more extensive treatments of these methods and the empirical findings associated with them.

Production Methods

Thought listing is one of the most common forms of assessing self-statements. In this assessment method, the subject is asked to write thoughts that occurred either while anticipating a social situation or during a social interaction. The subject usually is given a short amount of time to recall the thoughts; the thoughts are listed on a sheet that allows for one thought per line. Judges usually rate each thought as either positive (facilitating social interaction), negative (inhibiting social interaction), neutral, or irrelevant. Subjects also may rate their thoughts, so that discrepancies between the subject's ratings and the judge's (or clinician's) ratings can be computed and discussed. Table 6–2 provides an example of a thought-listing protocol for a socially phobic subject.

Table 6–2.   Examples of statements elicited using thought listing method of cognitive assessment

Client: 25-year-old socially phobic male, first-year graduate student in engineering

Situation: Attending lab staff meeting during which each student talks about research

Thoughts derived from thought listing while imagining the situation in therapy	Valence of thoughts	
	Client	Therapist
1. I'll freeze up and not be able to say anything.	–	–
2. My face will turn bright red.	–	–
3. I'll feel like a fool.	–	–
4. I know I'm smart, but I just can't seem to feel comfortable saying what I know.	–	+/–
5. It always comes out jumbled.	–	–
6. People look bored.	–	–
7. Damn, I wish I didn't feel this way, I feel like such a jerk.	–	–
8. Other new students seem kind of uptight and were able to do OK.	0	+
9. Maybe it's not so bad after all.	+	+
10. Yeah, but they're probably not as uptight as I am.	–	–
11. I always seem to find the panic button.	–	–

Note.   + = facilitating (positive) self-statement; – = inhibiting (negative) self-statement; 0 = neutral self-statement.

In the *videotape-aided thought recall* method, subjects are asked to recall their thoughts with the help of cues provided by a videotape replay of a social interaction in which the subject was engaged in a role-play or a naturalistic interaction. Generally, the clinician records the subject's thoughts on audio-tape as the subject speaks them aloud while watching the videotape. A variation on this method allows subjects to stop the videotape at various points and recall their thoughts; the clinician also may stop the videotape.

In this method, subjects have ample cues to use in thought recall; the problem, however, is that subjects may reconstruct thoughts consistent with their post hoc interpretation of the events on the videotape. That is, the recorded thoughts may represent a subject's reevaluation of his or her performance rather than the subject's true thoughts in that situation.

In the *think aloud* procedure, subjects are asked to express their thoughts as they are performing a task. Socially anxious subjects typically are unable to express their thoughts while taking part in a social interaction; if some form of desensitization or imagery is used during the course of treatment, however, the subject may be able to express thoughts while imagining the difficult situation. *Articulated thoughts* are acquired by having the subject listen to a prerecorded social interaction in which several pauses occur—during which the subject is asked to "think aloud" and record thoughts on audiotape (Davison et al. 1983).

Endorsement Methods

Perhaps the most common endorsement-type measure of self-statements is the Social Interaction Self-Statement Test (SISST) (Glass et al. 1982). This instrument contains 15 positive and 15 negative self-statements that relate to social interaction. Subjects are asked to read each statement and rate on a 5-point Likert scale how often they had that thought in a situation or in anticipation of a social situation. Negative SISST scores generally are more predictive of social anxiety and performance in social situations than positive SISST scores. However, as the states of mind model suggests, the ratio of negative to positive may be the best descriptor of psychopathology. Unfortunately, evidence for the convergent validity of the SISST and thought listing methods is weak (Arnkoff and Glass 1989).

One distinct advantage of the endorsement method is that an instrument such as the SISST is easy to administer and score. The disadvantage is that endorsement-type instruments usually are designed for a specific situation. Moreover, the thoughts provided for the subject to rate may not represent the thoughts the subject actually had in the social situation; thus, this assessment method may miss some idiosyncratic thoughts. Production methods are more versatile, but they require scoring by trained judges, and the reliability of scoring must be assessed.

Expectations

As noted above with regard to self-presentation, socially anxious individuals may have certain goals for social interactions and, at the same time, doubt their ability to meet those goals. This analysis is consistent with social learning theory because the expectation for social interaction may include behavior expectancies and outcome expectancies.

Behavior expectancy is the probability that the socially anxious individual can perform the behavior in question—for example, giving a presentation to co-workers. Outcome expectancy is the probability that the co-workers will like the presentation and, perhaps, be persuaded by the ideas presented. Behavior expectancy is what Bandura (1986) referred to as a self-efficacy expectation. In terms of self-presentation theory, a socially anxious individual is motivated to engage in behaviors in order to make a good impression. Outcome expectancy is the expectation that others will have a favorable impression and behave in a way that confirms the desired impression. The Self-Efficacy Questionnaire for Social Skills (Moe and Zeiss 1982) is one measure of efficacy expectations for social interaction.

Self-Consciousness

As I noted above with regard to public self-consciousness, socially anxious persons are chronically self-focused and tend to be publicly rather than privately self-conscious. That is, they view themselves as social objects. The Self-Consciousness Scale (Scheier et al. 1978) measures private self-consciousness, public self-consciousness, and social anxiety; psychologists have used this instrument extensively in research on self-focused attention. Researchers also have manipulated self-consciousness in a laboratory setting by using video cameras to stimulate public self-consciousness and by placing mirrors in front of subjects to stimulate private self-consciousness.

Reaction Time

Mattia et al. (1993) used a Stroop color-naming task in which socially phobic individuals were shown socially threatening words (e.g., boring), physically threatening words (e.g., fatal), and color words (e.g., blue). In all instances, the subject was asked to identify the colors of letters used to spell the words. Individuals with social phobia demonstrated longer response latencies to socially threatening words than to other words, compared with a nonphobic control group. Socially phobic individuals who had been treated successfully had significantly reduced latencies compared with nonphobic control subjects. Thus, the Stroop test demonstrates how the salience of certain words may provoke or activate anxiety that results in longer processing time for that stimulus. Treatment apparently corrects that defensive processing.

General Measures of Social Phobia

The Social Phobia and Anxiety Inventory (SPAI) (Turner et al. 1989) is an empirically derived measure of social phobia, with items that cover the major areas in social phobia: somatic symptoms, cognition, escape, and avoidance. This inventory appears to have good reliability, discriminant validity, and concurrent validity (Beidel et al. 1989). Herbert et al. (1991) endorsed the concurrent validity of the SPAI, reporting significant correlations with other self-report and behavioral measures of social anxiety.

   The Social Phobia Scale (SPS) (Mattick and Peters 1988) assesses anxiety experienced in situations that involve scrutiny by others. The reliability of the

SPS has received mixed reviews: Mattick and Peters (1988) reported relatively high reliability estimates, but Heimberg et al. (1992) indicated that the reliability of the instrument was not as strong.

Treatment Strategies for Social Phobia

Cognitive Therapy

Cognitive Behavioral Group Treatment for Social Phobia (CBGT) is administered in groups of 5–6 subjects in 12 weekly 2-hour sessions (Heimberg 1989; Heimberg and Barlow 1988). Treatment components include the following:

1. Developing a cognitive-behavioral explanation of social phobia and a rationale for the effectiveness of CBGT.
2. Training patients in the skills of identification, analysis, and disputation of problematic cognitions through the use of structured exercises.
3. Exposing patients to simulations of anxiety-provoking situations in the context of the treatment group.
4. Using cognitive restructuring procedures, such as those mentioned in Step 2 above, to teach patients to control their maladaptive thinking before and during exposure simulations.
5. Using similar procedures to teach patients to engage in rational self-analysis rather than negative self-evaluation after completing an exposure simulation.
6. Assigning homework in which patients expose themselves to real anxiety-provoking events after they have confronted these events in exposure simulations.
7. Teaching patients a self-administered cognitive restructuring routine so that they can engage in cognitive preparation for homework assignments and rational self-analysis after the completion of treatment.

In early sessions of CBGT, patients are encouraged to talk about the situations they fear; the therapist notes similarities among the situations that different patients cite. This process promotes universality among the participants and provides some encouragement for otherwise socially fearful persons to talk about their dire fear of evaluation and scrutiny.

Patients also learn about the sequence of events in social situations for socially phobic individuals. That is, there is an implicit or explicit demand for social interaction, which is followed by negative affect and expectations, lack of control, and anxiety. Preoccupation with self-presentation leads to attentional focus on negative consequences and negative thoughts—which, in turn, lead to lack of perception or misperception of social cues. Increased arousal tends to heighten awareness of expectations of poor performance or negative evaluation of performance. The result of the sequence is that the individual's social performance suffers, creating an interpersonal situation in which the socially phobic individual attempts to minimize rejection and thereby actually creates the consequence that the individual fears.

Next, patients are taught some cognitive-behavioral concepts through the use of structured exercises. The goals of this part of the treatment are for the patients to:

1. Reconceptualize their thoughts as hypotheses to be tested rather than facts to be accepted.
2. Develop an awareness of the frequency with which they engage in maladaptive thinking.
3. Develop skills to identify distortions or logical errors in their own thinking.
4. Develop an awareness of the connection between distorted thinking and social phobic anxiety.
5. Develop skills for challenging and changing their negative thinking patterns.

During this phase of the treatment, there is a great deal of emphasis on the identification and modification of automatic thoughts. Automatic thoughts are elicited, rebutted, and replaced with more rational and facilitating thoughts. In particular, automatic thoughts are analyzed as they relate to particular types of cognitive distortions. Patients discuss the consequences (behavioral and physiological) of dysfunctional automatic thoughts in contrast to rational or facilitative thoughts.

The middle sessions of the treatment program are devoted to simulated exposures, cognitive restructuring, and homework assignments. Patients select target situations, which therapists and other group members simulate through role-playing. The patient is asked to imagine the situation and indicate the kinds of thoughts that occur in that situation. Patients are encouraged to rebut negative thoughts and expectations and to use their new thoughts in the simulations. At times during these simulations, the role players (the other members of the group and the leaders) are encouraged to play out the patient's worst fear (humiliation, embarrassment, rejection, etc.). After each simulation, the patient is encouraged to talk about his or her performance and any problematic cognitions that may have occurred during the simulation.

Patients are encouraged to try the same process in real-life social situations that they may have avoided in the past. They are instructed to anticipate the situation, uncover dysfunctional thoughts, and replace them with coping thoughts. Patients are expected to analyze the situation afterward, evaluating their performance and any negative thoughts that may have interfered with their performance. The final therapy sessions are devoted to a critique of the homework assignments and a review of what the patients learned during the course of treatment.

In the following section, I describe a CBGT case study. This example includes typical CBGT features, such as anticipation of situations, disputing and replacing dysfunctional thoughts, simulations of difficult social situations, homework, and feedback, and illustrates how patients are encouraged to help each other throughout the course of therapy.

CBGT Case Example

M., a 27-year-old woman, described herself as a shy child who read a lot, did well in school, but never dated in high school. She attended a 2-year college in her community and specialized in computer applications. After college, she moved into an apartment by herself. She was employed at a small accounting firm as a computer operator and systems analyst. She spent most of her spare time by herself: reading, riding her bicycle, walking, and window shopping through the mall a couple of times a week. She usually chose to go to the mall during the busiest time, in order to watch people. She said she felt like an observer of life, rather than a full participant. She lived in fear that someone might actually approach her at the mall and ask her a question, and she usually conducted herself so as to minimize that possibility. She often felt uncomfortable at work, tended to be very anxious in groups, and tried to be so efficient and thorough that she would not need to speak at staff meetings. She thought of herself as competent but a loner; she recognized that her social fears and inhibitions prevented her from advancing in her work and having friendships.

M. came to therapy with some fear about the process, but she seemed quite motivated to "change her life." She was tired of always feeling like an "outsider," merely "watching the world go by." In the first therapy session, she mentioned the desire to have a friend as one of her primary goals. She thought that if she could spend some time with a friend, she could enjoy things such as shopping or going to a movie and still feel safe. She was far more reticent about her relationships with men, although she admitted that she eventually wanted to work on that as well.

After the initial sessions—in which she learned about the inhibiting nature of automatic thoughts and how those thoughts fostered and maintained her fear—M. was ready to work on a simulation. The situation she chose to work on was asking one of her co-workers, C., to lunch. She had known C.

for about two years but had avoided spending any social time with her, outside of work. On more than one occasion, C. had asked M. to join her and others for lunch, but the prospect of being in an "unstructured" situation with 4 or 5 people was too frightening for M.

For the simulation exercise, M. was asked to think through the situation from beginning to end and to report any thoughts she might have during the imagined interaction. She reported the following thoughts:

1. If C. says "yes," I'll be in a panic state just anticipating what lunch will be like.
2. I'll be a nervous wreck.
3. I'm afraid C. is just being polite but really doesn't like me.
4. C. probably thinks I'm dull and boring.
5. I feel like such a nerd.

Each thought was written on a large pad and analyzed in terms of the meanings and distortions it contained. For example, thought 4 is what Burns (1980) called a "fortune telling error." M. had no evidence that C. considered her dull and boring, yet she chose to anticipate that negative outcome. M was encouraged to dispute this thought and consider the possibility that C. might like her. In fact, M had more information indicating that C. might like her—namely, C.'s requests that M. join her group for lunch—than she had that C. did not like her. M. was urged to think about alternatives to the negative automatic thought and to replace it with the following: "She might like me, and we might become friends."

Statement 2 reflected M.'s assumption that she would be nervous—a safe assumption, given M.'s social history. Replacing that thought with a positive thought such as "I will be calm, cool, and collected" would not be appropriate because M. probably would experience anxiety. The goal in dealing with thought 2 would be to acknowledge the anxiety but not let it determine whether M. would "fail" as a lunch partner or a friend. A more functional replacement for thought 2 would be a coping statement such as "I may be nervous, but that doesn't mean I can't enjoy going to lunch with C."

To help M. prepare for the simulation exercise, a coping or facilitating thought was written on the pad opposite each dysfunctional thought. After each thought was analyzed, disputed, and replaced, a simulation was enacted. M. first stated what she hoped to accomplish with the simulation. She indicated that she merely wanted to spend an hour with C. and get to know her better. This goal seemed realistic and rational, so the simulation proceeded, with M. describing the situation in which she might ask C. to lunch, followed by the actual lunch.

During both the invitation and the lunch simulations, the interaction was interrupted to assess M.'s anxiety level and to encourage her to use the coping or facilitating thoughts that were suggested as alternatives to the dysfunctional thoughts. M. appeared to be quite anxious during the simulation and had some awkward moments during which she was unable to say anything, but she persisted with the enactment and was able to get through the situation. M. reported that she felt more confident as the interaction progressed—which was a new feeling for her.

Afterward, M. agreed to repeat the simulation, with the same format. During the second simulation, she was more fluent, had fewer awkward moments, and reported feeling somewhat more calm than she had during the first simulation.

After one more session, M. was given the homework assignment of asking C. to lunch. Although M.'s anticipatory anxiety about initiating the invitation was quite high, she did ask, and C. accepted. M. reported that the lunch was not the calmest experience she had ever had; however, she was able to reattribute a portion of her arousal to excitement at having accomplished something that she had thought about for a long time.

CBGT Outcome Studies

Several outcome studies have tested the efficacy of CBGT for social phobia. In Heimberg et al. (1985), 7 subjects who met the DSM-III criteria for social phobia were treated with the CBGT package using a multiple baseline design. Over the course of treatment, patients demonstrated significant reductions on self-report measures of anxiety while performing in simulated anxiety-provoking situations. In addition, judges' ratings of the subjects' performance anxiety decreased as a function of treatment. Finally, heart rate prior to, but not during, behavioral assessments tended to decrease in most subjects. In general, the treatment effects were substantial; 6 of the 7 subjects had maintained their gains at the 6-month follow-up assessment.

In a more elaborate study, Heimberg et al. (1990b) compared CBGT with a credible control treatment that included group discussion and support but none of the specific CBGT treatment components. At the post-treatment assessment, both groups had improved on a number of measures—including a clinician's rating of phobic severity, self-statement scores, and commonly used measures of social anxiety. In fact, on most measures there were no differences between the CBGT group and the discussion/support group, although statistical means indicated an advantage for CBGT. At the 6-month follow-up assessment, however, the CBGT group had maintained the changes, whereas the control group had not. This study had one major limitation, however: The measure that differentiated the treatment conditions most—the clinicians' ratings—was not blind; the raters aware of which treatment regimen the patients were enrolled in.

Gelernter et al. (1991) compared the efficacy of CBGT with pharmacological treatments. Sixty-five socially phobic patients were treated with CBGT, alprazolam, phenelzine sulfate, or a placebo pill and provided with instructions encouraging exposure to phobic situations. The patients showed gains for all treatment protocols, as well as the placebo; no single treatment, however, emerged as superior to the others. In general, patients reported less fearfulness of negative evaluation, less social avoidance, less work and social impairment, less general anxiety, less depression, and fewer negative self-statements. The phenelzine group tended to include more treatment responders than the other groups; that tendency was not statistically significant, however.

The fact that neither the drugs nor CBGT produced better results than the placebo is notable. One explanation for the lack of substantial differences between the placebo control and the active therapies is that all patients were encouraged to engage in self-directed exposure. Because the subjects in the placebo condition showed interest in volunteering for treatment, were in an experimental protocol, and were encouraged to engage in self-directed exposure, they may have initiated exposure to feared situations on their own—which boosted the efficacy of that "treatment." Moreover, there were several problems with this study, including the low number of subjects in each group and the fact that only one CBGT group was conducted.

Exposure Treatment With Cognitive Restructuring

Another treatment that clinicians have used with social phobia is exposure with cognitive restructuring. In one study using this approach (Mattick and Peters 1988), patients were treated in small groups (4–7 subjects) for 2 hours per week for 6 weeks. In the initial session, the patients were offered a rationale for the treatment, including information on the role of avoidance in the maintenance of social phobia as well as the role of irrational and negative thoughts. The patients were told that to overcome their phobia, they must enter phobic situations and engage in "challenging and altering their maladaptive beliefs and attitudes" (Mattick and Peters 1988, p. 253).

In group sessions, the patients were exposed to anxiety-producing situations, in a graduated fashion: moderately difficult situations were followed by a progression to more difficult situations. The patients were encouraged to remain in the feared situations until they no longer wished to avoid them. In the first couple of sessions, the therapist guided and directed the exposure situations; by the third session, however, the patients were managing the exposure situations, and the therapist's direction faded substantially.

To increase the study's generalizability, more difficult tasks were introduced, and homework was assigned. For these assignments, the patients were to write down the situation in which they were engaged, the level of anxiety they experienced, the amount of time they spent in the situation, their anxiety level after the situation, any negative or inhibiting thoughts, and their rational reappraisal of the situation. In each session, the therapists reviewed the homework assignments for about 15 minutes and conducted exposure exercises for about an hour.

The cognitive restructuring component of the treatment included a didactic portion in which the therapists spoke about the importance of identifying irrational thoughts and replacing them with rational thoughts. The patients were encouraged to analyze their automatic thoughts before, during, and after exposure situations to determine if their functioning was rational and realistic. Various irrational beliefs were discussed and incorporated into subsequent sessions and homework.

One group of patients in the study participated in cognitive restructuring as well as exposure exercises; the other group did exposure exercises only, without cognitive restructuring. Based on the patients' homework and in-session training, the amount of actual exposure was similar in the two conditions.

Patients in both groups—exposure-plus-cognitive restructuring and exposure-only—improved their functioning, as evidenced by substantial treatment gains. Judges' ratings of behavioral avoidance showed significant change. Patients in both groups also reported significant reductions in anxiety, avoidance, and depression. These gains were enhanced between post-test and follow-up assessments.

More critical, however, were the differences between the two groups: On actual behavioral performance and on self-rated avoidance, exposure plus cognitive restructuring was superior to exposure alone. Moreover, on a composite measure of improvement, the exposure-plus-cognitive restructuring group did better than the exposure-only group.

Summary

Despite the relatively recent inclusion of social phobia in the *Diagnostic and Statistical Manual of Mental Disorders*, there has been quite a bit of work on the description of social phobia. The most critical distinction among the subtypes of social phobia appears to be between generalized social phobia and all other types. Another critical distinction is between social phobia and Axis

II avoidant personality disorder. Empirical analyses of these two disorders seem to indicate that there is a high degree of comorbidity for generalized social phobia but not for more situational social phobias, such as public speaking. Conceptually, social phobia is characterized by a number of social cognitive processes and features that may emerge in late adolescence but may be fostered by early experiences.

Treatment studies that are beginning to appear in the literature seem to favor cognitive therapies for psychological treatment. More controlled comparative treatment studies with differential diagnosis are essential for progress in understanding social phobia.

References

Alden LE, Teschuk M, Tee K: Public self-awareness and withdrawal from social interactions. Cognitive Therapy and Research 16:249–267, 1992

American Psychiatric Association: Diagnostic and Statistical Manual of Mental Disorders, 3rd Edition. Washington, DC, American Psychiatric Association, 1980

American Psychiatric Association: Diagnostic and Statistical Manual of Mental Disorders, 3rd Edition, Revised. Washington, DC, American Psychiatric Association, 1987

American Psychiatric Association: Diagnostic and Statistical Manual of Mental Disorders, 4th Edition. Washington, DC, American Psychiatric Association, 1994

Arnkoff DB, Glass CR: Cognitive assessment in social anxiety and social phobia. Clinical Psychology Review 9:61–74, 1989

Bandura A: Social Foundations of Thought and Action: A Social Cognitive Theory. Englewood Cliffs, NJ; Prentice-Hall, 1986

Barlow DH: Anxiety and its Disorders. New York, Guilford, 1988

Beidel DC, Borden JW, Turner SM, et al: The Social Phobia and Anxiety Inventory: concurrent validity with a clinic sample. Behav Res Ther 5:573–576, 1989

Bruch MA: Familial and developmental antecedents of social phobia: issues and findings. Clinical Psychology Review 9:37–47, 1989

Bruch MA, Heimberg RG, Berger PA, et al: Social phobia and perceptions of early parental and personal characteristics. Anxiety Research: An International Journal 2:57–65, 1989

Burns DD: Feeling Good: The New Mood Therapy. New York, Signet, 1980

Buss AH: Self-Consciousness and Social Anxiety. San Francisco, CA, WH Freeman, 1980

Cloitre M, Heimberg RG, Liebowitz MR, et al: Perceptions of control in panic disorder and social phobia. Cognitive Therapy and Research 16:569–577, 1992

Davison GC, Robins C, Johnson MK: Articulated thoughts during simulated situations: a paradigm for studying cognition in emotion and behavior. Cognitive Therapy and Research 7:17–40, 1983

DiNardo PA, O'Brien GT, Barlow DH, et al: Reliability of DSM-III anxiety disorder categories using a new structured interview. Arch Gen Psychiatry 40:1070–1074, 1983

Gelernter CS, Uhde TW, Cimbolic P, et al: Cognitive-behavioral and pharmacological treatments of social phobia. Arch Gen Psychiatry 48:938–945, 1991

Glass CR: A little more about cognitive assessment. Journal of Counseling and Development 71:546–548, 1993

Glass CR, Merluzzi, TV: Cognitive assessment of social evaluative anxiety, in Cognitive Assessment. Edited by Merluzzi TV, Glass CR, Genest M. New York, Guilford, 1981, pp 233–269

Glass CR, Merluzzi TV, Biever JL, et al: Cognitive assessment of social anxiety: development and validation of a self-statement questionnaire. Cognitive Therapy and Research 6:37–55, 1982

Heimberg RG: Cognitive and behavioral treatments for social phobia: a critical analysis. Clinical Psychology Review 9:107–128, 1989

Heimberg RG, Barlow DH: Psychosocial treatments for social phobia. Psychosomatics 29:27–37, 1988

Heimberg RG, Becker RE, Goldfinger K, et al: Treatment of social phobia by exposure, cognitive restructuring and homework assignments. J Nerv Ment Dis 173:236–245, 1985

Heimberg RG, Bruch MA, Hope DA, et al: Evaluating the states of mind model: comparison to an alternative model and effects of method of cognitive assessment. Cognitive Therapy and Research 14:543–557, 1990a

Heimberg RG, Dodge CS, Hope DA, et al: Cognitive behavioral group treatment for social phobia: comparison with a credible placebo control. Cognitive Therapy and Research 14:1–23, 1990b

Heimberg RG, Hope DA, Dodge CS, et al: DSM-III-R subtypes of social phobia: comparison of generalized social phobics and public speaking phobics. J Nerv Ment Dis 178:172–179, 1990c

Heimberg RG, Mueller GP, Holt CS, et al: Assessment of anxiety in social interaction and being observed by others: the Social Interaction Anxiety Scale and the Social Phobia Scale. Behavior Therapy 23:53–73, 1992

Herbert JD, Bellack AS, Hope DA: Concurrent validity of the Social Phobia and Anxiety Inventory. Journal of Psychopathology and Behavioral Assessment 13:357–368, 1991

Herbert JD, Hope DA, Bellack AS: Validity of the distinction between generalized social phobia and avoidant personality disorder. J Abnorm Psychol 101:332–339, 1992

Holt CS, Heimberg RG, Hope DA: Avoidant personality disorder and the generalized subtype of social phobia. J Abnorm Psychol 101:318–325, 1992

Hope DA, Rapee RM, Heimberg RG, et al: Representations of the self in social phobia: vulnerability to social threat. Cognitive Therapy and Research 14:177–189, 1990

Ingram RE: Depressive cognition: models, mechanisms, and methods, in Contemporary Psychological Approaches to Depression. Edited by Ingram RE. New York, Plenum, 1990, pp 169–195

Ingram RE, Kendall PC: The cognitive side of anxiety. Cognitive Therapy and Research 11:523–536, 1987

Lazarus PJ: Incidence of shyness in elementary-school age children. Psychol Rep 56:367–374, 1982

Malone EM, Bruch MA, Heimberg RG: Focus of attention and social anxiety: the role of negative self-thoughts and perceived positive attributes of the other. Cognitive Therapy and Research 17:209–224, 1993

Marks IM: Behavioral treatment of social phobia. Psychopharmacol Bull 21: 615–618, 1985

Martzke JS, Anderson BL, Cacioppo JT: Cognitive assessment of anxiety disorders, in Anxiety and Stress Disorders: Cognitive-Behavioral Assessment and Treatment. Edited by Michelson L, Ascher LM. New York, Guilford, 1987, pp 62–88

Mattia JI, Heimberg RG, Hope DA: The revised Stroop color-naming task in social phobics: diagnostic and treatment outcome implications. Behav Res Ther 31:305–313, 1993

Mattick RP, Peters L: Treatment of severe social phobia: effects of guided exposure with and without cognitive restructuring. J Consult Clin Psychol 56:251–260, 1988

Meleshko KGA, Alden LE: Anxiety and self-disclosure: toward a motivational model. J Pers Soc Psychol 64:1000–1009, 1993

Merluzzi TV: Clinical applications of self-statement assessment. Journal of Counseling and Development 71:539–545, 1993

Merluzzi TV, Boltwood MD: Cognitive assessment, in Testing in Counseling Practice. Edited by Watkins CE, Campbell VL. Hillsdale, NJ, Lawrence Erlbaum, 1990, pp 135–176

Moe KO, Zeiss AM: Measuring self-efficacy expectations for social skills: a methodological inquiry. Cognitive Therapy Research 6:191–205, 1982

Pollard CA, Henderson JG: Four types of social phobia in a community sample. J Nerv Ment Dis 176:440–445, 1988

Sarason IG, Sarason BR, Pierce GR: Anxiety, cognitive interference, and performance. Journal of Social Behavior and Personality 5:1–18, 1990

Scheier MF, Buss AH, Buss DM: Self-consciousness, self-report of aggressiveness, and aggression. Journal of Research in Personality 12:133–140, 1978

Schlenker BR, Leary MR: Social anxiety and self-presentation: a conceptual model. Psychol Bull 92:641–669, 1982

Schlenker BR, Weingold MF: Interpersonal processes involving impression regulation and management. Annu Rev Psychol 43:133–168, 1992

Schneier FR, Spitzer RL, Gibbon M, et al: The relationship of social phobia subtypes and avoidant personality disorder. Compr Psychiatry 32:496–502, 1991

Schwartz RM, Garamoni GL: A structural model of positive and negative states of mind: asymmetry in the internal dialogue, in Advances in Cognitive-Behavioral Research and Therapy, Vol 5. Edited by Kendall PC. New York, Plenum, 1986, pp 1–62

Strauman TJ: Self-discrepancies in clinical depression and social phobia: cognitive structures that underlie emotional disorders? J Abnorm Psychol 98:14–22, 1989

Turner SM, Beidel DC: Social phobia: clinical syndrome, diagnosis, and comorbidity. Clinical Psychology Review 9:3–18, 1989

Turner SM, Beidel DC, Dancu CV, et al: An empirically derived inventory to measure social fears and anxiety: the Social Phobia and Anxiety Inventory. Psychol Assessment, 1:35–40, 1989

Turner SM, Beidel DC, Townsley RM: Social phobia: relationship to shyness. Behav Res Ther 28:497–505, 1990

Wallace ST, Alden LE: A comparison of social standards and perceived ability in anxious and nonanxious men. Cognitive Therapy and Research 15: 237–254, 1991

Zimbardo PG: Shyness: What is it and What to do About it. Reading, MA, Addison-Wesley, 1977

Part II

Interventions for Severe Neuropsychological Disorders

Chapter 7

Cognitive Rehabilitation for Cerebrovascular Accidents and Alzheimer's Disease

Neil H. Pliskin, Ph.D., Joseph M. Cunningham, Ph.D., Jacqueline Remondet Wall, Ph.D., and Jeffrey E. Cassisi, Ph.D.

T he achievements of modern medicine and the emphasis placed on lifestyle changes over the past several decades are increasing the percentage of Americans older than age 65, from 8% in 1950 to a predicted 13% of the total population by the year 2000 (U. S. Bureau of the Census 1989; U. S. Department of Health and Human Services 1990). Over the past 15 years, the death rate from cardiovascular disease has decreased by 50%, but the incidence of dementing disorders resulting from cerebrovascular accidents (CVAs) and Alzheimer's disease increases dramatically with advancing age. More than 20% of individuals older than age 80 are affected by CVAs or Alzheimer's disease (U.S. Department of Health and Human Services 1990). Therefore, cognitive rehabilitation strategies geared toward the remediation of cognitive impairments in this population has become critical, and the amount of research in this area has grown dramatically.

In this chapter we describe and critically review the cognitive rehabilitation techniques that have been developed for the two most common causes of dementia, CVAs and Alzheimer's disease. We summarize the most effective rehabilitation techniques and suggest future research in this area.

Cognitive Rehabilitation for Cerebrovascular Accidents

CVAs are the third leading cause of death in the United States (National Center for Health Statistics 1992). CVA mortality has been declining since the 1970s because of primary prevention efforts, such as hypertension education and control programs (McGovern et al. 1992). The decline in the CVA mortality rate has increased the number of patients who require long-term rehabilitation efforts focused on the cognitive and physical sequelae of CVAs.

The cognitive sequelae of CVAs include various intellectual and motor deficits that tend to be more specific than traumatic brain injuries. For example, CVAs involving the area served by the middle cerebral artery create specific deficits such as contralateral weakness, sensory loss, visual field defects, impaired spatial perception, or language disturbance. In addition to functional impairments, discrete personality changes can also result from CVAs (Stuss 1992). Finally, CVAs are not necessarily progressive conditions; the Framingham Study found that 58%–76% of all individuals who experience CVAs will not have a recurrence (Sacco 1982).

Because of the high incidence of CVAs, the specificity of associated deficits, and the potentially static (nonprogressive) nature of the illness, CVA patients provide an ideal population for studying cognitive rehabilitation efforts. Given the specific neuropsychological impairments that usually follow a CVA, long-term cognitive rehabilitation typically addresses specific post-CVA deficits. Cognitive functions most often affected by CVA include language, attention and concentration, perceptual functioning, and memory. Studies associated with each area are discussed in this chapter.

Language

One of the main areas addressed in rehabilitative efforts is language dysfunction, in part because of the frequency of language disorders after CVA. Twenty to 30% of all CVAs result in aphasia (Leske 1981). Aphasic patients have difficulty either comprehending language or formulating language, or both. In particular, difficulties occur with fluency, comprehension, repetition, and naming. Most aphasias develop after CVAs that involve the middle cerebral artery.

Types of aphasias.   Language difficulties in aphasic patients range from mild to very severe and can include a number of areas, such as understanding both spoken and written language and oral and written communication. Obviously, it is instructive to understand the relationship between deficit symptomatology and the affected cerebral area. For example, posterior CVAs may lead to aphasia. These patients may have impaired comprehension, visual agnosia, and reading deficits but may not have problems in writing, spelling, and oral speech. In these individuals, alexia may occur without agraphia, the latter resulting from a disconnection between the left occipital cortex and the angular gyrus and language areas. These patients would be able to write a sentence without being able to read what was written. Therefore, a clear understanding of an individual's post-CVA strengths and weaknesses through neuropsychological or speech evaluation is essential to the development of an effective rehabilitation plan.

Several systems have been developed to classify types of aphasias. One system categorizes aphasias based on an assessment of impaired language functions (e.g., fluency, comprehension, repetition, and naming). In this system, which includes both functional difficulties and cerebral impairments, the primary forms of aphasia include Broca's, Wernicke's, conduction, global, anomic, transcortical-motor, transcortical-sensory, and transcortical-mixed. Table 7–1 lists the symptoms of the different types of aphasia and the anatomical sites believed to be involved.

Other categorization systems classify aphasia on expressive and receptive dimensions. Patients with expressive aphasias have difficulty expressing themselves, but typically have few problems comprehending language. Patients with receptive aphasias generally have few problems with language production, but

Table 7–1.   Characteristics of cortical aphasias

Type	Verbal output	Repetition	Comprehension	Naming
Broca's	Nonfluent	Impaired	Normal	Slightly impaired
Wernicke's	Fluent	Impaired	Impaired	Impaired
Conduction	Fluent	Impaired	Normal	Impaired
Global	Nonfluent	Impaired	Impaired	Impaired
Anomic	Fluent	Normal	Normal	Impaired
Transcortical Motor	Nonfluent	Normal	Normal	Impaired
Sensory	Fluent	Normal	Impaired	Impaired
Mixed	Nonfluent	Normal	Impaired	Impaired

Type	Common lesion locations
Broca's	Left posterior inferior frontal
Wernicke's	Left posterior superior temporal
Conduction	Left parietal
Global	Left frontal temporal parietal
Anomic	Left posterior inferior temporal or temporal occipital
Transcortical	
Motor	Left medial frontal or anterior border zone
Sensory	Left medial parietal or posterior border zone
Mixed	Left medial frontal parietal or complete border zone

Source.   Adapted from Mayeux R, Kandel ER: "Disorders of Language: The Aphasias," in *Principles of Neuroscience*, 3rd Edition. Edited by Kandel ER, Schwartz SH, Jessell TM. Norwalk, CT, Appleton & Lange, 1991. Used with permission.

their speech content is inappropriate, and even unintelligible in severe cases, be-cause of difficulty understanding language. Another categorization system that is based on the receptive/expressive dimension classifies the aphasia by the por-tion of the brain that has been damaged and differentiates between anterior (front) and posterior (back) regions of the brain. Anterior aphasias are usually expres-sive aphasias, whereas posterior aphasias are usually receptive aphasias.

Aphasias are assessed by both standardized psychometrically based instru-ments and clinical acumen. Several widely used tests have proven to be reliable and valid. The most commonly used screening test is the Reitan-Indiana Apha-sia Screening Test (Reitan and Wolfson 1993). The individual taking this test is asked to copy, name, and spell simple figures, such as a square and a Greek cross. The test also includes a screening of reading skills, calculation ability, and right-left orientation. The test is widely used because it is short, usually taking patients less than 20 minutes to complete. However, it is not sufficiently comprehensive to detect some subtle language disturbances. Once a test such as the Reitan-Indiana Aphasia Screening Test identifies a possible language prob-lem, more in-depth tests such as the Boston Diagnostic Aphasia Examination (Goodglass and Kaplan 1983) or the Western Aphasia Battery (Kertesz 1980) can more accurately determine the nature and extent of the impairment. (See Lezak 1995 for a comprehensive review of language testing.)

Speech therapy.   Luria (1970) advanced the notion of prescribing specific language rehabilitation treatments based on carefully analyzed functional defi-cits. Two distinct approaches have evolved that address the rehabilitation of speech disorders: the classical and the neurolinguistic models. Classical ap-proaches typically focus on restoration of speech and language performance. Such approaches use tasks to attempt to restore lost skills. Common treatment techniques include repetition, cueing, and answering dichotomous (yes or no) questions. For example, a common therapy technique of the classical approach is to teach patients to respond to questions by having the therapist repeat the patients' answers. The classical approach to language rehabilitation emphasizes syntax as an important part of therapy. Syntax defines the rules for interrela-tionship between words in a sentence. For example, the verb in a sentence de-scribes the action of the subject of the sentence. The sentence, "The man is walking the dog," must be analyzed syntactically to understand who is walking whom. Classical approaches use exercises that require a patient to understand the meaning of a sentence and then limit understanding to the literal meaning of the sentence.

Neurolinguistic approaches in aphasia rehabilitation focus on differenti-ating between comprehension and expression in language. These approaches recognize that comprehension and expression are active processes that need to be addressed in the development of treatment plans. For example, both comprehension and expression are affected in expressive aphasia, and the rules required to comprehend a sentence are also the rules needed to express it (see Sarno 1992 for a review). Neurolinguistic approaches also address the issue of linguistic competence. Linguistic competence refers to the patient's ability to decipher meaning beyond the literal interpretation of the words in a sentence. For example, a restaurant patron with disturbances in linguistic competence who hears his or her companion say "pick up the check" will literally reach out and pick up the bill. He or she would not associate the expression with the idea of paying the bill, as is usually intended by the expression. Linguistic competence is critical to conversational language, which requires assumed logical linkages, contextual information, and implied meanings. An impairment in linguistic competence renders most conversational language meaningless to many aphasic patients.

Two models are followed in most neurolinguistic treatments of aphasia: 1) a substitute skill model and 2) a direct treatment model. Substitute skill methods attempt to find other ways to produce the lost skill. An example of this method is teaching a patient to use gestures to augment verbal communication. Direct treatment methods attempt to restore a function by repeated practice. Learning to move the lips to create sounds is an example of this method.

In cases where both comprehension and expression are affected (i.e., global aphasia), rehabilitation should first focus on comprehension as a precursor to performance rehabilitation (Basso 1987). Alternatively, substitute symbols benefit expressive aphasic patients who cannot communicate through natural language. Teaching patients sign language is an example of this method of treatment. One study showed that patients who were unable to effectively communicate orally were able to learn to communicate using American Sign Language (Moody 1982). Other approaches that are similar include Melodic Intonation Therapy (Sparks et al. 1974) and Melodic Rhythm Therapy (Van Eeckhout et al. 1983). These methods facilitate speech output using music and rhythm. An example of rhythm therapy is teaching Broca's aphasics to chant rhythms to facilitate the return of normal speech.

In contrast to the classic approach, neurolinguistic approaches also focus on helping patients decipher the contextual meaning of language. For example, in the phrase "pick it up" the patient must understand the sentence and the situation in which it is used. The phrase could imply the need to speed up one's pace (if said by a drill sergeant) or actually to lift an object (if said by an assembly line supervisor at work). The therapeutic approach must be shaped to the particular deficits experienced by each patient to increase his or her understanding of such phrases.

Most experts agree that functional recovery of language is stabilized in the 12- to 18-month period after a CVA. However, some believe that recovery of function can continue for the rest of the patient's life on a more subtle basis (Harrington 1975; Sarno 1992). Also, the effects of retraining may be multisensory, using kinesthetic and tactile input along with the more commonly used visual and verbal techniques. A study by Loughery (1992) employed multisensory methods with patients with Broca's aphasia in which words were presented orally, visually, and tactually (by tracing them out on the patient's hand). Although this form of treatment was not significantly more effective than a traditional visual-verbal presentation of the words, both forms of presentation were effective for increasing word knowledge and improving recognition.

The benefits of providing patients with speech therapy are supported in a few studies (Poeck et al. 1989; Wertz et al. 1986). For example, Poeck et al. (1989) found significant improvements resulting from intensive language therapy (450 minutes per week for 6–8 weeks). Furthermore, one recent review of the CVA rehabilitation literature by de Pedro-Cuesta et al. (1992) concluded that aphasia rehabilitation is effective.

The results of other outcome studies, however, suggest that speech therapy typically does not improve the language abilities of aphasic patients, beyond what would occur with spontaneous recovery. Lincoln et al. (1984) found no significant differences in language recovery between treatment and no-treatment groups because spontaneous recovery occurred for a significant portion of aphasic patients in the no-treatment group. A study by Wertz et al. (1986) indicated that the effectiveness of treatment cannot be demonstrated when variables that influence recovery are tightly controlled (e.g., age, number and location of CVAs, premorbid psychological condition, premorbid physiological condition, and social support). Other studies suggest that treatment by trained speech therapists produces no greater gains than interventions by volunteer therapists in language retraining with CVA patients (David et al. 1982; Hartman and Landau 1987; Meikle et al. 1979).

Attention

The most obvious behavioral and cognitive changes after CVA relate to the individual's arousal level and his or her ability to attend to and respond to the environment. For example, CVA patients who have extreme reductions in arousal do not respond to environmental stimuli regardless of intensity. Additionally, even mild attention deficits can reduce or impair memory, learning, perception, communication, and executive functions.

Attentional processes.   Posner and Rafal (1987) outlined three basic components of attention: alertness, selective attention, and vigilance or sustained attention. *Alertness* refers to the individual's physical and mental arousal level and his or her readiness to respond to environmental or bodily stimuli. Alertness can be further subdivided into tonic arousal and phasic arousal. *Tonic arousal* refers to the person's general level of alertness and incorporates normal daily fluctuations associated with sleep and waking patterns. *Tonic arousal* is relatively stable such that any change from the baseline level of alertness occurs at a slow rate. In contrast, *phasic arousal* refers to the body's capacity to quickly increase its level of alertness in response to warning stimuli. Phasic arousal is considered a general alerting mechanism.

Selective attention involves overt and covert orienting processes. Overt orientation refers to observable responses to stimuli that indicate shifts in attention, such as moving the body, head, or eyes. Covert orientation refers to cognitive shifts in attention; for example, shifting the reader's thoughts away from the abstract definitions previously discussed to think about this example. Both types of orienting can occur together, and these processes frequently are automatic and unconscious. Aspects of orienting responses include disengaging from previous stimuli, shifting to new stimuli, engaging new stimuli, and inhibiting return to old stimuli.

Vigilance or sustained attention refers to a person's ability to maintain his or her attention on specific stimuli over an extended period of time. Although selective attention often involves automatic and unconscious cognitive processing, sustained attention can be described as "deliberate and effortful attention" (p. 74) and involves conscious and controlled cognitive processing (Weber 1990). Sustained attention is necessary in remembering and learning new information, performing job tasks, playing a game, or driving a car safely.

Attention deficits.   The more common impairments in attention associated with CVA can be addressed by using Posner's concepts of attentional processes. Insufficient general alertness, a common consequence of CVA, can be viewed as an impairment in tonic arousal. As a result of brain stem lesions or compression from edema, the individual may be at the lowest level of tonic arousal and, therefore, be comatose and unable to respond to the environment. The victim may be confused, disoriented, and unable to respond effectively to environmental cues at less severe levels of impairment. Reductions in the CVA patient's response speed can be interpreted as the behavioral manifestation of deficits in the individual's phasic arousal. Response rates will be delayed because of decreases in the body's ability to prepare itself to react despite warning stimuli.

A CVA can affect an individual's ability to selectively attend or orient to specific stimuli, Posner's second level of attentional processes. The individual may perseverate in one aspect of the environment or task demand and be unable to disengage to focus on other environmental stimuli. For example, a CVA patient with deficits in selective attention may not be able to shift attention from the oral message presented by a physician to the written message printed on the instruction sheet. If the patient were writing notes, he or she may repeat the first letter or the first word over and over again and be unaware that he or she is perseverating.

The CVA patient may also be unable to inhibit a return to the old stimuli. For example, the patient may not be able to prevent himself or herself from continually looking back at the written medical instructions (overt orientation) or the patient may not be able to prevent his or her thought processes from continually shifting back to the information first presented by the physician (covert orientation). Because of the unconscious and automatic nature of most orienting processes, these individuals may report difficulties with the different tasks they are trying to perform, without being aware of the nature of their problems.

The CVA patient may also experience a number of deficits that can be described as an inability to sustain attention or maintain vigilance, Posner's third level of attentional processes. Impairments in control can result in the inability to focus consciously on a single task, maintain focus on a task, or shift to new tasks on demand. For example, a CVA patient may not be able to direct attention to the physician because he or she may be distracted by the pictures on the wall, the plants in the corner of the room, or the color of the physician's shirt. The individual may also have problems shifting from taking notes to responding to the physician's questions. Although some of the resulting functional impairments are similar to those caused by selective attention deficits (e.g., reduced memory and learning), sustained attention deficits always involve problems with conscious and intentional cognitive processes.

The prognostic implications of attentional problems vary with the different types of deficits. Higher levels of consciousness after CVA are significantly correlated with better rehabilitation outcomes (Henley et al. 1985). Conversely, length of coma, confusion, and perseveration problems are associated with poorer rehabilitation outcomes. Generally, limited attentional processes decrease the individual's ability to take advantage of rehabilitation efforts.

Cognitive rehabilitation of attention deficits.   The most comprehensive and systematic method for remediating attention deficits was developed by Ben-Yishay et al. (1987) at the New York University Medical Center Institute of Rehabilitation Medicine. Their Orientation Remedial Model (ORM) was designed to improve deficits at all three levels of attentional processing. The ORM evolved out of years of clinical research and recently was computerized to improve consistency, add graded cues, establish minimum guidelines for training, and make the program available to more patients.

Their ORM consists of five training components or stages that are systematically introduced to the patient. In the first stage, the patient is trained "to attend and react to environmental 'signals'" (Ben-Yishay et al. 1987, p. 168). This test is a computer program that presents a series of visual stimuli, allows the patient to respond, and then provides feedback on his or her performance. The goal is to engage the patient directly with his or her environment to increase overall arousal, attention, and responsiveness.

In the second stage, the patient is trained "to time his or her responses in relation to changing environmental cues" (Ben-Yishay et al. 1987, p. 168). In this training component, the patient is taught to stop the sweep of the arm of a clocklike device at a specified point. This stage emphasizes phasic arousal through response preparation, overt orientation to external stimuli, and response speed.

The next three stages focus more on controlled attentional processes. The patient is trained "to be actively vigilant" (Ben-Yishay et al. 1987, p. 168) during the third phase. The program teaches the patient to locate, identify, and discriminate among different stimuli that display colors, numbers, or both. The exercise at this level requires scanning, stimulus identification, and discrimination and is intended to improve the patient's concentration and ability to consciously shift attention.

In the fourth stage, the patient is trained "in time estimation" (Ben-Yishay et al. 1987, p. 169). Patients are taught to estimate how much time has passed and then instructed to activate a specially designed stopwatch. Focus is shifted away from the external environment to internal stimuli. Patients are progressively taught to rely on more internalized cues such as timed body movements, counting aloud, and counting silently to predict the passage of time. The goal is to teach the patient to sustain his or her attention on cognitively mediated tasks.

In the final stage of the ORM, the patient is trained "to synchronize responding with complex rhythms" (Ben-Yishay et al. 1987, p. 169). The patient is presented with a series of rhythmic tones that he or she must attend to, learn, internalize, and anticipate so that the proper key can be pressed at the right time and the right duration. This stage requires the integration of previous training, including responding to the environment, orienting to external and internal cues, and actively controlling attentional processes.

The developers of the ORM have attempted to validate their program primarily with traumatic brain injury patients. In a group design study, Ben-Yishay et al. (1987) reported that patients displayed significant improvements on several evaluation measures, including Visual Reaction Time (Ben-Yishay et al. 1987), Wechsler Adult Intelligence Scale (WAIS) (Wechsler 1955), Digit Span and Picture Completion, and Picture Description Test (Ben-Yishay et al. 1987). Although the authors reported improvements in overall patient functioning in case study presentations, no controlled studies were cited regarding generalization beyond the neuropsychological tests listed above. The ORM represents a comprehensive and well-designed rehabilitation technique for attention deficits. However, further research is needed to validate training effects and to determine whether generalization occurs. Additionally, future studies should include CVA patients with attention deficits.

Sohlberg and Mateer (1987) also developed a multilevel system to address attention deficits that used modified, commercially available computer programs. Their Attention-Training Program (ATP) primarily addressed aspects of controlled attention including what they describe as focused, sustained, selective, alternating, and divided attention. Several different training tasks were selected from commercially available materials and several were designed specifically for each attentional area. These tasks were introduced in increasing complexity and difficulty as patients' training progressed. For a complete description of their rehabilitation program, refer to *Attention Process Training* (Sohlberg and Mateer 1986).

In their single-subject experimental design study, Sohlberg and Mateer (1987) trained four patients with the ATP. Although they found that their patients displayed significant improvements in attention processes, they reported no consistent gains in visual processing. Additionally, although patients achieved more global rehabilitation goals in vocational and independent living areas, the experimenters indicated that improvements could not be directly attributed to the ATP. More studies are needed that include CVA patients, considering that the Sohlberg and Mateer (1987) study included three traumatic brain injury patients and one aneurysm patient. Additionally, Sohlberg and Mateer (1987) indicated that the effects of the treatment levels could not be individually separated; therefore, studies are needed that isolate and compare the effects of the different training procedures.

In contrast to the ORM and ATP approaches, Wood (1986) presented several single-subject experimental design studies applying behavior modification techniques to the rehabilitation of attentional deficits. In the first study, Wood (1986) demonstrated that reinforcement can improve attentional behavior, as measured by head and eye orientation to a visual stimuli presented by the trainer. Patients in this reinforcement program displayed greater sustained attention compared with baseline.

In the second remediation program, four patients were trained to improve attending to visual and auditory stimuli as measured by frequency of errors. The patients were given positive and negative feedback in addition to rewards or punishments for correct and incorrect responses. Wood (1986) reported that the number of errors decreased for all patients. However, lack of improvement in performance on memory tasks indicates limited generalizability.

Wood (1986) argued that complex machines, computers, or other technological devices may not be necessary when reinforcement techniques improve attention deficits. This idea is important because these devices are often very expensive, which may prohibit their general access by patients who may benefit from treatment. In addition, Wood (1986) stated that the simplicity of the remediation program that uses reinforcement reduces the level of staff skills required to train patients. Because staff members would require less training, more individuals would be qualified and available to train CVA patients.

Webster and Scott (1983) used Meichenbaum's (Meichenbaum and Cameron 1973) self-instructional training (SIT) in the remediation of attention deficits. This training follows the premise that an individual can provide his or her own attentional controls through verbal self-regulation. Training proceeded from repeating step-by-step instructions aloud, to subvocalizing instructions, to private speech. In the Webster and Scott (1983) single-subject design study, the traumatic brain injury patient displayed great improvement in the amount of information recalled, a measure of attention.

In summary, of the several different approaches to the remediation of attentional deficits, ORM is the most comprehensive and well-researched. However, most research has focused on traumatic brain-injury patients, and there appear to be few attention remediation studies that include CVA patients. In addition, much of the published research in the area is limited to case studies and single-subject experimental design studies. Therefore, although some encouraging signs exist regarding the remediation of attentional deficits, much more research is needed in the area.

Perception

Sensation involves the reception of information by the different senses (sight, taste, and so forth), whereas perception involves the active processing of information received through the senses. Perceptual functions are generally associated with the right hemisphere of the brain; in particular, more complex visual perceptual operations (e.g., visual-spatial integration) are believed to occur in the right parietal lobe (Hier et al. 1983; Vallar and Perrani 1986). As defined here, sensory deficits can impair perceptual functioning, but perceptual deficits cannot be solely the result of sensory deficits. For example, cortical blindness, as a result of bilateral occipital lobe infarcts, is considered a sensory and not a perceptual deficit because of pure dysfunction of the sensory system. In comparison, visual-spatial impairments caused by right parietal lobe lesions are considered perceptual in nature because of the processing problems that arise from distortions in the received information, not from dysfunction of the sensory system.

Perceptual deficits.   Impairments in perceptual functioning can be subdivided into three major groups based on their clinical significance: modality-specific perceptual deficits, modality-nonspecific perceptual deficits, and behavioral consequences of perceptual deficits (Bechinger and Tallis 1986). Modality-specific perceptual deficits affect only one sensory system. For example, left visual imperception or neglect involves only the visual system and can lead to the inability to perceive information in the left visual field. An individual with this deficit may have difficulty with reading, writing, scanning, or other tasks that require the visual perception of the whole stimulus field while other systems remain intact.

In contrast, modality-nonspecific perceptual deficits can involve multiple sensory systems including auditory, visual, and somatosensory functions. For example, left hemi-imperception or neglect includes deficits of both the somatosensory and visual systems. Persons with this impairment will have difficulty perceiving physical and visual stimuli on their left side and may not even recognize that the left side is part of their own body. The individual with left hemi-imperception may have difficulty with motor skills such as dressing and walking, as well as with visual skills such as reading, writing, and scanning.

Behavioral consequences of perceptual deficits refer to specific functional impairments that result from one or more perceptual deficits. For example, constructional dyspraxia is a possible behavioral consequence of visual-spatial deficits, visual-perceptual deficits, or visual motor planning and organization deficits, or any combination of the three. A person with constructional dyspraxia may have difficulty manually reproducing visual stimuli, such as a block design or a complex figure, because of problems in the perception of the stimuli, the spatial organization of the information, or the planning of the motor activities necessary to reproduce the stimuli. This category of perceptual deficits represents an attempt to further classify the behavioral consequences that commonly result from one or more perceptual deficits.

The literature indicates that the majority of perceptual recovery occurs within the first 6 months after the CVA (Meerwaldt 1983; Thorngren and Westling 1990). However, many factors can affect the amount and speed of recovery and the patient's overall prognosis. The size of the lesion and the severity of the CVA influence recovery of perceptual functions. For example, Meerwaldt (1983) found a negative correlation between the size of the lesion and speed of recovery. Hier et al. (1983) found that recovery of some perceptual functions was faster with smaller lesions. Levine et al. (1986) found that the size of the lesion helped determine the severity of neglect and degree of improvement after CVA.

The location of the lesion can also affect recovery. Stone et al. (1991) found that visual imperceptions were common to both left-hemisphere (72%) and right-hemisphere (62%) damage 3 days after CVA. However, 3 months after the CVA, they reported that 75% of right-hemisphere CVA patients still experienced visual hemi-imperception compared with only 33% of those with left-hemisphere CVAs. Swindell et al. (1988) found that drawing abilities recovered better for left-hemisphere CVA patients compared with right-hemisphere CVA patients. The importance of perceptual operations, especially visual-perceptual functioning, has been well-documented in research. For example, visual-perceptual functioning in CVA patients has been shown to be related closely to the ability to perform activities of daily living (e.g., personal hygiene, cleaning, cooking) and independent living skills (e.g., mobility, shopping, laundry) (Edmans and Lincoln 1990; Edmans et al. 1991; Titus et al. 1991). Similarly, visual-spatial functions were shown to be important predictors of rehabilitation outcome (Jongbloed 1986; Kaplan and Hier 1982; Kotila et al. 1984). More severe visual-perceptual deficits are associated with poorer functioning in activities of daily living (Jesshope et al. 1991). Therefore, improving visual-perceptual functioning may lead to a better prognosis and a better overall rehabilitation outcome for CVA patients.

Cognitive rehabilitation of perceptual deficits.   Because of the strong relationship between visual-perceptual operations and overall functioning, the majority of the studies examining the cognitive rehabilitation of perception have focused on the remediation of visual-perceptual deficits. Initial cognitive rehabilitation studies of visual-perceptual dysfunction focused on the remediation of scanning deficits in patients with right hemisphere lesions (Carter et al. 1983; Webster et al. 1984; Weinberg et al. 1977, 1979; Young et al. 1983). Aspects of scanning training include: 1) compelling the patient to turn his or her head to the neglected side, 2) anchoring the patient's vision to the neglected side, 3) decreasing the density of stimuli, and 4) pacing the patient's tracking patterns (Gordon et al. 1985; Weinberg et al. 1977).

In the scanning training studies, the trainers used a scanning machine and graded visual material. The scanning machine was a wooden board with two parallel rows of colored lights. These lights could be lit in any order or pattern the experimenters desired. Additionally, another stimulus or "target" could be moved mechanically to any location around the edge of the board. The graded visual material consisted of letters, words, paragraphs, or arithmetic problems.

The first step in training required the patient to learn to locate the stationary target on the scanning board. After the patient had acquired this skill, he or she was trained to track the target as it moved around the board. Once this skill had been mastered, the patient was trained to search systematically from left to right by locating lights as they were lit on the board. To assist in this process, the patient was instructed to "anchor" his or her scan to the far left target.

Anchoring taught patients to begin their search pattern from the far left side, which is often not perceived or is neglected by patients with right-hemisphere injuries. As training progressed, the experimenters used increasingly dimmed lights to improve the patient's perceptual skills.

In conjunction with the scanning training described above, patients practiced with 13 types of graded visual-perception tasks such as reading, writing, and performing paper-and-pencil arithmetic (Weinberg et al. 1977). These stimuli varied in density (distance between targets) and complexity (from large trigrams to *New York Times* print). The number of cues provided in the written materials, such as numbers or anchoring lines, decreased, and the task difficulty increased as training progressed and the patients' abilities improved.

Subjects in an experimental group that involved visual scanning and graded visual materials displayed significantly greater improvements in cancellation tasks and academic skills compared with the improvements of the control group (Weinberg et al. 1977). Furthermore, the largest improvements were observed in the experimental subgroup with the most severe deficits. These results suggested that the cognitive rehabilitation program was better than no treatment or normal recovery and that the largest, treatment-related improvements in scanning abilities occurred with severely impaired individuals with the poorest rehabilitation prognosis.

Weinberg et al. (1979) added somatosensory awareness and size estimation training to their scanning training in another study. To increase the effects of the cognitive remediation program, the experimenters addressed nonvisual awareness issues and visual-spatial functions that were not affected by scanning training alone. Somatosensory training involved the identification of tactile stimulation at various locations on the patient's back. To teach the patient visual-spatial skills, the experimenters had the patient estimate the size of different rods placed on his or her back. To reduce the length of training, letter cancellation tasks were introduced to replace some of the graded visual materials. Cancellation tasks involved locating and crossing out predetermined stimuli (e.g., the letter H) located on a sheet of paper covered with random stimuli. Weinberg et al. (1979) found that their patients showed significantly greater improvements in visual scanning, academic skills, body awareness, and spatial organization than standard rehabilitation control subjects.

Researchers have attempted also to address comprehension problems, disorganization, and visual problem-solving deficits that were still evident in CVA patients after visual scanning training (Weinberg et al. 1982). The treatment program included training patients to impose a system on dispersed meaningful and meaningless stimuli and training patients to systematically appraise visual stimuli. Significant improvements were found in experimental subjects' performance on complex visual-cognitive tasks, such as the WAIS Block Design and Embedded Figures Test, compared with no-treatment control subjects. Block design augments training for patients with left hemi-imperception problems (Young et al. 1983). This task was believed to improve complex visual integration and to increase visual-motor integration compared with occupational therapy alone or to scanning training, letter cancellation training, and occupational therapy.

Despite the initially positive results of earlier studies, some subsequent studies of the cognitive remediation of perceptual deficits have produced less positive findings, especially regarding generalization. Researchers linked the different treatments outlined here in a logical fashion beginning with scanning training, proceeding to somatosensory and size estimation training, and finishing with training in organization and systematic appraisal (Gordon et al. 1985). However, no significant differences were found between experimental and control groups after treatment. Gordon et al. (1985) hypothesized that the combined and abbreviated treatment programs progressed too rapidly for patients to learn and become adequately skilled at each method. The investigators noted that the duration (4 weeks) of the complete treatment package used in this study was equivalent to that of earlier studies using individual treatments.

Subsequent studies attempted to replicate the visual scanning program using single-subject experimental designs to identify and measure individual changes (Gouvier et al. 1984, 1987; Webster et al. 1984). In addition, these researchers added training in a wheelchair obstacle course to examine generalization of training. The combined results indicated that learning occurred in the scanning tasks but that generalization was less clear for wheelchair navigation. Gouvier et al. (1984) found that two patients improved in wheelchair navigation, although Webster et al. (1984) found only one of their three patients showed dramatic improvement in wheelchair navigation. Additionally, Gouvier et al. (1987) stated that measures of reading, writing, and wheelchair navigation during and after training produced inconsistent results for their five patients.

In an attempt to use technology in rehabilitation, Robertson et al. (1988) developed a computer program to present the scanning training tasks that remediate visual neglect. In their single-subject experimental design study they found that patients improved in computer-trained skills. However, the investigators found little generalization to other untrained tasks, suggesting that generalization was limited by the specificity of training materials.

In contrast to cognitive retraining research, some clinicians have promoted stimulus manipulation, which directly modifies environmental or task stimuli to improve the patient's perceptual functioning. Heilman and Watson (1978) found that symptoms of neglect in right-hemisphere CVA patients were reduced when using visual-spatial stimuli (e.g., line orientation) as opposed to verbal stimuli (e.g., words) in cancellation tasks. The authors hypothesized that the use of visual stimuli, as opposed to verbal stimuli, increased the general arousal of the damaged right hemisphere, thereby reducing neglect. However, no direct measures of cortical activity were used in the study, and more research is needed to validate this conclusion.

Riddoch and Humphreys (1983) found that visual cuing can also reduce symptoms of neglect in right-hemisphere CVA patients. They found that cues placed on the contralateral side of a line bisection task improved performance more than cues on the ipsilateral side or on both sides. This improvement was observed when patients were forced to report the left cue. In a related study, Nichelli and Rinaldi (1989) found that cues placed on the contralateral side of the lesion reduced line bisection errors. They also showed that line bisecting errors decreased when the *task* was shifted from the contralateral hemispace to the center and further reduced when the task was shifted to the ipsilateral hemispace. Ishiai et al. (1990) examined the use of numbering during cancellation tasks. They found that when patients were asked to number the lines canceled, the amount of spatial neglect was significantly reduced compared with simply crossing out the lines. These results and the above studies in stimulus manipulation suggest that alterations in task demands and environmental stimuli can reduce visual-perceptual deficits and improve functioning.

Based on the group cognitive retraining studies described above, the cognitive remediation of perceptual deficits has had some early successes, and some of these successes have generalized to real-world applications. Generalization has been demonstrated in reading, writing, and paper-and-pencil math (Weinberg et al. 1977), somatosensory and spatial awareness (Weinberg et al. 1979), comprehension, organization, systematic visual appraisal (Weinberg et al. 1982), and wheelchair navigation (Gouvier et al. 1984). However, other research has resulted in less conclusive results. In a combined treatment approach, Gordon et al. (1985) found no treatment effects compared with control subjects.

Cognitive Rehabilitation for Alzheimer's Disease

Alzheimer's disease is currently classified in the DSM-IV (American Psychiatric Association 1994) under the Axis I cognitive disorders subcategory of dementia. The diagnostic criteria for dementia of the Alzheimer's type listed in the DSM-IV are presented in Table 7–2.

The Consortium to Establish a Registry for Alzheimer's Disease (CERAD) was formed to assist in the development of a standard process for diagnosing the illness. CERAD gathered together a number of clinical and neuropsychological assessment instruments to more reliably diagnose Alzheimer's disease (J. C. Morris et al. 1989). The CERAD battery consists of a dementia rating scale and measures of verbal fluency, naming, mental status, verbal learning, word recall and recognition, and constructional praxis. The purpose of this battery is to give researchers and clinicians around the world the same systematic procedure to diagnose Alzheimer's disease (J. C. Morris et al. 1989).

Table 7–2. Diagnostic criteria for Dementia of the Alzheimer's Type

A. The development of multiple cognitive deficits manifested by both:
  (1) Memory impairment (impaired ability to learn new information or to recall previously learned information)
  (2) One (or more) of the following cognitive disturbances:
      (a) Aphasia (language disturbance)
      (b) Apraxia (impaired ability to carry out motor activities despite intact motor function)
      (c) Agnosia (failure to recognize or identify objects despite intact sensory function)
      (d) Disturbance in executive functioning (e.g., planning, organizing, sequencing, abstracting)
B. The cognitive deficits in Criteria A1 and A2 each cause significant impairment in social or occupational functioning and represent a significant decline from a previous level of functioning.
C. The course is characterized by gradual onset and continuing cognitive decline.
D. The cognitive deficits in Criteria A1 and A2 are not caused by any of the following:
  (1) Other central nervous conditions that cause progressive deficits in memory and cognition (e.g., cerebrovascular disease, Parkinson's disease, Huntington's disease, subdural hematoma, normal-pressure hydrocephalus, brain tumor)
  (2) Systemic conditions that are known to cause dementia (e.g., hypothyroidism, vitamin B_{12} or folic acid deficiency, niacin deficiency, hypercalcemia, neurosyphilis, HIV infection)
  (3) Substance-induced conditions
E. The deficits do not occur exclusively during the course of a delirium.
F. The disturbance is not better accounted for by another Axis I disorder (e.g., major depressive disorder, schizophrenia).

Source. Reprinted with permission from American Psychiatric Association: *Diagnostic and Statistical Manual of Mental Disorders,* 4th Edition. Washington, DC, American Psychiatric Association, 1994, pp 142–143. Copyright 1994, American Psychiatric Association.

The growing consensus is that Alzheimer's disease is a heterogeneous group of disorders (Mayeux et al. 1985). The distinct subtypes of this disorder appear to differ in their rate of the deterioration. For example, some individuals show little functional decline for many years, whereas others rapidly progress to a vegetative state in just a few years. Miller et al. (1991) discuss two possible subgroups, those with early age onset and those with extrapyramidal symptoms. Both subtypes are associated with a more severe course, greater intellectual decline, and a larger number of symptoms. Specific subtypes, however, have not yet been established on a histochemical level (Galasko et al. 1990).

Memory

Memory impairment is usually the first observable symptom of Alzheimer's disease (Chui 1989). For example, Alzheimer's patients often misplace items or forget the names of significant others. As the disease progresses, judgment and reasoning deficits emerge, and eventually, language deficits and apraxia appear. The memory is targeted for early intervention because memory deficits are the first to appear and most other cognitive functions remain intact in the early stages of Alzheimer's disease.

Memory processes.   Information processing theory proposes that memory is divided into two main components: working memory and remote memory (Salmon and Butters 1987). *Working* or *short-term memory* is the hypothetical process in which information is briefly but actively processed or held before encoding. Rehearsing a telephone number before dialing is an example of working memory. Information processing theory also proposes that memory is divided into three primary operations: encoding, storage, and retrieval (Salmon and Butters 1987). For example, if the information is sufficiently rehearsed, it can be encoded or consolidated into remote or long-term memory. In *remote memory,* the information is believed to be organized, categorized, and stored for later use. For example, the telephone number rehearsed earlier can be organized and then stored by individual called, place called, or strictly as a number. Encoding and storage processes are strongly interrelated and, therefore, are difficult to isolate. Encoding processes also vary with the type of information. Evidence suggests that auditory and visual memories are encoded differently (Wilson 1982) and, therefore, may be affected differently by Alzheimer's disease.

Retrieval is the process by which information previously stored in remote memory is brought forth to working memory on demand. Recalling a telephone number and the person called at a later date is an example of retrieval. Theorists have hypothesized that different types of remote memory exist (Cushman and Caplan 1987) and that these types are accessed through retrieval processes. *Semantic memory* (also referred to as declarative or explicit memory) involves the storage of factual information and learned knowledge. This type of memory is illustrated by asking the person to answer the question, "Who was President of the United States during the Civil War?" *Episodic memory* is related to semantic memory but involves personal facts or events directly related to the individual. This type of memory is illustrated by asking the person to answer the question, "What did you do on your vacation?" Procedural or implicit memory involves acquired skills or actions. This type of memory can be inferred from the observation of behaviors or activities such as sewing, cooking, or brushing hair.

Memory deficits.   Every memory component and process can be affected by Alzheimer's disease. Patients may have reductions in the amount of information they can hold within their working memory. Instead of being able to handle seven bits of information (the memory capacity of the average individual), an Alzheimer's patient may be able to handle only one or two bits of information. From the example used earlier, an Alzheimer's patient with working memory deficits may not be able to actively process and remember the seven digits of a telephone number.

Encoding and storage processes can also be disrupted by Alzheimer's disease. Patients may have trouble categorizing and organizing information, or they may have difficulty transferring information from working memory to remote memory. A patient who cannot remember new information regardless of the number of rehearsals may be experiencing either encoding or storage problems, or both. For example, a patient may be able to remember a telephone number while he or she is actively processing it, but once rehearsal stops, the information is lost.

Alzheimer's disease may also result in impairments in retrieval from remote memory. In this situation, information can be encoded and stored, but patients have difficulty accessing that information. For example, a patient is said to be experiencing a retrieval problem when he or she cannot remember a specified word in free recall, but can recognize it when presented with a multiple choice format. The fact that he or she can recognize the information demonstrates that the information was stored somewhere within remote memory.

The extent and severity of memory deficits vary with each individual, and not every memory area is impaired. For example, patients with early Alzheimer's disease often have intact working memory but have problems encoding information into remote memory. Thus, the patient may be able to state his or her physician's name after introduction as long as the patient is rehearsing it. This information will be lost, however, if the patient stops rehearsing or is distracted. Alzheimer's patients also have retrieval problems with information from semantic and episodic stores but commonly have intact procedural memory. They may be unable to recall factual information or personal events, but perform overlearned tasks such as walking, combing hair, or brushing teeth.

As with other cognitive functions, memory operations depend on adequate attentional processes. Often attention deficits appear as memory problems. For example, not being able to attend to stimuli may lead to inadequate or incomplete encoding and storage of information. Therefore, before attempting to remediate apparent memory impairments, trainers should carefully assess the patient neuropsychologically to ensure that the patient's memory problems are not solely the result of attentional disruption.

Cognitive rehabilitation of memory deficits.   A variety of interventions for the remediation of memory impairments have been attempted, including repetition and practice (e.g., rehearsal), strategy learning (e.g., mnemonics and paired associate learning), and external aids (e.g., memory books) (Glisky and Schacter 1986). Although these interventions have been used to treat memory problems resulting from other neurological disorders, the majority of the published research with clinical populations in this area has used Alzheimer's patients.

Repetition and practice techniques are based on the premise that "exercising" a person's memory will improve memory functioning overall. These techniques have received a large amount of research attention and, generally, the results have not been positive. Weingartner et al. (1993) found that repetition exercises did not enhance the memory of words for Alzheimer's patients. Beck et al. (1988) found that memory training improved patients' recall of numbers but not their recall of a story. Little et al. (1987) found that unsystematic rehearsal alone is ineffective in the treatment of memory deficits for Alzheimer's patients. Goldstein et al. (1985) found that rehearsal improved memory for training lists of words and numbers, although generalization did not occur and overall memory function did not improve. The results of these studies suggest that repetition and practice generally do not improve memory. However, on occasions where some minimal improvement is evident, these improvements do not generalize to information other than that specifically used in the training materials.

A notable exception to the findings cited above is a series of studies conducted by Glisky and Schacter (1986, 1987) and Glisky et al. (1986a, 1986b). Although their research does not directly address patients with Alzheimer's disease, their findings are important regarding memory rehabilitation. Glisky and Schacter (1986) acknowledged that repetition and practice is effective only for improving memory of the actual tasks involved in training. They proposed that remediation should focus on the "acquisition of domain-specific knowledge" (p. 58) that is relevant to the patient's impairments (Glisky and Schacter 1986). Instead of teaching random lists of information, they taught memory-impaired patients information that may improve their functioning in particular deficit areas.

In their studies, Glisky et al. demonstrated that patients could learn both simple and complex information related to computer operations, such as computer-related vocabulary and basic computer operations (e.g., running programs, manipulating disk information, and simple programming). Because patients are learning the specific tasks required of them, generalization and overall memory improvements are not required. Applying this concept to Alzheimer's patients, training could involve tasks related to individual deficits rather than abstract and meaningless information such as number lists, stories, or words. Additionally, the acquisition of domain-specific knowledge involves teaching at two levels of processing, semantic and procedural memory. Training at multiple memory levels is believed to enhance encoding and retrieval processes and forms the basis of some of the strategy-learning techniques (e.g., pairing visual images with verbal information).

Strategy learning involves the use of different techniques to improve the encoding and retrieval of information. Some evidence suggests that the encoding and retrieval of information is a greater problem than storage in Alzheimer's disease (Zandi and Woods 1988). For example, memory accuracy is enhanced in Alzheimer's patients when researchers test recognition as opposed to recall of information (Finley et al. 1990; Kopelman 1991; Zandi and Woods 1988). In addition, it is apparent that the different aspects of memory function are affected to varying degrees by Alzheimer's disease. Therefore, a great amount of emphasis has been given to the study of strategy learning and the maximization of intact memory functions.

Mnemonics are memory strategies that encompass a variety of techniques. Mnemonics provide patients with a fixed method of categorizing and organizing new information on more than one cognitive level to assist in the encoding and retrieval of that information. The most common mnemonic technique used with Alzheimer's patients involves the pairing of visual imagery or mental images with other information that is intended to be remembered. For example, name-face associations involve the pairing of names with faces to improve a patient's recall (Backman et al. 1991; Byrd 1990; Hill et al. 1987; Zandi and Woods 1988). These studies found that pairing visual images with other forms of information can improve the patient's recall. In addition to visual imagery, verbal associations were found to improve Alzheimer's patients' recall of object locations (Camp and Stevens 1990).

Other memory improvement strategies include embedded sentences, verbal labeling, and "chunking" information (Parenté and DiCesare 1991). In embedded sentences, seemingly unrelated words are strung together to integrate them into a functional unit, making them easier to remember. For example, *pencil, computer, door, hand, lightbulb, statue,* and *dog* could form the sentence, "When the *lightbulb* over the *computer* broke, the *dog* took the *pencil* out of the *statue's hand* and ran out the *door*." Verbal labeling involves associating the unfamiliar with something familiar. For example, the operating instructions of a facsimile machine may become easier to learn if they are associated with the operations of a photocopier and a telephone. Chunking is a commonly used mnemonic that groups information into a smaller number of bits that are easier to remember. Telephone numbers represent a chunking process in which 10 individual numbers are chunked into two groups of three and one group of four (e.g., 123-456-7890) to improve recall. It is important to note that the acquisition of any of the mnemonic techniques cited above requires repetition and practice.

Although mnemonic techniques have met with some initial success (Byrd 1990; Hill et al. 1987; Zandi and Woods 1988), some criticisms have been raised (Glisky and Schacter 1986; Goldstein et al. 1985). None of the studies described above have demonstrated any generalization of memory improvements to other areas. Similar to the more direct repetition and practice studies, the effects of mnemonic training appear to be specific to the area trained. Mnemonic techniques also require effort by the individual; the strategy has to be remembered and then applied in the appropriate situation. Learning the mnemonic technique can be a difficult process. This effort, which is inconsequential for a healthy individual, is taxing for someone who is cognitively impaired. Additionally, as the disease process progresses, patients will experience further losses in executive function or will be unable to recognize their memory deficits, both of which can impair their ability to use these effortful techniques in appropriate situations. These demands may limit the usefulness of this technique for patients with dementia (Glisky and Schacter 1986).

Retrieval practice, another memory improvement strategy, is based on the premise that repeatedly recalling recently learned material will improve overall retrieval functioning. Along with practice, researchers have employed spaced retrieval, or increasing intervals between recall, to improve long-term retention (Camp and Stevens 1990) and the pairing of multiple forms of information (similar to mnemonics) to improve encoding and retrieval. This combined strategy has met with some success with Alzheimer's patients (Camp 1989; Camp and Stevens 1990). Camp (1989) found that two patients were able to learn the associations between the names and photographs of staff persons. In another study, patient memory was improved by verbally associating the name of objects with the names of different locations (Camp and Stevens 1990). The primary limitations of retrieval practice is that treatment generalization and improvement in overall retrieval processes have yet to be demonstrated.

External aids have been proposed as a method for improving the memory of Alzheimer's patients. This approach acknowledges that memory deficits cannot be directly remediated and, therefore, require external compensatory interventions. Bourgeois (1990) found that conversation skills of Alzheimer's patients could be improved with external memory aids. Hanley (1981) placed signs around a nursing home ward to prompt the patients' memory of objects and locations. These prompts proved successful in decreasing disorientation on the ward. Glisky et al. (1986a, 1986b) have proposed that computers serve as external memory aids. In previous research, they have demonstrated that some memory-impaired patients can learn the skills necessary to operate computers. Sohlberg and Mateer (1989) hypothesized that memory books in conjunction with behavioral training could improve adaptive skills. A memory book contains information pertinent to the individual. Sohlberg and Mateer (1989) presented a case study in which a head injury patient with severe memory and other cognitive impairments could increase his independence and work-related skills through behavioral training and use of a memory book.

Although relatively simple compared with other memory training programs, these external memory aids are useful because they target behaviors that may improve patients' adaptive functioning. For example, a memory book can remind a person of any number of critical details including his or her daily activities, work tasks and responsibilities, or medication schedule. Unfortunately, only case studies have been presented, and more research is needed to demonstrate the effectiveness of these aids. In addition, because of the severe impairments that Alzheimer's patients experience in other cognitive areas, their ability to learn and appropriately use this strategy is questionable. This strategy, described as "remembering to remember," or metamemory, is an important prerequisite for using an external memory aid, and metamemory has been shown to be impaired in Alzheimer's patients (R. G. Morris and Kopelman 1986).

Summary

The development of cognitive rehabilitation strategies geared toward the adaptation and remediation of disorders affecting cognitive function in older adults is extremely critical. Much of the research in this area has been devoted to the rehabilitation of specific postCVA deficits, including language, attention, perceptual functioning, and memory.

Two distinct approaches are currently used in language rehabilitation: the classical and the neurolinguistic models. The classical approach focuses on restoring language expression using techniques such as repetition, cueing, or answering dichotomous questions. The neurolinguistic model addresses the important issue of language comprehension by helping patients decipher the contextual meaning of language. However, the effectiveness of speech therapy in language rehabilitation has not yet been conclusively established. Future studies must use larger and more homogenous groups of patients with clearly defined lesions and well-characterized language deficits that have been determined during a formal assessment.

Disorders affecting attentional processes are a major rehabilitation concern because of the secondary deficits that can be produced in memory, learning, and problem solving. Impairments in alertness, selective attention, and vigilance are commonly seen in CVA and the latter stages of Alzheimer's disease. Among the different approaches reviewed in this chapter, ORM seems to be the most comprehensive and promising, although much of the research in this area has been limited to case studies and single-subject experimental design studies with traumatic brain injury patients. Further controlled research with other clinical populations, such as CVA and Alzheimer's patients, will be needed before the usefulness of cognitive rehabilitation techniques for attentional disorders can be established.

The majority of studies examining the cognitive rehabilitation of perceptual deficits in CVA patients has focused on the remediation of problems regarding visual scanning, somatosensory awareness, comprehension, disorganization, and visual problem solving. Despite initially positive results, subsequent controlled studies have produced equivocal results, especially regarding generalization of improvement outside of the laboratory.

Studies in rehabilitation of patients with Alzheimer's disease have emphasized the remediation of memory impairment through the use of rehearsal techniques, strategy learning (mnemonics), and external aids. However, consistent improvement in overall memory function beyond the specific domain being addressed has not been demonstrated. Considering the fact that rehabilitation strategies will not be able to reverse the neuronal damage that underlies degenerative disorders in older adults, external memory aids may ultimately prove to be the most effective of the rehabilitation aids used in treating Alzheimer's patients.

References

American Psychiatric Association: Diagnostic and Statistical Manual of Mental Disorders, 4th Edition. Washington, DC, American Psychiatric Association, 1994

Backman L, Josephsson S, Herlitz A, et al: The generalizability of training gains in dementia: effects of an imagery-based mnemonic on face-name retention duration. Psychol Aging 6:489–492, 1991

Basso A: Approaches to neuropsychological rehabilitation: language disorders, in Neuropsychological Rehabilitation. Edited by Meier M, Benton A, Diller L. New York, Guilford, 1987, pp 294–314

Bechinger D, Tallis R: Perceptual disorders in neurological diseases, I: British Journal of Occupational Therapy 49:282–284, 1986

Beck C, Heacock P, Mercer S, et al: The impact of cognitive skills remediation training on persons with Alzheimer's disease or mixed dementia. J Geriatr Psychiatry 21:73–88, 1988

Ben-Yishay Y, Piasetsky EB, Rattok J: A systematic method for ameliorating disorders in basic attention, in Neuropsychological Rehabilitation. Edited by Meier M, Benton A, Diller L. New York, Guilford, 1987, pp 165–181

Bourgeois MS: Enhancing conversation skills in patients with Alzheimer's disease using a prosthetic memory aid. J Appl Behav Anal 23:29–42, 1990

Byrd M: The use of visual imagery as a mnemonic device for healthy elderly and Alzheimer's disease patients. The American Journal of Alzheimer's Care and Related Disorders and Research 5:10–15, 1990

Camp CJ: Facilitation of new learning in Alzheimer's disease, in Memory and Aging: Theory, Research, and Practice. Edited by Gilmore G, Whitehouse P, Wykle M. New York, Springer, 1989, pp 212–225

Camp CJ, Stevens AB: Spaced-retrieval: a memory intervention for dementia of the Alzheimer's type (DAT). Clin Gerontol 10:58–60, 1990

Carter LT, Howard BE, O'Neil WA: Effectiveness of cognitive skill remediation in acute stroke patients. Am J Occup Ther 37:320–326, 1983

Chui HC: Dementia: a review emphasizing clinicopathologic correlation and brain-behavior relationships. Arch Neurol 46:806–814, 1989

Cushman L, Caplan B: Multiple memory systems: evidence from stroke. Percept Mot Skills 64:571–577, 1987

David R, Enderby P, Bainton D: Treatment of acquired aphasia: speech therapists and volunteers compared. J Neurol 45:957–961, 1982

de Pedro-Cuesta J, Widen-Holmqvist L, Bach-y-Rita P: Evaluation of stroke rehabilitation by randomized controlled studies: a review. Acta Neurol Scand 86:433–439, 1992

Edmans JA, Lincoln NB: The relation between perceptual deficits after stroke and independence in activities of daily living. British Journal of Occupational Therapy 53:139–142, 1990

Edmans JA, Towle D, Lincoln NB: The recovery of perceptual problems after stroke and the impact on daily life. Clinical Rehabilitation 5:301–309, 1991

Finley GE, Sharp T, Agramonte R: Recall and recognition memory for remotely acquired information in dementia patients. J Genet Psychol 151:267–268, 1990

Galasko D, Kwo on Yuen PF, Klauber MR, et al: Neurological findings in Alzheimer's disease and normal aging. Arch Neurol 47:625–627, 1990

Glisky EL, Schacter DL: Remediation of organic memory disorders: current status and future prospects. Journal of Head Trauma Rehabilitation 1: 54–63, 1986

Glisky EL, Schacter DL: Acquisition of domain-specific knowledge in organic amnesia: training for computer-related work. Neuropsychologia 25: 893–906, 1987

Glisky EL, Schacter DL, Tulving E: Computer learning by memory-impaired patients: acquisition and retention of complex knowledge. Neuropsychologia 24:313–328, 1986a

Glisky EL, Schacter DL, Tulving E: Learning and retention of computer-related vocabulary in memory-impaired patients: method of vanishing cues. J Clin Exp Neuropsychol 8:292–312, 1986b

Goldstein G, Ryan C, Turner SM, et al: Three methods of memory training for severely amnestic patients. Behav Modif 9:357–373, 1985

Goodglass H, Kaplan E: The Assessment of Aphasia and Related Disorders. Philadelphia, PA, Lea & Febiger, 1983

Gordon W, Hibbard M, Egelko S, et al: Perceptual remediation in patients with right brain damage: a comprehensive program. Arch Phys Med Rehabil 66:353–359, 1985

Gouvier WD, Cottam G, Webster JS, et al: Behavioral interventions with CVA patients for improving wheelchair navigation. International Journal of Clinical Neuropsychology 6:186–190, 1984

Gouvier WD, Bua BG, Blanton PD, et al: Behavioral changes following visual scanning training: observations of five cases. International Journal of Clinical Neuropsychology 9:74–80, 1987

Hanley IG: The use of signposts and active training to modify ward disorientation in elderly patients. J Behav Ther Exp Psychiatry 12:241–247, 1981

Harrington R: Communication for the aphasic stroke patient: assessment and therapy. J Am Geriatr Soc 23:254–257, 1975

Hartman J, Landau WM: Comparison of formal language therapy with supportive counseling for aphasia caused by acute vascular accident. Arch Neurol 44:646–649, 1987

Heilman KM, Watson RT: Changes in the symptoms of neglect induced by changing task strategy. Arch Neurol 35:47–49, 1978

Henley S, Pettit S, Todd-Pokropek A, et al: Who goes home? Predictive factors in stroke recovery. J Neurol Neurosurg Psychiatry 48:1–6, 1985

Hier DB, Mondlock J, Caplan LR: Recovery of behavioral abnormalities after right hemisphere CVA. Neurology 33:345–350, 1983

Hill RD, Evankovich KD, Sheikh JI, et al: Imagery mnemonics training in a patient with primary degenerative dementia. Psychol Aging 2:204–205, 1987

Ishiai S, Sugishita M, Odajima N, et al: Improvement of unilateral spatial neglect with numbering. Neurology 40:1395–1398, 1990

Jesshope HJ, Clark MS, Smith DS: The Rivermead Perceptual Assessment Battery: its application to stroke patients and relationship with function. Clinical Rehabilitation 5:115–122, 1991

Jongbloed L: Prediction of function after stroke: a critical review. Stroke 17: 765–776, 1986

Kaplan J, Hier DB: Visuospatial deficits after right hemisphere stroke. Am J Occup Ther 36:314–321, 1982

Kertesz A: The Western Aphasia Battery. London, Ontario, University of Western Ontario, 1980

Kopelman MD: Frontal dysfunction and memory deficits in the alcoholic Korsakoff syndrome and Alzheimer's type dementia. Brain 114:117–137, 1991

Kotila M, Waltimo O, Miemi M, et al: The profile of recovery from stroke and factors influencing outcome. Stroke 15:1039–1044, 1984

Leske MC: Prevalence estimates of communication disorders in the United States: language, hearing, and vestibular disorders. ASHA 23:229–237, 1981

Levine DN, Warach JD, Benowitz L, et al: Left spatial neglect: effects of lesion size and premorbid brain atrophy on severity and recovery following right cerebral infarction. Neurology 36:362–366, 1986

Lezak MD: Neuropsychological Assessment, 3rd Edition. New York, Oxford University Press, 1995

Lincoln NB, McGuirk E, Mulley GP, et al: Effectiveness of speech therapy for aphasia patients: a randomized controlled trial. Lancet 1:1197–1200, 1984

Little A, Hemsley D, Bergmann K, et al: Comparison of the sensitivity of three instruments for the detection of cognitive decline in elderly living at home. Br J Psychiatry 150:808–814, 1987

Loughery L: The effects of two teaching techniques on recognition and use of function words by aphasic stroke patients. Rehabil Nurs 17:134–137, 1992

Luria AR: Traumatic Aphasia. The Hague, Mouton Press, 1970

Mayeux R, Kandel ER: Disorders of language: the aphasias, in Principles of Neuroscience, 3rd Edition. Edited by Kandel ER, Schwartz JH, Jessell TM. Norwalk, CT, Appleton & Lange, 1991, pp 839–851

Mayeux R, Stern Y, Sano M: Heterogeneity and prognosis in dementia of the Alzheimer's type. Bull Clin Neurosci 50:7–10, 1985

McGovern PG, Burke GL, Sprafka JM, et al: Trends in mortality, morbidity, and risk factor levels for stroke from 1960 through 1990: the Minnesota heart survey. JAMA 268:753–759, 1992

Meerwaldt JD: Spatial disorientation in right-hemisphere infarction: a study of speed of recovery. J Neurol Neurosurg Psychiatry 46:426–429, 1983

Meichenbaum D, Cameron R: Training schizophrenics to talk to themselves: a means of developing attentional controls. Behavior Therapy 4:515–534, 1973

Meikle M, Wechsler E, Tupper A, et al: Comparative trial of volunteer and professional treatments of dysphasia after stroke. BMJ 2:87–89, 1979

Miller TP, Tinklenberg JR, Brooks JO III, et al: Cognitive decline in patients with Alzheimer's disease: differences in patients with and without extrapyramidal signs. Alzheimer Dis Assoc Disord 5:251–256, 1991

Moody EJ: Single case study: sign language acquisition by a global aphasic. J Nerv Ment Dis 170:113–116, 1982

Morris JC, Heyman A, Mohs RC, et al: The Consortium to Establish a Registry for Alzheimer's Disease (CERAD), I: clinical and neuropsychological assessment of Alzheimer's disease. Neurology 39:1159–1165, 1989

Morris RG, Kopelman MD: The memory deficits in Alzheimer-type dementia: a review. Q J Exp Psychol [A] 38:575–602, 1986

National Center for Health Statistics: Advance report of final mortality statistics 1986. Mon Vital Stat Rep 40 (suppl 2):1–55, 1992

Nichelli P, Rinaldi M: Selective spatial attention and length representation in normal patients and in patients with unilateral spatial neglect. Brain Cogn 9:57–70, 1989

Parenté R, DiCesare A: Retraining memory: theory, evaluation, and applications, in Cognitive Rehabilitation for Persons with Traumatic Brain Injury. Edited by Kreutzer JS, Wehman PH. Baltimore, MD, Brookes, 1991, pp 147–162

Poeck K, Huber W, Willmes K: Outcome of intensive language treatment in aphasia. J Speech Hear Disord 54:471–479, 1989

Posner MI, Rafal RD: Cognitive theories of attention and the rehabilitation of attentional deficits, in Neuropsychological Rehabilitation. Edited by Meier M, Benton A, Diller L. New York, Guilford, 1987, pp 182–201

Reitan RM, Wolfson D: The Halstead-Reitan Neuropsychological Test Battery Theory and Clinical Interpretation. Tucson, Arizona, Neuropsych Press, 1993

Riddoch MJ, Humphreys GW: The effect of cuing on unilateral neglect. Neuropsychologia 21:589–599, 1983

Robertson I, Gray J, McKenzie S: Microcomputer-based cognitive rehabilitation of visual neglect: three multiple-baseline single-case studies. Brain Inj 2:151–163, 1988

Sacco RL, Wolf PA, Kannel WB, et al: Survival and recurrence following stroke: the Framingham study. Stroke 13:290–295, 1982

Salmon DP, Butters N: Recent developments in learning and memory: implications for the rehabilitation of the amnesic patient, in Neuropsychological Rehabilitation. Edited by Meier M, Benton A, Diller L. New York, Guilford, 1987, pp 280–293

Sarno MT: Preliminary findings in a study of age, linguistic evolution and quality of life in recovery from aphasia. Scand J Rehabil Med 26 (suppl):43–59, 1992

Sohlberg MM, Mateer CA: Attention Process Training. Puyallup, WA, Center for Cognitive Rehabilitation, 1986

Sohlberg MM, Mateer CA: Effectiveness of an attention-training program. J Clin Exp Neuropsychol 9:117–130, 1987

Sohlberg MM, Mateer CA: Training use of compensatory memory books: a three stage behavioral approach. J Clin Exp Neuropsychol 11:871–891, 1989

Sparks R, Albert ML, Helm N: Aphasia rehabilitation resulting from melodic intonation therapy. Cortex 10:303–316, 1974

Stone SP, Wilson B, Wroot A, et al: The assessment of visuospatial neglect after acute stroke. J Neurol Neurosurg Psychiatry 54:345–350, 1991

Stuss DT, Crow CA, Hetherington CR: "No longer Gage": frontal lobe dysfunction and emotional change. J Consult Clin Psychol 60:349–359, 1992

Swindell CS, Holland AL, Fromm D, et al: Characteristics of recovery of drawing ability in left and right brain-damaged patients. Brain Cogn 7:16–30, 1988

Thorngren M, Westling B: Rehabilitation and achieved health quality after stroke: a population-based study of 258 hospitalized cases followed for one year. Acta Neurol Scand 82:374–380, 1990

Titus MN, Gall NG, Yerxa EJ, et al: Correlation of perceptual performance and activities of daily living in stroke patients. Am J Occup Ther 45:410–418, 1991

U.S. Bureau of the Census: Projections of the United States by age, sex, and race: 1988 to 2080, in Current Population Reports, Population Estimates, and Projections. Washington, DC, U.S. Bureau of the Census, 1989

U.S. Department of Health and Human Services: Healthy People 2000: National Health Promotion and Disease Prevention Objectives. Washington, DC, U.S. Department of Health and Human Services, 1990

Vallar G, Perrani D: The anatomy of unilateral neglect after right-hemisphere stroke lesions: a clinical/CT-scan correlation study in man. Neuropsychologia 24:609–622, 1986

Van Eeckhout P, Horando C, Bhatt, et al: De la T.M.R. et de sa pratique. Reeducation Orthophonique 21:305–316, 1983

Weber AM: A practical clinical approach to understanding and treating attentional problems. Journal of Head Trauma Rehabilitation 5:73–85, 1990

Webster JS, Scott RR: The effects of self-instructional training on attentional deficits following head injury. Clinical Neuropsychology 5:69–74, 1983

Webster JS, Jones S, Blanton P, et al: Visual scanning training with stroke patients. Behavior Therapy 15:129–143, 1984

Wechsler D: Manual for Wechsler Adult Intelligence Scale (WAIS). New York, The Psychological Corporation, 1955

Weinberg J, Diller L, Gordon WA, et al: Visual scanning training effect on reading-related tasks in acquired right brain damage. Arch Phys Med Rehabil 58:479–486, 1977

Weinberg J, Diller L, Gordon WA, et al: Training sensory awareness and spatial organization in people with right brain damage. Arch Phys Med Rehabil 60:491–496, 1979

Weinberg J, Piasetsky E, Diller L, et al: Treating perceptual organizational deficits in nonneglecting RBD stroke patients. J Clin Neuropsychol 4:59–75, 1982

Weingartner H, Eckardt M, Grafman J, et al: The effects of repetition on memory performance in cognitively impaired patients. Neuropsychology 7:385–395, 1993

Wertz RT, Weiss DC, Aten JL, et al: Comparison of clinic, home, and deferred language treatment for aphasia: a Veterans Administration cooperative study. Arch Neurol 43:653–658, 1986

Wilson B: Success and failure in memory training following a cerebral vascular accident. Cortex 18:581–594, 1982

Wood RL: Rehabilitation of patients with disorders of attention. Journal of Head Trauma Rehabilitation 1:43–53, 1986

Young GC, Collins D, Hren M: Effect of pairing scanning training with block design training in the remediation of perceptual problems in left hemiplegics. J Clin Neuropsychol 5:201–212, 1983

Zandi T, Woods S: Alzheimer's memory strategies. The American Journal of Alzheimer's Care and Related Disorders and Research 3:7–11, 1988

Chapter 8

Cognitive Rehabilitation After Traumatic Brain Injury

George P. Prigatano, Ph.D., Elizabeth L. Glisky, Ph.D., and Pamela S. Klonoff, Ph.D.

W hen external forces are applied to an individual's cranium with such impact that the individual's brain is disturbed and permanently damaged, the question naturally arises: Can anything be done to restore impaired brain function and thereby rehabilitate the individual? This question obviously is important for the patient who has suffered brain damage, the family that cares for that patient, and rehabilitation therapists of various disciplines. It also is important for psychologists and psychiatrists who may work as part of the patient's treatment team.

Although the terms *cognitive retraining* and *cognitive rehabilitation* have been used to note different activities (Berrol 1990), the two terms are used interchangeably in this chapter. Elsewhere, the concept of cognitive rehabilitation has been put into historical perspective (Prigatano et al. 1986), and guidelines for working with traumatically brain injured (TBI) patients from a cognitive rehabilitation point of view have been suggested (Prigatano 1987). In this chapter, we attempt to reconsider the concept of cognitive rehabilitation from both a "specific" and "broad" point of view. The specific problem of memory disorder, which is quite common following significant TBI (Levin et al. 1990), is considered in light of the theoretical underpinnings of cognitive rehabilitation and the empirical evidence in favor of certain forms of retraining. Discussion of these issues may help shed light on how to proceed effectively in rehabilitation following TBI.

At a broader level: What can practically be done to help TBI patients understand their higher cerebral deficits and make a reasonable psychosocial adjustment in the face of permanent residual neurological and neuropsychological disturbances? Does cognitive rehabilitation in any way fit into this process? We address this question in the second portion of the chapter.

A Clinically Relevant Historical Observation

When faced with young adult TBI patients who are referred for "cognitive rehabilitation," one is often impressed with the variability of symptoms and the variability of the degree of neuropsychological impairments (Ben-Yishay and Prigatano 1990). Despite the nature and severity of the problems, however, one is also impressed that the patient can learn to improve performance on some specific tasks, even though underlying (hypothesized) cerebral functions may not be substantially improved with time and/or training.

In 1938, Karl S. Lashley (1938) pointed this out in the second John Hughlings Jackson lecture at the Montreal Neurological Institute. His lecture was entitled, "Factors Limiting Recovery After Central Nervous Lesions." He noted a striking difference between "the acquisition of specific associations and of general capacities" (p. 747). For example, an animal may be retrained to learn certain experimental tasks, but the underlying capacity referred to as "memory" appeared permanently damaged despite the passage of time or various "training procedures."

This presents perhaps the central problem faced when attempting cognitive rehabilitation. Moreover, even when a specific memory deficit becomes the focus of rehabilitation activities, seldom is there a single cognitive impairment present. In fact, one is impressed with the wide variety of cognitive disturbances not to mention emotional and motivational impairments in TBI patients (Prigatano 1992). Although there is no definitive list that documents all relevant changes in higher cerebral functioning associated with TBI, several authors have attempted to describe common cognitive and behavioral disturbances and their associated psychosocial consequences (Ben-Yishay and Prigatano 1990; Brooks 1990; Prigatano and Fordyce 1986). Table 8–1 summarizes many of these problems. Memory disturbances and speed of information processing deficits are perhaps the most common cognitive disturbances associated with this form of brain dysfunction in young adults (Levin et al. 1990). Also present are subclinical language disturbances, which are frequently documented when measuring rapid word retrieval and confrontation naming. There is also evidence of tangentiality of thought expressed in free speech (Prigatano et al. 1986).

Lack of insight into residual neuropsychological deficits and their social impact is common in this patient group (Prigatano 1991). Finally, impairments in various aspects of thinking and reasoning are noted, particularly the problem of "integrating" information in the appropriate sequence and/or in the most logical manner.

For the purposes of this chapter, however, we will begin by focusing on the literature dealing with cognitive rehabilitation for memory disorders.

Table 8–1.   Some common sequelae of moderate and severe brain damage

Assumed generic deficits	Clinical variants
Disturbances in the balance between excitatory and inhibitory processes	a. Adynamic or impulse-control problems b. Reduced stamina and/or energy levels c. Organically based tendencies to "flood" emotionally, even when engaged in emotionally "neutral" (i.e., cognitive or problem-solving) tasks d. Lowered tolerance for frustration and/or "irritability"
Disturbances in basic attentional functions	a. Suboptimal alertness and/or arousal b. Inadequate focusing of attention and/or c. Inadequate concentration (i.e., ability to sustain train of thought) d. Psychomotor impersistence
Impaired memory functions	a. Problems in registering and coding, hence, in the acquisition and retention of new verbal or nonverbal information b. Problems in the retrieval (free recall; cued or context-bound recall; recall by recognition) of newly acquired or old verbal or nonverbal information
Impaired "integrative" functions	Problems in the adequate or time-efficient execution of various perceptual-motor-spatial-sequential tasks
Impaired speed of information processing	Impaired or slowed-down sensory-motor skills (i.e., disrupted "kinetic melodies" and/or habituated functional "algorithms")
Impaired language and communications skills	a. Problems in comprehension of word meaning or "labeling" (i.e., word finding) in oral communications b. Impaired academic skills (reading, spelling, writing, arithmetic) c. Impaired ability to "stick" to the topic and tendency to become fragmented in free speech
Thinking disorders	a. Problems in convergent reasoning (e.g., abstracting the core or main idea)

(continued)

Table 8–1.   Some common sequelae of moderate and severe brain damage *(continued)*

Assumed generic deficits	Clinical variants
	b. Problems in divergent reasoning (e.g., ability to flexibly shift one's perspective and consider alternatives)
	c. Problems in the area of "executive functions" (e.g., ability to plan, prioritize, formulate "action plans"; implement, self-monitor, and self-correct actions; and evaluate results)
Inadequate awareness	a. Problems related to unrealistic expectations* concerning the recovery of functions and the possibility and/or prospect of resuming one's preinjury lifestyle
	b. Problems in assessing the severity of one's deficits (i.e., understanding their implications)
	c. Problems related to poor compliance in treatments and/or resistance to inputs/ guidance by rehabilitation professionals
Reactive affective responses	a. Agitation and/or depression in response to perceived "losses"
	b. Poor morale and/or sense of "hopelessness" regarding the future
Damaged self-esteem and "ego-identity"	Low self-esteem and impaired sense of "self" (i.e., viewing oneself as "diminished" or "devalued" by the injury); inability to deal with/accept the situation with a measure of "calm resignation"; inability to find any solace in present life

Note.   Naturally, unrealistic expectations or resistance to rehabilitation can be caused by purely psychological factors (e.g., "denial") as well. In the traumatically head-injured person, however, the underlying causes very frequently are caused by interactions between organic and psychogenic factors.

Source.   Reprinted with permission from Ben-Yishay Y, Prigatano GP: "Cognitive Remediation," in *Rehabilitation of the Adult and Child With Traumatic Brain Injury.* Edited by Rosenthal M, Griffith ER, Bond MR, et al. Philadelphia, PA, FA Davis, 1990, p. 399.

Cognitive Rehabilitation for Memory Impairments

As we noted earlier, an impaired ability to remember recent events and acquire new information is one of the most prevalent and debilitating consequences of TBI. The extent of memory deficit usually is related to the severity of brain trauma (Bond 1986; Van Zomeren and Van Den Berg 1985); the impact of the deficit may lead to considerable restriction of patients' daily life activities. In the context of rehabilitation, TBI patients may forget their therapy sessions and/or the content or purpose of therapy—and consequently question why they are in need of rehabilitation.

Theories of Rehabilitation

Cognitive rehabilitation for specific impairments generally has focused on one of two goals: repairing damaged cognitive processes or alleviating functional disabilities resulting from brain damage (Harris 1984; Howard and Patterson 1989; Luria 1948/1963; Miller 1978; Rothi and Horner 1983; Schacter and Glisky 1986). The former approach assumes that patients can reestablish impaired *abilities*, thereby reattaining functional competence and accomplishing the goal of mitigating impairments. The latter approach does not necessarily presuppose that patients' damaged processes will be repaired; it focuses instead on directly affecting functional behaviors or *performance*.

With regard to memory disorders, rehabilitation theories and the treatment methods that have evolved from those theories implicitly emphasize either ability or performance as the target of treatment. Although a comprehensive neuropsychological theory of rehabilitation ultimately must address not only the ability/performance distinction but also the relationship between cognitive and neural mechanisms (see Caramazza 1989), most theories of memory rehabilitation have been formulated at only one level of analysis. In the discussion to follow, we adopt a primarily cognitive perspective, although we note behavioral and neural implications when appropriate. We outline three theories of memory rehabilitation: One proposes restoration of function, one focuses on compensation for lost function, and one suggests the substitution of intact functions for damaged ones.

Restoration of function.   The notion of restoration of function generally implies that with appropriate treatment, patients' cognitive abilities or processes can be restored close to premorbid levels. This theory suggests that memory processes that are damaged or lost through injury can be repaired so that they function at pre-TBI levels.

From this perspective, rehabilitation involves the activation or stimulation of damaged mechanisms through extensive exercise and relearning or retraining of memory skills and strategies presumed to have been intact before trauma. Psychologists frequently advocate interventions "that place demands on the brain to use the disrupted processes . . . so that continued stimulation and activation of the objective cognitive processes can occur" (Sohlberg and Mateer 1989, p. 24). This view also entails an expectation that treatment may effect neural changes, speeding spontaneous recovery (Rothi and Horner 1983), or that other undamaged brain structures may assume the roles of lesioned areas (Luria 1948/1963).

Compensation for lost function.   An alternative theory of rehabilitation assumes that damaged cognitive or neural mechanisms cannot be restored and that the appropriate focus of rehabilitation therefore involves functional outcome. This framework emphasizes improving patients' memory performance or behavior rather than restoring their memory ability.

Based on the assumption that normal memory processes cannot be reactivated, therapists direct their rehabilitation efforts toward enabling impaired individuals to use compensatory devices to function more effectively in everyday life (Glisky and Schacter 1989b; Harris 1984; Wilson and Moffat 1984). In this context, behavioral rehabilitation may be accomplished without the restoration of cognitive or neural function. Psychologists most often adopt this approach, which usually is associated with the use of external aids or other environmental supports, when brain damage is extensive and memory deficit is severe (Kirsch et al. 1987).

Substitution of intact functions.   A third theory of rehabilitation accepts the proposition that damaged cognitive mechanisms that normally are involved in memory cannot be restored but proposes that patients can exploit other *intact* functions that are not normally used in the performance of memory tasks (Luria 1948/1963; Miller 1978). Although the ultimate goal in this approach emphasizes behavioral outcome, rehabilitation focuses at a cognitive level. This approach further assumes that the reconstitution of cognitive structures will be accompanied by a corresponding reorganization of neuronal structures (Luria 1948/1963; Rothi and Horner 1983).

Rehabilitation Methods

Each of the three theories of memory rehabilitation discussed earlier is associated with a number of rehabilitation techniques. In this section, we review those methods, along with empirical evidence concerning their efficacy.

Exercises and drills.   Exercise and drill therapies have been the most prevalent rehabilitation techniques for the restoration of memory. In many rehabilitation settings, patients spend hours trying to remember arbitrary lists of words, pictures, digits, locations, and shapes (Harris and Sunderland 1981). Such treatment may help patients to learn specific words, pictures, and so forth; there is no evidence, however, that such exercises improve memory in any general sense. That is, patients are no more likely to show improved memory performance on a new set of items than they were before treatment (Berg et al. 1991; Godfrey and Knight 1985; Schacter and Glisky 1986).

Researchers also have failed to demonstrate that non-TBI subjects derive general mnemonic benefits from practice. For example, after months of practice, a college student was able to increase the number of digits he could recall in order immediately after presentation from 7 to 80 digits; his ability to recall letters, however, remained unchanged (Chase and Ericcson 1981). Practice had enabled him to develop a complex system of codes for remembering numbers, but the strategy did not generalize to other materials. As William James hypothesized more than a hundred years ago, practice can affect "the retention of particular things" but has no bearing on "general physiological retentiveness" (James 1890, p. 665).

Mnemonic strategies.   Rehabilitation professionals have devoted an extensive amount of energy to training memory-impaired patients in the use of mnemonic strategies such as visual imagery or semantic elaboration (Glisky and Schacter 1989b); the results, however, have been variable and, for the most part, disappointing. Although mildly impaired patients are able to learn and use strategies to acquire specific pieces of information (Cermak 1975; Wilson 1987), there is little evidence that such training generalizes to new information or that subjects use such strategies spontaneously in everyday life (Cermak 1975; Crovitz et al. 1979; Wilson 1981; but see Berg et al. 1991). Mnemonic training typically has been confined to the learning of word lists or paired associates (e.g., Cermak 1975; Crovitz 1979; Kovner et al. 1985; Lewinsohn et al. 1977); the presumed goal of such interventions has been the restoration or reacquisition of memory processes or skills impaired by trauma. Researchers have not found generalization beyond the training materials, however; there is therefore no evidence for general restoration of function.

On the other hand, mnemonic strategies may be beneficial to the extent that they can help a patient acquire specific useful information, such as the names of people in the individual's environment (Glasgow et al. 1977; Wilson 1982). In this case, remediation is directed toward optimizing the patient's use of residual skills to achieve a functional outcome (Prigatano 1990)—a notion consistent with the finding that mnemonic strategies are most effective when used with high-functioning patients who have suffered mild-to-moderate brain injuries.

Often, however, rehabilitation professionals use these techniques with the implicit hope that continued exercise of residual processes will lead to some general memory improvement—perhaps via regeneration of neural structures or reorganization of other, undamaged parts of the brain (Luria 1948/1963). Although researchers increasingly have focused on the possibility of recovery of anatomical or physiological function following injury (Meier et al. 1987), such research has not yet provided convincing evidence of changes in neural structures beyond the stage of spontaneous recovery.

External aids.   Because many internal strategies are ineffective in achieving long-term benefits for TBI patients, many rehabilitation professionals have turned to the development and use of external aids in attempting to help these patients compensate for lost memory function and achieve meaningful behavioral outcomes (Harris 1984; Wilson and Moffat 1984). These aids include relatively simple environmental restructurings—for example, labels on cupboards and instructions on appliances—as well as aids that require more active participation by the individual, such as alarm watches and notebooks. For the most part, patients have been able to take advantage of these environmental supports to improve their functioning in everyday life; many of these aids, however, require extensive patient training (e.g., Sohlberg and Mateer 1987).

Microcomputers may have the greatest potential for beneficial use by memory-impaired patients. Unfortunately, rehabilitation professionals have left this potential largely untapped. Early attempts to teach amnesic patients how to use a simple computing device were unsuccessful (Wilson and Moffat 1984); although other researchers demonstrated that patients with severe memory deficits were able to learn and apply simple computer commands (Glisky and Schacter 1988b; Glisky et al. 1986a, 1986b), little subsequent research in the use of the computer as a compensatory device has been reported.

Notably, however, Kirsch et al. (1987) and Kirsch et al. (1992) demonstrated that, with very little training, some patients with severe memory disorders were capable of using a microcomputer as an "interactive task guidance system" to cue their performance of real-world tasks, such as baking cookies or doing a janitor's job. In these demonstrations, the computer served a strictly compensatory function, providing a sequence of steps for patients to follow when performing tasks. The researchers pointed out, however, that such cuing also might be effectively accomplished by the use of index cards or other nontechnological means; they noted that there is nothing inherently therapeutic about a computer.

Acquisition of domain-specific knowledge.   Another approach that attempts to alleviate problems associated with memory disability involves teaching patients things that are relevant to various domains of everyday life (Glisky and Schacter 1989b; Mayer et al. 1986; Wilson 1987). For example, patients have learned the names of people in their immediate environment (Dolan and Norton 1977; Jaffe and Katz 1975; Wilson 1982), activities of daily living (Cermak 1976), and information concerning their illness and prognosis (Wilson 1987).

Although rehabilitation professionals have used a variety of strategies to help patients acquire these pieces of information, the goal in each case is functional: enabling patients to improve their performance within the context of their daily lives. No particular assumptions concerning underlying cognitive or neural functions necessarily are implied. The success of these interventions may result either from the use of residual memory processes available to mildly impaired patients or from the reconstitution of other, undamaged cognitive processes (Luria 1948/1963).

Two findings from cognitive neuropsychology are relevant in this context. First, although amnesic patients are severely impaired in their acquisition of factual or *declarative* knowledge, they are able to acquire *procedural* knowledge such as motor, perceptual, and cognitive skills in a normal fashion (e.g., Brooks and Baddeley 1976; Charness et al. 1988; Cohen and Squire 1980; Milner et al. 1968; Squire 1987). Second, amnesic patients show normal repetition priming: They are as likely as nonamnesic subjects to produce previously encountered information in response to partial cues, even though they fail to recollect the prior encounter (Warrington and Weiskrantz 1968, 1974). Psychologists believe that priming relies on *implicit* memory processes, which are preserved in amnesia and do not require conscious recollection of prior occurrence (Graf and Schacter 1985; Schacter and Graf 1986). On the other hand, *explicit* memory processes, which are used to consciously retrieve information from a study episode, are impaired in amnesic patients.

Inspired partly by Luria's views concerning substitution of function and partly by the foregoing empirical findings regarding preserved memory abilities in amnesic patients, Glisky and her colleagues embarked on a series of experiments to explore whether patients' intact memory abilities could be exploited to facilitate their acquisition of complex information. Glisky et al. (1986b) proposed that memory-impaired patients might be able to acquire complex knowledge by using the implicit memory processes underlying priming, particularly if such knowledge had a strong procedural component. To test this possibility, the researchers devised a faded cuing technique—the *method of vanishing cues*—that was designed to take advantage of memory-impaired patients' preserved ability to respond normally to partial cues.

The method of vanishing cues provides subjects with as much cue information as they need (usually in the form of initial letters of target words) to make a correct response and then gradually withdraws information across learning trials. Using this technique, Glisky and her colleagues demonstrated that patients with memory disorders of varying severities and etiologies (including TBI) were able to learn large amounts of factual and procedural information that could be applied both at home and in the workplace (Glisky 1992a): basic computer operations (Glisky and Schacter 1988b; Glisky et al. 1986a), computer data entry (Glisky and Schacter 1987, 1989a; Glisky 1992b), database management (Glisky 1993), and word processing (Glisky 1995). All of these studies involved computer-controlled learning; materials were presented in a consistent fashion across trials, and patients were able to work independently at their own pace. Computer presentation is not required for the delivery of the technique, however. Glisky and Schacter (1988a) and Heinrichs et al. (1992) have reported successful use of vanishing cues without computers and for noncomputer tasks.

Glisky et al. (1986b) speculated that patients were able to learn complex knowledge and skills through their use of preserved implicit memory. They suggested that the method of vanishing cues induced these patients to make use of memory processes that are not normally used in explicit remembering. Learning proceeded at a much slower rate for memory-impaired patients than for subjects who were not memory-impaired, however; the latter presumably relied on explicit memory processes, which were more efficient.

Memory-impaired patients' learning also seemed to result in internal representations of knowledge unlike those acquired by subjects who were not memory-impaired (Glisky et al. 1994). Their representations seemed to be hyperspecific such that the patients were less likely than subjects who were not memory-impaired to produce target responses to changed cues (but see Shimamura and Squire 1988). Although memory-impaired patients may fail to access newly acquired knowledge explicitly when cues are altered; nevertheless, they may be able to use that knowledge implicitly to facilitate their performance in new situations (Glisky 1992b). They also show increased evidence that the probability of transfer or generalization increases with greater degrees of overlearning (Butters et al. 1993).

Evidence for the generalization of new learning to real-world contexts has been sparse, however; researchers more commonly have reported failures of transfer. For example, Cermak (1976) found that although a severely impaired amnesic patient learned to recite many instructions concerning the activities of his daily life, he never actually carried out the instructions (see also Dolan and Norton 1977).

Although researchers still have much to learn about the conditions under which successful learning and transfer occur in memory-impaired patients, the aforementioned studies of acquisition of domain-specific knowledge offer a promising beginning. They demonstrate that brain-injured patients are capable of learning even very complex materials, thereby improving their ability to function independently at home and in the workplace. This research illustrates the advantages of basing rehabilitation methods on a sound theoretical and empirical rationale, and it provides suggestive evidence for substitution of function. These studies make no claim regarding the restoration of general memory and learning ability; rather, they suggest that rehabilitation may achieve meaningful behavioral outcomes by encouraging memory-impaired patients to use alternate, intact processes.

In sum, although restoration of function is the ultimate treatment goal for patients with memory impairments, researchers have found little evidence that cognitive rehabilitation can restore general memory ability. Treatment programs that emphasize functional outcomes have produced more promising results than approaches that focus on general memory skills. Researchers continue to search for cognitive processes that may be unaffected by brain trauma and effective ways to help memory-impaired patients exploit preserved functions to compensate for damaged or lost abilities.

Cognitive Rehabilitation in the Context of a Holistic Neuropsychological Rehabilitation Program

A "holistic" approach to neuropsychological rehabilitation focuses on much more than a specific cognitive deficit such as a memory disorder. The approach attempts to help patients cope with persistent cognitive deficits within the broader context of their lives. This ultimately means that rehabilitation activities attempt, at some level, to deal with the psychosocial consequences of the neuropsychological disturbance, patients' personal reaction to the disturbance in light of their psychosocial background and history, and the environmental factors that may facilitate or impede the greatest level of adjustment.

Cognitive rehabilitation has become an important part of this process. Cognitive rehabilitation is not used so much to restore lost higher cerebral functioning, but to use residual functions to maximum capacity. In this regard, one specific goal of cognitive rehabilitation is to help the patient attend to and process information more effectively. This in turn helps patients positively respond to feedback from individual therapists as well as from others in various group settings. This capacity to learn from small group interaction has been reported to be an important predictor for vocational outcome in TBI patients (Ben-Yishay and Prigatano 1990). The goal of holistic, neuropsychologically oriented rehabilitation therefore is not restoration of function per se, but greater personal and interpersonal adaptation to lost higher cerebral abilities. An example of how cognitive retraining activities are incorporated in this approach will be briefly described.

The cognitive rehabilitation process utilized within a broadly defined neuropsychological rehabilitation program has been described in several publications (Ben-Yishay et al. 1985; Klonoff et al. 1989; Prigatano et al. 1986). Patients work on a variety of tasks in these programs. Some tasks include simple drills or exercises aimed at improving efficiency and speed of information processing, while other tasks are used to help individuals learn external or compensatory techniques (e.g., note taking). In all cases of cognitive rehabilitation, however, the patient is 1) engaged in the rehabilitation activity; 2) helped to become aware of residual deficits as well as strengths; and 3) helped to recognize how these deficits impact everyday activities including job or work responsibilities. Thus, patients are encouraged (and reinforced) to look at the "big picture" regarding their neuropsychological status and the specific and broad purposes of any given cognitive retraining task. Always, the relationship between skill level and work performance is evaluated and discussed with the patient. Compensatory strategies are developed and patients are encouraged to utilize them. Therapists monitor the home, community, and work environments to ensure that learned compensations are applied by the patient.

In addition, the patient's personal reaction to his or her cognitive deficits is discussed and/or handled within the context of individual psychotherapy, group psychotherapy, and the milieu treatment time (Klonoff and Lage 1991; Klonoff et al. 1993; Prigatano 1987, 1991, in press; Prigatano et al. 1986). The cognitive retraining sessions, by their nature, provide a rich source of data with respect to the patient's ability to learn and accept injury-related problems. Some patients are able to accept and adapt to their deficits, whereas others may become overwhelmed and intolerant of imperfections and limitations imposed by their injury.

Cognitive rehabilitation sessions can serve as the "training ground" for self-acceptance and pursuit of realistic, attainable goals. To this end, it is important for rehabilitation staff to develop and utilize therapeutic techniques that educate the patient, but in the context of clinical attunement with their needs and emotional reactions. This enables patients to develop renewed self-esteem and competency, despite their limitations. The staff's clinical sensitivity and capacity to form a true working alliance with the patient are integral for the holistic or milieu-oriented rehabilitation—a process that tends to foster long-term adjustment and productivity.

Case Example

TBI patients enrolled in the Work Reentry Program at the Barrow Neurological Institute at St. Joseph's Hospital and Medical Center work on a variety of tasks aimed at trying to improve their efficiency in speed of information processing. Figure 8–1 shows how two TBI patients in this program performed on one such task.

Patient AB had suffered moderate TBI and had an admission Glasgow Coma Scale (GCS) (Teasdale and Jennett 1974) score of 11. CT scan showed that patient AB had a left temporal lobe contusion. Patient CD had sustained a more severe injury, with an admitting GCS score of 8. CT findings revealed that patient CD had damage to the brain stem and both cerebral hemispheres. Patient CD suffered from diplopia, dysarthria, and motor ataxia, in addition to a variety of cognitive deficits.

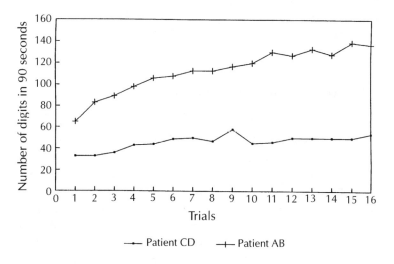

Figure 8-1.   Digit symbol exercise.

Both patients were asked to perform a speed of information processing task derived from the Digit Symbol subtest of the Wechsler Adult Intelligence Scale-Revised (WAIS-R) (Wechsler 1981). The patients were provided with a list of 10 digit-symbol relations and were given 90 seconds to fill in the matched digit as quickly as possible. The data depicted in Figure 8–1 were obtained approximately 3 months postinjury for patient AB and 2.2 years postinjury for patient CD. As Figure 8–1 shows, patient AB showed clear improvement over time, whereas patient CD did not.

This type of data provides an important source of feedback for the patient. The results demonstrated, for example, that with practice, patient AB was able to improve performance on this basic task. This patient was responsive to suggestions from therapists and used compensatory strategies. In contrast, patient CD did not show a learning curve and frequently resisted therapists' suggestions concerning compensatory techniques.

This information also provides therapists with a more realistic understanding of what patients can do in new learning settings. A positive learning curve for simple tasks suggests that, with practice, patients may be able to learn a variety of work-related skills. In contrast, patients who do not show improvement with time on such repetitive tasks may be less likely to benefit from certain work trial experiences.

Thus, the use of specific cognitive retraining activity tasks provides valuable feedback to patients and therapists about how practice may or may not influence patients' level of performance on certain basic tasks. This information is important for practical decision making and provides a milieu in which patients can discuss their feelings concerning residual neuropsychological deficits.

Programmatic Outcome Findings

Researchers have progressively evaluated the efficacy of neuropsychologically oriented rehabilitation. For example, Prigatano et al. (1986) reported the effects of this form of rehabilitation on specific neuropsychological functions (such as speed of information processing), as well as on broader psychosocial outcomes (such as the patient's work status). Patients who underwent this form of rehabilitation showed a higher percentage of productivity, and their relatives reported that they showed less emotional distress than nontreated patients. A study by Scherzer (1986) that did not emphasize the role of small-group interaction and psychotherapy (which Prigatano and colleagues have repeatedly emphasized) produced a less favorable outcome.

Ben-Yishay et al. (1985) reported that approximately 50% of treated patients in a noncontrolled study returned to work. This figure was similar to findings by Prigatano et al. (1984). These results are impressive because less than one-third of severe TBI patients appear to get back to a productive lifestyle without some form of specialty training program (Prigatano et al. 1987). Ben-Yishay et al. (1987) provided additional data in support of this claim. They demonstrated that patients' ability to benefit from small-group interactions, to be involved with others, and to control their emotions contributed significantly to outcome status. Ben-Yishay et al. (1987), along with Prigatano et al. (1986), further emphasized that patients' improved awareness and acceptance of their higher cerebral deficits following TBI contribute significantly to a positive psychosocial outcome.

In a recent study, Prigatano et al. (1994) observed a significant relationship between the working or therapeutic alliance (reported by treatment staff with 38 TBI patients) and work outcome 12 months to 3 years after program discharge. The researchers defined *working alliance* operationally as the patient's capacity to comply with program rules, follow through with staff recommendations (e.g., use compensatory strategies), and develop a realistic view of the effects of brain injury. Prigatano et al. (1994) also replicated the percentage of productive individuals that Prigatano et al. (1984) reported.

Summary and Conclusions

To date, empirical studies suggest that cognitive retraining does not restore impaired higher cerebral functions, particularly memory. These findings do not imply that cognitive retraining lacks clinical utility, however. Teaching TBI patients specific skills has been effective in memory rehabilitation—especially when patients can use preserved procedural learning capacities. For some patients, this retraining can mean the difference between employment and nonemployment.

Moreover, outcome studies continue to demonstrate that holistic, neuropsychology oriented rehabilitation enables a higher proportion of TBI patients to be productive, compared with nontreated TBI patients. Rehabilitation professionals must keep in mind, however, that the cohort of TBI patients who can benefit from this form of rehabilitation is limited. Not all TBI patients can be equally helped using this approach (Prigatano et al. 1986).

Cognitive rehabilitation clearly is developing its place in the rehabilitation of TBI patients. Helping patients to recognize and compensate for residual disturbances and training patients in specific skills are the major contributions of such rehabilitation.

References

Ben-Yishay Y, Prigatano GP: Cognitive remediation, in Rehabilitation of the Adult and Child with Traumatic Brain Injury, 2nd Edition. Edited by Rosenthal M, Griffith ER, Bond MR, et al. Philadelphia, PA, FA Davis, 1990, pp 393–409

Ben-Yishay Y, Rattok J, Lakin P, et al: Neuropsychologic rehabilitation: quest for a holistic approach. Sem Neurol 5:252–258, 1985

Ben-Yishay R, Silver SL, Piasetsky E, et al: Relationship between employability and vocational outcome after intensive holistic cognitive rehabilitation. Journal of Head Trauma Rehabilitation 2:35–40, 1987

Berg IJ, Koning-Haanstra M, Deelman BG: Long-term effects of memory rehabilitation: a controlled study. Neuropsychological Rehabilitation 1:97–111, 1991

Berrol S: Issues in cognitive rehabilitation. Arch Neurol 47:219–220, 1990

Bond MR: Neurobehavioral sequelae of closed head injury, in Neuropsychological Assessment of Neuropsychiatric Disorders. Edited by Grant I, Adams KM. New York, Oxford University Press, 1986, pp 347–373

Brooks DN: Cognitive deficits, in Rehabilitation of the Adult and Child with Traumatic Brain Injury, 2nd Edition. Edited by Rosenthal M, Griffith ER, Bond MR, et al. Philadelphia, PA, FA Davis, 1990, pp 163–178

Brooks DN, Baddeley AD: What can amnesic patients learn? Neuropsychologia 14:111–122, 1976

Butters MA, Glisky EL, Schacter DL: Transfer of learning in memory-impaired patients. J Clin Exp Neuropsychol 15:219–230, 1993

Caramazza A: Cognitive neuropsychology and rehabilitation: an unfulfilled promise? in Cognitive Approaches in Neuropsychological Rehabilitation. Edited by Seron X, Deloche G. Hillsdale, NJ, Lawrence Erlbaum, 1989, pp 383–398

Cermak LS: Imagery as an aid to retrieval for Korsakoff patients. Cortex 11: 163–169, 1975

Cermak LS: The encoding capacity of a patient with amnesia due to encephalitis. Neuropsychologia 14:311–322, 1976

Charness N, Milberg W, Alexander MP: Teaching an amnesic a complex cognitive skill. Brain Cogn 8:253–272, 1988

Chase WG, Ericcson KA: Skilled memory, in Cognitive Skills and Their Acquisition. Edited by Anderson JR. Hillsdale, NJ, Lawrence Erlbaum, 1981, pp 141–190

Cohen NJ, Squire LR: Preserved learning and retention of pattern-analyzing skill in amnesia: dissociation of "knowing how" and "knowing that." Science 210:207–209, 1980

Crovitz HF: Memory retraining in brain-damaged patients: the airplane list. Cortex 15:131–134, 1979

Crovitz HF, Harvey MT, Horn RW: Problems in the acquisition of imagery mnemonics: three brain-damaged cases. Cortex 15:225–234, 1979

Dolan MP, Norton JC: A programmed training technique that uses reinforcement to facilitate acquisition and retention in brain-damaged patients. J Clin Psychol 33:495–501, 1977

Glasgow RE, Zeiss RA, Barrera M, et al: Case studies on remediating memory deficits in brain-damaged individuals. J Clin Psychol 33:1049–1054, 1977

Glisky EL: Acquisition and transfer of declarative and procedural knowledge by memory-impaired patients: a computer data-entry task. Neuropsychologia 30:899–910, 1992a

Glisky EL: Computer-assisted instruction for patients with traumatic brain injury: teaching of domain-specific knowledge. Journal of Head Trauma Rehabilitation 7:1–12, 1992b

Glisky EL: Training persons with traumatic brain injury for complex computer jobs: the domain-specific learning approach, in Community-Based Employment Following Traumatic Brain Injury. Edited by Thomas DF, Menz FE, McAlees DC. Menomonie, WI, University of Wisconsin–Stout Research and Training Center, 1993, pp 3–27

Glisky EL: Acquisition and transfer of word processing skill by an amnesic patient. Neuropsychological Rehabilitation 5:299–318, 1995

Glisky EL, Schacter DL: Acquisition of domain-specific knowledge in organic amnesia: training for computer-related work. Neuropsychologia 25:893–906, 1987

Glisky EL, Schacter DL: Acquisition of domain-specific knowledge in patients with organic memory disorders. J Learn Disabil 21:333–339, 1988a

Glisky EL, Schacter DL: Long-term retention of computer learning by patients with memory disorders. Neuropsychologia 26:173–178, 1988b

Glisky EL, Schacter DL: Extending the limits of complex learning in organic amnesia: computer training in a vocational domain. Neuropsychologia 27:107–120, 1989a

Glisky EL, Schacter DL: Models and methods of memory rehabilitation, in Handbook of Neuropsychology, Vol 3. Edited by Boller F, Grafman J. Amsterdam, Elsevier, 1989b

Glisky EL, Schacter DL, Tulving E: Computer learning by memory-impaired patients: acquisition and retention of complex knowledge. Neuropsychologia 24:313–328, 1986a

Glisky EL, Schacter DL, Tulving E: Learning and retention of computer-related vocabulary in amnesic patients: method of vanishing cues. J Clin Exp Neuropsychol 8:292–312, 1986b

Glisky EL, Schacter DL, Butters MA: Domain-specific learning and remediation of memory disorders, in Cognitive Neuropsychology and Cognitive Rehabilitation. Edited by Riddoch MJ, Humphreys GW. Hove, England, Lawrence Erlbaum, 1994, pp 527–548

Godfrey HPD, Knight RG: Cognitive rehabilitation of memory functioning in amnesic alcoholics. J Consult Clin Psychol 53:555–557, 1985

Graf P, Schacter DL: Implicit and explicit memory for new associations in normal and amnesic subjects. J Exp Psychol Learn Mem Cogn 11:501–518, 1985

Harris JE: Methods of improving memory, in Clinical Management of Memory Problems. Edited by Wilson B, Moffat N. London, Aspen, 1984, pp 46–62

Harris JE, Sunderland A: A brief survey of the management of memory disorders in rehabilitation units in Britain. International Journal of Rehabilitation Medicine 3:206–209, 1981

Heinrichs RW, Levitt A, Arthurs A, et al: Learning and retention of a daily activity schedule in a patient with alcoholic Korsakoff's syndrome. Neuropsychological Rehabilitation 2:43–58, 1992

Howard D, Patterson K: Models for therapy, in Cognitive Approaches in Neuropsychological Rehabilitation. Edited by Seron X, Deloche G. London, Lawrence Erlbaum, 1989, pp 36–43

Jaffe PG, Katz AN: Attenuating anterograde amnesia in Korsakoff's psychosis. J Abnorm Psychol 34:559–562, 1975

James W: Principles of Psychology, Vol 1. New York, Dover, 1890

Kirsch NL, Levine SP, Fallon-Krueger M, et al: The microcomputer as an "orthotic" device for patients with cognitive deficits. Journal of Head Trauma Rehabilitation 2:77–86, 1987

Kirsch NL, Levine SP, Lajiness-O'Neill R, et al: Computer-assisted interactive task guidance: facilitating the performance of a simulated vocational task. Journal of Head Trauma Rehabilitation 7:13–25, 1992

Klonoff PS, Lage GA: Narcissistic injury after traumatic brain injury. Journal of Head Trauma Rehabilitation 6:11–21, 1991

Klonoff PS, O'Brien K, Prigatano GP, et al: Cognitive retraining after traumatic brain injury and its role in facilitating awareness. Journal of Head Trauma Rehabilitation 4:37–45, 1989

Klonoff PS, Lage GA, Chiapello DA: Varieties of the catastrophic reaction after traumatic brain injury: a self-psychology perspective. Bulletin of the Menninger Clinic 57:227–241, 1993

Kovner R, Mattis S, Pass R: Some amnesic patients can freely recall large amounts of information in new contexts. J Clin Exp Neuropsychol 7:395–411, 1985

Lashley KS: Factors limiting recovery after central nervous lesions. J Nerv Ment Dis 88:733–755, 1938

Levin HS, Gary HE, Eisenberg HM, et al: Neurobehavioral outcome 1 year after severe head injury. J Neurosurg 73:699–709, 1990

Lewinsohn PM, Danaher BG, Kikel S: Visual imagery as a mnemonic aid for brain-injured persons. J Consult Clin Psychol 45:717–723, 1977.

Luria AR: Restoration of Function After Brain Trauma (in Russian) (1948). London, Pergamon, 1963

Luria AR: Restoration of Function After Brain Injury. New York, Macmillan, 1963

Mayer NH, Keating DJ, Rapp D: Skills, routines, and activity patterns of daily living: a functional nested approach, in Clinical Neuropsychology of Intervention. Edited by Uzzell B, Gross Y. Boston, MA, Martinus Nijhoff, 1986, pp 205–222

Meier MJ, Strauman S, Thompson WG: Individual differences in neuropsychological recovery: an overview, in Neuropsychological Rehabilitation. Edited by Meier MJ, Benton AL, Diller D. London, Guilford, 1987, pp 71–100

Miller E: Is amnesia remediable? in Practical Aspects of Memory. Edited by Gruneberg MM, Morris, PE, Sykes, RN. London, Academic Press, 1978, pp 705–711

Milner B, Corkin S, Teuber HL: Further analysis of the hippocampal amnesic syndrome: 14-year follow-up study of H.M. Neuropsychologia 6:215–234, 1968

Prigatano GP: Recovery and cognitive retraining after craniocerebral trauma. J Learn Disabil 20:603–613, 1987

Prigatano GP: Recovery and cognitive retraining after brain injury, in Traumatic Brain Injury. Edited by Bigler ED. Austin, TX, Pro-Ed, 1990, pp 273–295

Prigatano GP: Disturbances of self-awareness of deficit after traumatic brain injury, in Awareness of Deficit After Brain Injury: Theoretical and Clinical Issues. Edited by Prigatano GP, Schacter DL. New York, Oxford University Press, 1991, pp 111–126

Prigatano GP: Personality disturbances associated with traumatic brain injury. J Consult Clin Psychol 60:360–368, 1992

Prigatano GP: Individuality, lesion location and psychotherapy after brain injury, in Brain Injury and Neuropsychological Rehabilitation. Edited by Uzzell B, Christensen AL. Hillsdale, NJ, Lawrence Erlbaum, 1994, pp 173–186

Prigatano GP, Fordyce DJ: The neuropsychological rehabilitation program at Presbyterian Hospital, Oklahoma City, in Neuropsychological Rehabilitation After Brain Injury. Edited by Prigatano GP, Fordyce DJ, Zeiner HK, et al. Baltimore, MD, Johns Hopkins University Press, 1986, pp 69–118

Prigatano GP, Fordyce DJ, Zeiner HK, et al: Neuropsychological rehabilitation after closed head injury in young adults. J Neurol Neurosurg Psychiatry 47:505–513, 1984

Prigatano GP, Fordyce DJ, Zeiner HK, et al: Neuropsychological Rehabilitation After Brain Injury. Baltimore, MD, Johns Hopkins University Press, 1986

Prigatano GP, Klonoff PS, Bailey I: Psychosocial adjustment associated with traumatic brain injury: statistics BNI neurorehabilitation must beat. BNI Quarterly 3:18–21, 1987

Prigatano GP, Klonoff P, O'Brien KP, et al: Productivity after neuropsychologically oriented milieu rehabilitation. Journal of Head Trauma Rehabilitation 9:91–102, 1994

Rothi LJ, Horner J: Restitution and substitution: two theories of recovery with application to neurobehavioral treatment. J Clin Neuropsychol 5:73–81, 1983

Schacter DL, Glisky EL: Memory remediation: restoration, alleviation, and the acquisition of domain-specific knowledge, in Clinical Neuropsychology of Intervention. Edited by Uzzell B, Gross Y. Boston, MA, Martinus Nijhoff, 1986, pp 257–282

Schacter DL, Graf P: Preserved learning in amnesic patients: perspectives from research on direct priming. J Clin Exp Neuropsychol 8:727–743, 1986

Scherzer BP: Rehabilitation following severe head trauma: results of a 3-year program. Arch Phys Med Rehabil 67:366–374, 1986

Shimamura AP, Squire LR: Long-term memory in amnesia: cued recall, recognition memory, and confidence ratings. J Exp Psychol Learn Mem Cogn 14:763–770, 1988

Sohlberg MM, Mateer CA: Training use of compensatory memory books: a three-stage behavioral approach. J Clin Exp Neuropsychol 11:871–887, 1987

Sohlberg MM, Mateer CA: Introduction to Cognitive Rehabilitation: Theory and Practice. New York, Guilford, 1989

Squire LR: Memory and Brain. New York, Oxford University Press, 1987

Teasdale G, Jennett B: Assessment of coma and impaired consciousness: a practical scale. Lancet 2:81–84, 1974

Van Zomeren AH, Van Den Berg W: Residual complaints of patients 2 years after severe head injury. J Neurol Neurosurg Psychiatry 48:21–28, 1985

Warrington EK, Weiskrantz L: New method of testing long-term retention with special reference to amnesic patients. Nature 217:972–974, 1968

Warrington EK, Weiskrantz L: The effect of prior learning on subsequent retention in amnesic patients. Neuropsychologia 12:419–428, 1974

Wechsler D: Wechsler Adult Intelligence Scale-Revised. San Antonio, TX, Psychological Corporation, 1981

Wilson B: Teaching a patient to remember people's names after removal of a left temporal tumor. Behavioral Psychotherapy 9:338–344, 1981

Wilson B: Success and failure in memory training following a cerebral vascular accident. Cortex 18:581–594, 1982

Wilson B: Rehabilitation of Memory. New York, Guilford, 1987

Wilson B, Moffat N: Rehabilitation of memory for everyday life, in Everyday Memory: Actions and Absentmindedness. Edited by Harris JE, Morris PE. London, Academic Press, 1984, pp 207–233

Chapter 9

Cognitive Rehabilitation for Seizure Disorders

Michael D. Franzen, Ph.D., and James Petrick, Ph.D.

Seizure disorders may occur as the result of many different etiologic agents or processes, including head injury (especially when associated with skull fracture), cerebral tumor, stroke, infectious disease, or endocrinological imbalances. Additionally, some forms of seizure disorders may occur without any identified cause (idiopathic seizures), although there may be a genetic influence on the development of the disorder. Various degrees of cognitive dysfunction are found in many patients with seizure disorder. The site of the seizure focus in specific areas of the brain is probably one of the key factors in determining the nature of the cognitive impairment.

Cognitive dysfunction associated with seizure disorders is fairly well documented when the seizure disorder is poorly controlled. Despite the prevalence of cognitive dysfunction, there are few published studies involving the treatment of these cognitive deficits. Although there is popular literature about improving cognitive skills in neurologically normal individuals and a few studies regarding treatment of cognitive dysfunction in general rehabilitation settings, there are few empirical reports of rehabilitation efforts with seizure disorder patients. Because the cognitive rehabilitation of patients with stroke or head injury is discussed in other chapters, in this chapter we will concentrate on the rehabilitation of patients with idiopathic seizure disorders. The purpose of this chapter is to provide an overview of the cognitive sequelae associated with seizure disorders, the psychological and psychosocial consequences of seizure disorders, and the various forms of rehabilitation that might be considered.

Impact of Seizures

For many years, high rates of psychological and social problems have been observed among individuals with seizure disorders. In one study, Rodin et al. (1972) discovered that more than half of the epileptic persons they sampled had some sort of psychological or social problem with behavioral manifestations. Furthermore, fewer than one of four individuals with seizure disorders were free of intellectual problems, neurological handicaps, or behavioral problems. Individuals with seizure disorder often have difficulties in psychosocial adaptation (Gregoriades 1972; Hodgman et al. 1979; Long and Moore 1979; Richardson and Friedman 1974), scholastic achievement (Hackney and Taylor 1976; Holdsworth and Whitmore 1974; Pazzaglia and Frank-Pazzaglia 1976; Stores et al. 1978), and vocational success (Karan 1972; Porter 1968; Rodin et al. 1972). However, the exact relationship among neurological, psychiatric, and social factors remains unclear.

Cognitive Sequelae

Seizure disorders may have associated cognitive impairments depending on the presence of different variables, including neurological, psychiatric, and social factors. Individuals with seizures secondary to head injury may show deficits in attention, memory, or abstraction skills, but these deficits may be more highly related to the etiology of the seizures than to their effects. The site of the seizure focus also plays a role in the manifestation of cognitive deficits. For example, individuals with temporal lobe epilepsy (TLE) may demonstrate impairments in the transfer of information from short-term memory to long-term memory (Martin et al. 1991). Childhood seizure disorders may be associated with lowered levels of academic skill due to identification of the child as different and resultant social isolation and lessened access to educational opportunities. The extent to which the seizures are controlled may play a role in whether children exhibit decrements in Performance IQ as measured by the Wechsler Intelligence Scale for Children but not decrements in Verbal IQ (Rodin et al. 1988). The reason for this last result is unclear, but it may be related to the greater number of timed tasks on the Performance subscales.

Etiology of Cognitive Deficits

The neuropsychological consequences of seizure disorders include all of the possible functions involved in brain-behavior relations. However, certain functions are more likely to be affected than are others. For example, memory impairment is probably one of the most common complaints associated with seizure disorders. Intellectual functions also are affected by seizure activity, and some individuals with seizure disorders may have lower IQs than other individuals (Klove and Matthews 1974). It appears that the severity of the seizure disorder—whether measured by number, frequency, duration, or intensity of seizures—plays a significant role in the effect of seizures on cognitive functions, because individuals with less severe seizure disorders do not show decrement in cognitive functions (Lesser et al. 1986). The type of seizure disorder also may play a role; patients with generalized seizure disorders may have greater cognitive deficits than patients with temporal lobe disorders (Stevens et al. 1972).

A number of types of cognitive dysfunction are associated with seizure disorders (see Table 9–1). These range from simple motor and sensory deficits to generalized reductions in intelligence and higher order executive functions. Furthermore, the cognitive sequelae of seizure disorder may vary from transient to persistent impairment. The foci of the seizure activity appear to play a significant role in the nature of the cognitive deficit. For example, somatosensory deficits usually do not occur when damage is confined to the temporal lobes; such deficits indicate abnormality extending beyond the frontal and anterior temporal lobes to involve the parietal cortex. Profound olfactory deficits, in contrast, implicate orbitofrontal damage (Jones-Gotman and Zatorre 1988), and a significant unilateral hand grip weakness also suggests contralateral frontal lobe abnormality. Memory functions seem to be affected by several different types of seizure disorder.

Memory

Research evidence has accumulated that gives support to the hypothesis that memory disturbance is present in patients with epilepsy. Individuals with seizure disorders have been reported to perform significantly worse than matched control subjects on various memory tests (Brittain 1980; Loiseau et al. 1983). Perhaps one of the most studied areas of cognitive dysfunction in patients with seizure disorder is the memory dysfunction characteristic of temporal lobe disorders. The temporal lobes, especially the anterior tips and medial surfaces, are highly involved in the transfer of information from short-term to long-term memory. As a result, it might be expected that patients with unilateral temporal lobe seizures would show differential effects on verbal versus nonverbal memory, at least in delayed recall. Within the group of patients with TLE, some discriminations have been made, comparing individuals who have left temporal lobe foci with individuals who have right temporal lobe foci. Several researchers reported that patients with left-sided foci did less well than

Table 9–1. Cognitive functions potentially affected in seizure disorders

Memory	Abstraction
Motor (unilateral strength or speed)	Executive functions
Somatosensory	Problem solving
Generalized intelligence	Language
Olfaction	

patients with right-sided foci on verbal memory tests and that those with right-sided foci did less well than those with left-sided foci on nonverbal memory tests (Berent et al. 1980; Delaney et al. 1980; Fedio and Mirsky 1969; Hermann et al. 1987).

Unfortunately, the relation between laterality of seizure activity and type of memory dysfunction does not appear to be simple. Although greater deficits in verbal memory for left temporal lobe patients (Hermann et al. 1987) and greater deficits in nonverbal memory for right temporal lobe patients were demonstrated, other reports indicated that the effect may not be robust; in other words, not all unilateral patients show this pattern (Jones-Gotman 1991; Thompson 1991). Part of the problem may be in the choice of single measures to examine the effect. Loring et al. (1988) used multiple measures of unilateral memory and found that an accurate determination of hemisphericity of seizure focus could be obtained when there was consistent dissociation between the verbal memory and visuospatial memory measures.

It should be noted that consistency of dissociation effects was found in only 5 of the 30 patients in the Loring et al. (1988) study. The short-term memory dysfunction associated with unilateral TLE may not be specific to the type of material. Delaney et al. (1986) reported that for both right and left temporal lobe seizure patients, there may a decrement in short-term recall of verbal material but not of nonverbal material. Evidently, abnormal activity of the temporal lobes may adversely affect the early stages of memorial processes.

Intelligence

As mentioned earlier, seizure disorders also may have adverse affects on intellectual functioning. However, the exact relationship between seizure disorder and IQ has not been clearly delineated. Type of seizure disorder, age of the patient at seizure onset, the degree to which seizures are controlled, and the social implications of seizure disorder all appear to play a role. Although the majority of children with seizure disorder attend ordinary schools, various studies (Cavazutti 1980; Ross et al. 1980) showed that learning disabilities and school problems are frequent. The average IQ of children with epilepsy has been found to be lower than that of a matched control group (Farwell et al. 1985). Furthermore, about one-sixth of children with epilepsy who have normal intelligence appear to be underachievers (Pazzaglia and Frank-Pazzaglia 1976). It is difficult to state the exact effects of seizure disorder on intelligence because of the heterogeneity of the disorders and their causes and because of methodological differences in the studies performed. However, it is clear that seizure disorders may affect overall intellectual functioning as well as specific types of learning abilities.

Executive Functions

In addition to memory and intelligence, some research has suggested impairments in higher order executive functioning in patients with seizure disorder. Hermann et al. (1988) demonstrated that a substantial proportion of patients with complex partial seizures with foci in the temporal lobe and associated limbic structures performed on the Wisconsin Card Sorting Test (Heaton 1985) in a manner suggestive of frontal lobe dysfunction. This finding was in contrast to that in patients with generalized epilepsy, suggesting that it is not merely attributable to the presence of seizures. Furthermore, Hermann et al. (1988) noted differences between patients with dominant versus nondominant foci in terms of problem-solving efficiency. Patients with nondominant foci manifested more errors (total and perseverative) and more perseverative responses than patients with dominant foci, who in turn performed in a more impaired fashion relative to epilepsy control subjects. These findings were explained in terms of a dysfunction in the frontal cortex caused by the propagation of "neural noise" from the temporal lobe–hippocampal epileptic focus.

Effects of Drugs on Cognitive Functions

An important consideration in the study of cognitive deficits and seizure disorders is the effect of treating the seizures. Frequently, treatment involves a pharmacologic agent, and many of these agents also may have effects on neuropsychological function. For example, barbiturates may inhibit psychomotor speed and sustained attention, and phenytoin may adversely affect psychomotor performance, memory, problem-solving skills, and concentration. On the other hand, carbamazepine and sodium valproate may have minimal cognitive effects (Bennett 1992). The potential effects of treatment should be kept in mind whenever attempting to determine the cognitive effects of the seizure disorders for which the drugs are prescribed.

Psychopathology and Seizure Disorders

There exists a large body of clinical lore implicating seizure disorders in the development of psychiatric problems. Behavioral changes reported to be associated with epilepsy are listed in Table 9–2. The empirical data for such associations are equivocal; however, Manchanda et al. (1992) reported that 45% of patients admitted to an inpatient epilepsy service were diagnosed as having a psychiatric disorder. However, no data were presented regarding the prevalence of psychiatric disorders in the larger population of all individuals with seizure disorders. There may be no adequate comparison group to determine

Table 9–2.   Reported interictal behavioral changes

Obsessiveness	Aggression
Viscosity	Anger
Depression	Altered sexuality
Emotionality	Dependence
Paranoia	Hypergraphia
Hyperreligiosity	Circumstantiality

the prevalence of psychiatric disorders in the general population. Whitman et al. (1984) reviewed published studies of Minnesota Multiphasic Personality Inventory data for a total of 2,786 patients with seizure disorders, other neurological disorders, or chronic medical disorders. They found that the seizure patients did not have a significantly greater occurrence of psychopathology than the other subjects, but that the psychopathology that did occur in patients with epilepsy was related to a greater prevalence of psychotic disorders in both the group with seizures and the group with neurological disorders, compared with the group who had chronic medical disorders.

Because of the literature regarding the effects of psychopathology on performance on neuropsychological measures, it might be assumed that seizure disorder patients with substantial psychopathology would perform even worse on clinical measures of neuropsychological function. However, one of the early studies to investigate this hypothesis found no relation between the degree of psychopathology as measured by the Minnesota Multiphasic Personality Inventory and the degree of cognitive deficit as measured by the Wechsler Adult Intelligence Scale, the Wechsler Memory Scale, and (in a limited subsample) the Halstead-Reitan Neuropsychological Test Battery (Stevens et al. 1972).

The interictal emotional characteristics of patients with temporal lobe seizure disorders received a large amount of attention recently after the proposal of a "temporal lobe personality" (Bear and Fedio 1977). This personality includes features of hyperreligiosity, hyper- or hyposexuality, hypergraphia, irritability, and lack of humor. Although there is some controversy as to whether neurobiological or psychosocial features play a dominant role in the appearance of behavioral abnormalities in these patients, there is some intriguing evidence that these patients show altered emotional responsiveness (greater arousal), as measured by galvanic skin response, to both emotional and innocuous stimuli (Bear et al. 1981). This anomalous responsiveness may indicate an organic basis for the reported personality traits.

Although the exact characteristics of the symptoms found interictally in patients with TLE remain somewhat controversial, there is agreement that psychiatric symptoms are an important characteristic of these patients. In a review, Trimble (1992) reported that a schizophrenia-like psychosis can be found in approximately 7% of patients with epilepsy and that this proportion is even higher in patients with TLE. The schizophrenic-like symptoms can include paranoia or hebephrenia and tend to be chronic. A recent paper retrospectively investigated the occurrence of manic symptoms in a chart review of patients with TLE (Lyketsos et al. 1993) and found that 20% of the sample showed signs of mania.

A recently investigated and fascinating phenomenon involves the relation between seizures and anxiety disorders. Although part of the relation was first noted in patients with partial complex seizure disorders who reported anxiety interictally, as yet the relation is largely circumstantial. Other evidence includes the fact that substances such as caffeine are both anxiogenic and epileptogenic (Nickell and Uhde 1991). Hermann et al. (1992) reported that ictal fear is associated with a right hemisphere focus in TLE. Clearly, we do not yet have a reasonable understanding of the exact relation between seizure activity and psychopathology; however, clinicians working with this population should remain vigilant to the possibility of these disorders coexisting in their patients.

Psychosocial Consequences

Individuals with seizure disorders face the possibility of social isolation as the result of being labeled different. If the seizure disorder first occurs in childhood, these individuals may not develop adequate social skills, causing further social isolation. Social problems do not develop in a vacuum; for example, an interesting study by Hermann and colleagues (1992) identified some of the factors related to the development of social competence in children with seizure disorders. These investigators found that intact parental marriages, good seizure control, higher family income, later age of onset, and shorter duration of the disorder all facilitated the development of social competence, whereas the existence of multiple seizure types had a negative influence.

Yet another interaction between psychological and neurological features is contained in the context of pseudoseizures. Pseudoseizures occur when the clinical behavioral manifestations of seizure episodes appear, while ictal and immediately postictal electroencephalograms are usually not abnormal and prolactin serum levels do not increase (Delgado-Escueta et al. 1991). The issue is complicated by the fact that patients who have seizures also may have pseudoseizures (Gumnit and Gates 1986). There do not appear to be personality differences between patients with pseudoseizures and patients with other seizure disorders (Vanderzant et al. 1986). However, patients with pseudoseizures may be more likely to respond to psychological treatment with a reduction of behavioral seizure activity.

Typically, behavioral treatment of seizure disorders involves assessment and modification of either the events that tend to elicit seizure activity or the events that follow the seizure. For example, seizure activity may be elicited by certain situations that are stressful to the individual. Alternately, the occurrence of seizure activity may be followed by nurturant behavior on the part of significant others in the social environment of the patient. In either case, treatment involves reducing the frequency of associated events, thereby effecting a reduction in pseudoseizure episodes.

Let us consider a clinical example involving a school age child. A functional assessment indicates that seizure activity is more frequent on the mornings when a math test is scheduled at school. It may be that the stress associated with the impending test is eliciting the seizure, or the nurturant behavior of the mother, who allows the child to stay home from school after the seizure, may be responsible. Treatment could not realistically involve reducing the frequency of math tests; however, the mother could be instructed to care for the child but still ensure attendance at school, thereby reducing the frequency of seizures on math test days.

Rehabilitation

As mentioned earlier, empirical reports of rehabilitation efforts with seizure disorder patients are rare. Silfvenius (1990) described a program for assessing and treating children with seizure disorders. This program included neuropsychological assessment to determine the need for educational, psychosocial, or vocational interventions. Unfortunately, although a strong argument was made for a comprehensive treatment program, no data regarding the efficacy of these programs in the rehabilitation of seizure patients were presented. Strang (1990) described a program for treating the cognitive problems evidenced by children with seizure disorders and suggested that such treatment is beneficial to the development of adaptive behavior in these children, but again no empirical evaluation of the program was offered. Henriksen (1990) recommended that children with seizure disorders be evaluated to determine the need for special education services. An additional consideration is the possibility of detrimental effects of antiepileptic medications on learning; however, as in all of the above cases, definitive empirical data regarding the effects of such medications on academic performance are lacking.

The rehabilitation process involves multiple components that may vary across treatment programs. Components usually include a thorough evaluation to identify treatment targets, cognitive retraining for deficient skills, psychoeducation to provide an environment conducive to maintaining the treatment gains, psychotherapy to help facilitate adjustment to the life changes, and family therapy to help relatives adjust to the changes, as well as to provide a family environment that is optimal for recovery.

Assessment

Before the implementation of any formal rehabilitation strategy or program, specific areas of dysfunction must be identified. Proper assessment of cognitive dysfunction will likely require the collaborative effort of patients, family members, teachers, physicians, and psychologists. Various assessment strategies have been used to determine the cognitive, psychological, and psychosocial sequelae of seizure disorder. These strategies include neuropsychological examinations, self-report questionnaires, and functional assessments.

In recent years, data obtained from neuropsychological examinations have been used to identify cognitive strengths and weaknesses in patients with seizure disorder. Such data are used especially for predicting the potential risk of cognitive deficit after surgery (Chelune et al. 1991; Rausch et al. 1977; Wannamaker and Matthews 1976). The neuropsychological examination involves assessment of a variety of cognitive functions, ranging from simple motor and perceptual skills to complex abstraction and problem-solving skills. Specific domains of assessment include fine motor speed; dexterity and coordination; tactual and visuospatial perception; language; attention and concentration; memory and learning; and sequencing, abstraction, and reasoning skills.

Neuropsychological assessment may include complete battery approaches such as the Halstead-Reitan Neuropsychological Test Battery or the Luria Nebraska Neuropsychological Battery, which use set procedures with standardized scoring; process-oriented approaches that focus on qualitative aspects of performance; or flexible, adjustable approaches that use collections of shorter standardized tests that are different for each patient. Numerous psychometric tools are used in neuropsychological evaluations (see Table 9–3 for a partial list). Such an examination may assist the clinician in determining the association between specific areas of dysfunction and the site of the seizure focus. Additionally, this type of examination may assist the clinician in determining specific areas of strength that might be used to compensate for impairments.

In addition to identifying and quantifying specific neuropsychological deficits associated with seizure disorder, another approach to assessment involves self-report. A number of measures sensitive to psychosocial adjustment in assessment of seizure disorder patients have been suggested. These include

Table 9–3.   Psychometric instruments used in neuropsychological assessment

Wechsler Adult Intelligence Scale—Revised
Wechsler Memory Scale—Revised
California Verbal Learning Test
Knox Cube Test
Boston Diagnostic Aphasia Examination
Boston Naming Test
Multilingual Aphasia Examination
Visual Form Discrimination
Judgment of Line Orientation
Hooper Visual Organization Test
Stroop Color Word Test
Wisconsin Card Sorting Test

scales such as the Perceived Stigma and Perceived Limitations Scales (Ryan et al. 1980), Washington Psychosocial Seizure Inventory (Dodrill et al. 1991), Life Experiences Scale (Sarason et al. 1978), Social Support Questionnaire (Sarason et al. 1983), Center for Epidemiological Studies of Depression Scale (Radloff 1977), and the Internal-External Control of Reinforcement Scale (Rotter 1966). One caution concerning self-report questionnaires such as these concerns the nature of their standardization. These tests are often standardized with populations other than seizure disorder patients. Probably the most common example is the Minnesota Multiphasic Personality Inventory (Dahlstrom et al. 1972), which was developed entirely within a psychiatric context.

Finally, another area of assessment that deserves mention—but that has not been systematically investigated—is functional ability, or the capacity to perform ecologically relevant behaviors such as household tasks or job-related duties. Functional assessment requires use of multiple sources, including interview, history, tests, simulations and role playing, direct observation in contrived or natural environments, and specialized evaluations (vocational, speech, occupational therapy). Rating scales can provide relevant information about functional abilities and limitations. Examples are the Patient Competency Rating Scale and the Patient's Assessment of Own Functioning Inventory. Ratings completed by rehabilitation professionals also are useful, provided the instruments have sufficient specificity and meet basic psychometric properties for reliability and validity.

Cognitive Retraining

Cognitive retraining is a broad term used to refer to a variety of activities designed to help a patient improve specific higher cognitive functioning.

Individual or individualized (systematic) remedial training exercises are carried out in accordance with a set curriculum. One form of cognitive retraining is attention process training, which is designed to improve the patient's ability to attend, concentrate, and provide accurate responses. Dexterity training involves cognitive remediation techniques consisting of both retraining and compensatory training of hand-eye coordination and fine motor dexterity. Visual process training involves remediation techniques consisting of both retraining and compensatory training of visuospatial information processing, as well as visual-constructional, sequential, and integrational skills.

Memory skills training is directed toward developing techniques designed to counter problems of initial registration and learning, as well as retention problems associated with both short-term and long-term memory deficits. Memory skills training attempts to develop efficient information encoding with supplemental techniques to enhance both verbal and nonverbal memory and information processing. Basic academic retraining concerns orientation, the speed and efficiency of information processing, and basic academic skills (i.e., reading, writing, arithmetic). Finally, executive skills training is designed to improve the patient's higher order executive functions. This training is primarily focused on problem-solving abilities—for example, use of organizing, planning, and sequencing techniques; the ability to draw correct conclusions and make inferences; and the ability to order behaviors into priorities and to carry through solutions.

Let us consider how the neuropsychological evaluation might be used to develop a rehabilitation plan. For example, the patient's neuropsychological evaluation may uncover deficits in planning and abstract problem-solving skills, as well as deficits in retrieval of verbal information. The rehabilitation plan would include teaching the patient to use self-verbalization to guide problem solving. For example, when faced with a problem, the patient would ask himself a set of questions designed to identify possible solutions—for example, "What is the problem?" "Have I ever faced this problem before?" "What did I do that time?" Additionally, the patient may be taught to use cued retrieval procedures for memory deficits. The patient associates the verbal information with a single cue, such as associating the street address 317 Maple Road with syrup. When the patient has trouble remembering his physician's address, he is told to think of syrup and use that to cue retrieval of the address.

There are few empirical reports on the effectiveness of retraining efforts in remediating cognitive dysfunction secondary to seizure disorder. However, there have been some exemplary studies concerning psychosocial intervention. For example, Helgeson et al. (1990) demonstrated the efficacy of psychoeducational treatment programs aimed at increasing patient understanding of epilepsy, decreasing patient fear of seizures, decreasing hazardous medical self-management practices, and increasing patient compliance with medication. Another study by Freeman et al. (1984) demonstrated the positive impact of special intervention programs involving psychological assessment, counseling, and work experience placements on school dropout and unemployment rates. Specific rehabilitation strategies for cognitive deficits secondary to seizure disorder are rare, but several approaches were documented in the context of treating forms of cognitive dysfunction with etiologies other than seizure disorder (Franzen 1991).

A small group of investigators are examining the ability of behavioral techniques to reduce seizure activity. Although their focus is on reduction of seizure activity rather than on remediation of cognitive deficits, a recently reported study examined the effect of this treatment on cognitive performance and therefore is relevant here. Lantz and Sterman (1992) reported the results of using biofeedback to reduce seizure activity. The general idea was to provide positive reinforcement for increasing 11- to 15-Hz activity while suppressing 0- to 5-Hz activity, 20- to 25-Hz activity, and high-voltage transients. Compared with subjects who were given noncontingent (inaccurate) feedback, subjects who received accurate feedback were better able to reduce seizure activity. Not all subjects receiving the treatment were able to reduce seizure activity, and success in treatment was associated with higher levels of pretreatment performance on neuropsychological tests. Additionally, subjects who were successful in reducing seizure activity also demonstrated improvement in cognitive performance.

There has been much excitement regarding the use of psychological or behavioral methods to treat acquired memory impairments (Franzen and Haut 1991). Unfortunately, relatively little empirical work has assessed the efficacy of these treatment methods in seizure disorder patients. There are three basic forms of treatment for acquired neuropsychological impairment: retraining, alternate systems, and behavioral prosthetics (Franzen 1991). Retraining involves practice with the implicated skill. For example, if a person has a deficit in verbal memory, he or she may receive structured exercises aimed at improving that skill. Deficits in learning textual material are remediated by structured exercises in which audiotapes of short conversational stories are played for patients, and they are asked either to write down everything that they remembered or else to repeat everything they remembered.

The alternate-functional systems approach involves using an intact neurocognitive skill to compensate for the impaired skill. For example, if a person has a verbal memory deficit, he or she may receive treatment to learn to encode information visually by associating the information with visual imagery. Behavioral prosthetics involve using overt observable behaviors to overcome the functional impairment. For example, a person with a verbal memory deficit may be taught to use a memory notebook to record important information.

All these methods have been used in patients with different types of cognitive impairment, including memory impairment (Franzen and Haut 1991). However, there are very few reports on the use of these techniques in patients who have seizure disorders. In one study, Aldenkamp and Vermeulen (1991) reported results of using the alternate-functional-systems method in three patients with seizure disorders. The retraining method also was used in these same patients to help them learn specific bits of important information. The data presented are anecdotal and lack the rigor of controlled evaluations, but they suggest that these techniques may be useful in some patients.

As is the case with memory impairment, few empirical data have been presented on the usefulness of cognitive remediation techniques in the areas of abstract problem solving, language, and sequencing. Strategies for the remediation of problem-solving techniques have been proposed. For example, McCue et al. (1992) suggested the importance of teaching the individual to think aloud. The rationale underlying this technique is for the individual to make explicit what is usually known and used implicitly. The patient is taught to talk out loud while thinking through problems and to write things down in identified steps. By making the steps explicit, it is hoped that accuracy and efficiency will be improved. Speech and language pathologists often address issues related to speech, language, pragmatics, and cognitive communicative functions. This discipline stresses both remediation and compensation for the behavioral manifestations of deficits. Finally, occupational therapy is designed to address cognitive skills such as sequencing and planning.

Let us examine how these approaches might be implemented in a single patient. A patient might have deficits in word-finding skills, memory, planning, and sequencing. The neuropsychologist responsible for cognitive rehabilitation would develop a treatment plan that would include memory exercises and the use of visual encoding. The speech therapist would implement a treatment that uses practice in *visual confrontation naming* (eliciting the word name of an object presented visually or pictorially), vocabulary-building exercises, and structured practice in conversation. Finally, the occupational therapist would provide practice in planning and sequencing everyday activities such as shopping and cooking.

Generalizability

Generalization refers to the development of behavioral and cognitive strategies that are applicable in a variety of different contexts. Ideally, the therapist should strive to teach generalizable strategies because the patient who learns them becomes more autonomous and requires less supervision (Gifford et al. 1984; Horner et al. 1982). For example, teaching a memory-impaired patient to use speaking aloud to encode important material to be remembered may not be useful if the patient is unable to use the strategy in his or her environment because of embarrassment. Woolcock (1989) provided an exceptionally cogent discussion of generalization strategies for rehabilitation of the head-injured individual. Similarly, Ellis (1965) comprehensively documented the basic paradigms for transfer of learning, including similarity of task demands and explicit practice in adapting methods to new situations. These paradigms can be used to describe the similarity between the training and real-life settings. Although the term *generalization* is commonly used in the literature on cognitive rehabilitation, very little has been written about evaluating its application (Woolcock 1989).

At the very least, the therapist could provide encouragement and feedback on the patient's attempts to apply the newly learned behaviors in a variety of situations. More beneficial would be to program generalizability into the treatment by reinforcing generalization; patients could be provided with diverse examples of both appropriate new behaviors and appropriate situations in which to apply the new behaviors.

Managing Seizures

An interesting sideline to the discussion of psychological treatment for the cognitive and emotional-behavioral correlates of seizure disorders is the application of treatment methods for the seizure disorder itself. Previously, we discussed the application of behavioral methods in the treatment of pseudoseizures, but behavior therapy also has been presented in the context of treating seizure episodes. An early review of these studies (Mostofsky and Balaschak 1977) classified the methods into three categories: self-control and psychotherapy, operant behavioral programs, and psychophysiological techniques.

The self-control and psychotherapy approaches are predicated on the idea that levels of stress and emotional distress can affect the initiation of a seizure. The behavioral approaches are based on the idea that reports of seizures and behaviors surrounding seizures are partly influenced by environmental consequences. By controlling the environmental consequences, one could conceivably affect the incidence of seizures. For example, by decreasing the nurturant behavior directly elicited by seizure activity (removing social reinforcement), the therapist may help effect a decrease in seizure activity. The psychophysiological approaches are based on the idea that biofeedback can be used to favorably affect epileptogenic brain electromagnetic activity. Although there are positive reports in the literature on all three approaches, the research methodology involved was less than optimal.

Goldstein (1990) reviewed more recent studies that addressed some of the methodological criticisms raised by Mostofsky and Balaschak (1977) in their earlier review. These criticisms included failure to account for the placebo effect, lack of evidence that the treatment effect was generalizable, poor diagnosis, and uncontrolled changes in medications during treatment. Unfortunately, although these more recent studies indicated that improvement in seizure activity is possible as a result of the application of psychological techniques, methodological shortcomings (e.g., failure to match treatment to disorder type, lack of attention placebo groups in the experimental design) persist and continue to limit the generalizability of the findings.

Postsurgery Rehabilitation

There has been a recent increase in the number of medical facilities that provide surgical treatment for intractable seizure disorders. The typical outcome measure for evaluating the success of the surgery has been reduction in seizure activity. However, other variables such as vocational status, psychosocial functioning and adjustment, degree of independence, and quality of life also have been addressed (Dodrill et al. 1991). In general, improvement in any of these areas depends on successful reduction of seizure activity, and not all areas are uniformly benefited. The same issues involved in rehabilitation of the seizure patient also would apply to the postsurgery seizure patient. However, there would be additional issues for the postsurgery seizure patient, such as dealing with adverse effects of surgery and dealing with the disappointment if the surgery did not result in seizure reduction.

Summary

Seizure disorders may be associated with a host of cognitive and emotional difficulties. Complete treatment of the patient with a seizure disorder includes consideration of the medical, cognitive, and psychosocial aspects of remediation. Indeed, a unifying theme in the understanding of seizure disorders and their effects is the need to consider the diversity of domains. Unfortunately, there is little published empirical evidence to guide the selection of techniques for cognitive remediation. For the most part, clinicians will have to rely on the literature regarding cognitive remediation in patients with other etiologies. Studies specifically investigating seizure patients are needed because specific factors may be work in the development of the cognitive deficits in these patients. For example, group studies comparing rehabilitation interventions in both seizure patients and closed head injury patients would address the relative effectiveness of the interventions in these two populations. Intensive clinical studies would help address the issue of complicating factors particular to seizure disorder patients.

References

Aldenkamp AP, Vermeulen J: Neuropsychological rehabilitation of memory function in epilepsy. Neuropsychological Rehabilitation 1:199–214, 1991

Bear DM, Fedio P: Quantitative analysis of interictal behavior in temporal lobe epilepsy. Arch Neurol 34:454–467, 1977

Bear D, Schenk L, Benson H: Increased autonomic responses to neutral and emotional stimuli in patients with temporal lobe epilepsy. Am J Psychiatry 138:843–845, 1981

Bennett TL: Cognitive effects of epilepsy and anticonvulsant medications, in The Neuropsychology of Epilepsy. Edited by Bennet TL. New York, Plenum, 1992, pp 73–95

Berent S, Boll TS, Giordani B: Hemispheric site of epileptogenic focus: cognitive, perceptual and psychosocial implications for children and adults, in Advances in Epileptology: 11th International Symposium. Edited by Canger R, Angelini F, Penry JK. New York, Raven, 1980, pp 185–190

Brittain H: Epilepsy and intellectual functions, in Epilepsy and Behavior. Edited by Kulig BM, Meinardi H, Stores G. New York, Lisse, Swets & Zeitlinger, 1980, pp 2–13

Cavazutti GB: Epidemiology of different types of epilepsy in school-age children of Modena, Italy. Epilepsia 21:57–62, 1980

Chelune GJ, Naugle RI, Luders H, et al: Prediction of cognitive change as a function of preoperative status among temporal lobectomy patients seen at 6-month follow-up. Neurology 41:399–404, 1991

Dahlstrom WG, Welsh GS, Dahlstrom LE: An MMPI Handbook, Vol I. Minneapolis, University of Minnesota Press, 1972

Delaney RC, Rosen AJ, Mattson RH, et al: Memory function in focal epilepsy: a comparison of non-surgical, unilateral temporal lobe and frontal lobe samples. Cortex 16:103–117, 1980

Delaney RC, Prevey ML, Mattson RH: Short term retention with lateralized temporal lobe epilepsy. Cortex 22:591–600, 1986

Delgado-Escueta AV, Swartz BE, Walsh GO, et al: Frontal lobe seizures and epilepsies in neurobehavioral disorders, in Advances in Neurology: Neurobehavioral Problems in Epilepsy, Vol 55. Edited by Smith D, Treiman D, Trimble M. New York, Raven, 1991, pp 317–340

Dodrill CB, Batzel LW, Fraser R: Psychosocial changes after surgery for epilepsy, in Epilepsy Surgery. Edited by Luders H. New York, Raven, 1991, pp 661–667

Ellis HC: The Transfer of Learning. New York, Macmillan, 1965

Farwell JR, Dodrill CB, Batzel LW: Neuropsychological abilities of children with epilepsy. Epilepsia 26:395–400, 1985

Fedio P, Mirsky AF: Selective intellectual deficits in children with temporal lobe or centrocephalic epilepsy. Neuropsychologia 7:287–300, 1969

Franzen MD: Behavioral assessment and treatment of brain-impaired individuals, in Progress in Behavior Modification, Vol. 27. Edited by Hersen M, Eisler RM, Miller PM. Beverly Hills, CA, Sage, 1991, pp 56–85

Franzen MD, Haut MW: The psychological treatment of memory impairment: a review of empirical studies. Neuropsychol Rev 2:29–63, 1991

Freeman JM, Jacobs H, Vinning E, et al: Epilepsy and the inner city schools: a school based program that makes a difference. Epilepsia 25:438–442, 1984

Gifford J, Rusch F, Martin J, et al: Autonomy and adaptability: a proposed technology for maintaining work behavior, in International Review of Research on Mental Retardation, Vol 12. Edited by Ellis N, Bray N. New York, Academic Press, 1984, pp 285–314

Goldstein LH: Behavioural and cognitive-behavioral treatments for epilepsy: a progress review. Br J Clin Psychol 29:257–269, 1990

Gregoriades AD: A medical and social survey of 231 children with seizures. Epilepsia 13:13–20, 1972

Gumnit RJ, Gates JR: Psychogenic seizures. Epilepsia 27 (suppl 2):124–129, 1986

Hackney A, Taylor DC: A teacher's questionnaire description of epileptic children. Epilepsia 17:275–281, 1976

Heaton RK: Wisconsin Card Sorting Test Manual. Odessa, TX, Psychological Assessment Resources, 1985

Helgeson DC, Mittan R, Tan SY, et al: Sepulveda epilepsy education: the efficacy of a psychoeducational treatment program in treating medical and psychosocial aspects of epilepsy. Epilepsia 31:75–82, 1990

Henriksen O: Education and epilepsy: assessment and remediation. Epilepsia 31 (suppl 4):S21–S25, 1990

Hermann BP, Wyler AR, Richey ET, et al: Memory function and verbal learning ability in patients with complex partial seizures of temporal lobe origin. Epilepsia 28:547–554, 1987

Hermann BP, Wyler AR, Richey ET: Wisconsin card sorting test performance in patients with complex partial seizures of temporal-lobe origin. J Clin Exp Neuropsychol 10:467–476, 1988

Hermann BP, Whitman S, Anton M: A multietiological model of psychological and social dysfunction in epilepsy, in The Neuropsychology of Epilepsy. Edited by Bennett TL. New York, Plenum, 1992, pp 39–57

Hodgman CH, McAnarney ER, Meyers GT, et al: Emotional complications of adolescent grand mal epilepsy. J Pediatr 95:309–312, 1979

Holdsworth L, Whitmore K: A study of children with epilepsy attending ordinary schools, I: their seizure patterns, progress and behavior in school. Dev Med Child Neurol 16:746–758, 1974

Horner RH, Sprague J, Wilcox B: General case programming for community activities, in Design of High School Programs for Severely Handicapped Students. Edited by Wilcox B, Bellamy GT. Baltimore, MD, Paul H. Brookes, 1982, pp 61–98

Jones-Gotman M: Presurgical neuropsychological evaluation for localization and lateralization of seizure focus, in Epilepsy Surgery. Edited by Luders H. New York, Raven, 1991, pp 469–475

Jones-Gotman M, Zatorre R: Olfactory identification deficits in patients with focal cerebral excision. Neuropsychologia 26:387–400, 1988

Karan O: Epilepsy: the non-medical aspects. Rehabil Rec 13:37–40, 1972

Klove H, Matthews CG: Neuropsychological studies of patients with epilepsy, in Clinical Neuropsychology: Current Status and Applications. Edited by Reitan RM, Davison LA. Washington, DC, Hemisphere, 1974, pp 237–265

Lantz D, Sterman MB: Neuropsychological prediction and outcome measures in relation to EEG feedback training for the treatment of epilepsy, in The Neuropsychology of Epilepsy. Edited by Bennett TL. New York, Plenum, 1992, pp 213–231

Lesser RP, Luders H, Wyllie E, et al: Mental deterioration in epilepsy. Epilepsia 27 (suppl 2):105–123, 1986

Loiseau P, Strube E, Broustet D, et al: Learning impairment in epileptic patients. Epilepsia 24:183–192, 1983

Long CG, Moore JR: Parental expectations for their epileptic children. J Child Psychol Psychiatry 20:299–312, 1979

Loring DW, Lee GP, Martin RC, et al: Material-specific learning in patients with partial complex seizures of temporal lobe origin: convergent validation of memory constructs. J Epilepsy 1:53–59, 1988

Lyketsos CG, Stoline AM, Longstreet P, et al: Mania in temporal lobe epilepsy. Neuropsychiatry, Neuropsychology, and Behavioral Neurology 6:19–25, 1993

Manchanda R, Schaefer B, McLachan RS, et al: Interictal psychiatric morbidity and focus of epilepsy in treatment-refractory patients admitted to an epilepsy unit. Am J Psychiatry 149:1096–1098, 1992

Martin RC, Loring DW, Meador KJ, et al: Impaired long-term retention despite normal verbal learning in patients with temporal lobe dysfunction. Neuropsychology 5:3–12, 1991

McCue M, Pramuka M, Chase S: A model of applied cognitive rehabilitation: guidelines for implementation. Paper presented at the annual conference of the National Academy of Neuropsychology, Pittsburgh, PA, 1992

Mostofsky DI, Balaschak BA: Psychobiological control of seizures. Psychol Bull 84:723–750, 1977

Nickell PV, Uhde TW: Anxiety disorders and epilepsy, in Epilepsy and Behavior. Edited by Devinsky I, Theodore WH. New York, Wiley-Liss, 1991, pp 67–84

Pazzaglia P, Frank-Pazzaglia L: Record in grade school pupils with epilepsy: an epidemiological study. Epilepsia 17:361–366, 1976

Porter RJ: Epilepsy and employment. Ir J Med Sci 1:89–91, 1968

Radloff LS: The CES-D scale: a self-report depression scale for research in the general population. Applied Psychological Measurement 1:385–401, 1977

Rausch R, McCreary C, Crandall PH: Predictions of psychological functioning following successful surgical treatment of epilepsy. J Psychosom Res 21: 141–146, 1977

Richardson DW, Friedman SB: Psychosocial problems of the adolescent patient with epilepsy. Clin Pediatr 13:121–126, 1974

Rodin E, Rennick P, Dennerill R, et al: Vocational and educational problems of epileptic patients. Epilepsy 13:149–160, 1972

Rodin EA, Schmaltz S, Twitty G: Intellectual functions of patients with childhood-onset epilepsy. Dev Med Child Neurol 28:25–33, 1988

Ross EM, Peckham CS, West PB, et al: Epilepsy in childhood: findings from the National Child Development Study. Br Med J 1:207–210, 1980

Rotter JB: Generalized expectancies for internal versus external control of reinforcement. Psychol Monogr 80(609), 1966

Ryan R, Kempner K, Emlen AC: The stigma of epilepsy as a self-concept. Epilepsia 21:433–444, 1980

Sarason IG, Johnson JH, Siegel JM: Assessing the impact of life changes: development of the Life Experiences Survey. J Consult Clin Psychol 46: 932–946, 1978

Sarason IG, Levine HM, Basham RB, et al: Assessing social support: the social support questionnaire. J Pers Soc Psychol 44:127–139, 1983

Silfvenius H: Pre- and postoperative rehabilitation related to epilepsy surgery. Acta Neurochir (Wien) 21 (suppl 50):100–106, 1990

Stevens JR, Milstein V, Goldstein S: Psychometric test performance in relation to the psychopathology of epilepsy. Arch Gen Psychiatry 26:532–538, 1972

Stores G, Hart J, Piran N: Inattentiveness in school children with epilepsy. Epilepsia 19:169–175, 1978

Strang JD: Cognitive deficits in children: adaptive behavior and treatment techniques. Epilepsia 31 (suppl 4):S54–S58, 1990

Thompson PJ: Memory function in patients with epilepsy, in Advances in Neurology:Neurobehavioral Problems in Epilepsy, Vol 55. Edited by Smith D, Treiman D, Trimble M. New York, Raven, 1991, pp 369–384

Trimble MR: The schizophrenia-like psychosis of epilepsy. Neuropsychiatry, Neuropsychology, and Behavioral Neurology 5:103–107, 1992

Vanderzant CW, Giordani B, Berent S, et al: Personality of patients with pseudoseizures. Neurology 36:664–668, 1986

Wannamaker BB, Matthews CG: Prognostic implications of neuropsychological test performance for surgical treatment of epilepsy. J Nerv Ment Dis 163:29–34, 1976

Whitman S, Hermann BP, Gordon AC: Psychopathology in epilepsy: how great is the risk? Biol Psychiatry 19:213–236, 1984

Woolcock WW. Generalization strategies, in Vocational Rehabilitation for Persons with Traumatic Brain Injury. Edited by Wehman P, Kreuter JS. Rockville, MD, Aspen Publishers, 1989, pp 243–263

Chapter 10

Cognitive Rehabilitation for Children With Traumatic Brain Injury

Mark Ylvisaker, Ph.D., and Shirley F. Szekeres, Ph.D.

*B*rain injury has been used for several decades as a disability category in discussions of special education. Its original scope was extremely broad, including children with genetic neurological disorders and those with any type of brain injury, acquired before, during, or after birth. Therefore, this heterogenous group included children with mental retardation, learning disabilities, cerebral palsy, and a variety of other more specific disabilities resulting from a variety of causes.

Current discussions of acquired brain injury in children have been influenced by developments in rehabilitation for adults with head injury (e.g., Rosenthal et al. 1990) and by the new federal definition of traumatic brain injury (TBI) as a mandated special education disability category in P.L. 101–476, the Individuals with Disability Education Act of 1990. This definition restricts TBI to include only children with brain injury resulting from external causes (e.g., closed or open head injury). However, some state departments of education have adopted a broad definition that equates TBI with *acquired* (noncongenital) brain injury, including that resulting from stroke, tumor, anoxia, encephalitis, meningitis, and toxic encephalopathy, as well as from head injury. The value of a broad definition is that important characteristics of this group from an educational perspective are associated with the injury occurring after a substantial period of normal development. These characteristics include the following:

- *Neurological change* over an extended period of time after the injury (usually improvement, but possibly delayed deterioration)
- An *unusual profile* of strengths and needs, based on the juxtaposition of possibly high-level skills and knowledge, acquired before and recovered after the injury, with substantial deficits caused by the injury
- *Bursts of progress,* based on recovery of preinjury knowledge and skill, that may lead professionals to be overly optimistic about new learning

- Profound *emotional struggles,* based on loss of ability, friends, social status, and sense of self
- A need to shed possibly effective preinjury intellectual, academic, and social habits in order to learn new serviceable strategies
- A degree of confusion, disorientation, disinhibition, unawareness of deficits, and lack of self-control for which professionals in the educational system may be unprepared, particularly in the early months after the injured student returns to school

In this chapter, we use the term *TBI* to refer generally to children with acquired brain injury who may need specialized cognitive intervention. In discussing general aspects of outcome, our focus is further restricted to closed head injury (CHI), partly because this comprises the largest group of children and adolescents with acquired brain injury and partly because there are some interesting themes with this group that merit discussion.

Epidemiology of Head Injury in Children

Approximately 150,000 to 200,000 children and adolescents, school age and younger, are hospitalized annually in the United States with head injury (Eiben et al. 1984; Raphael et al. 1980). Using a narrower definition of pediatric (age 14 and younger) and a more conservative definition of brain injury, Kraus et al. (1987) estimated 100,000 pediatric hospital admissions annually for acute brain trauma. Incidence estimates vary with the age group, geographic area, and other variables but include a peak of approximately 400 to 600 per 100,000 in the highest risk group, 15- to 25-year-old men (Annegers et al. 1980). A secondary peak occurs for infants and young children. The cumulative risk of TBI from birth through age 15 is approximately 4% for boys and 2.5% for girls (Rivara and Mueller 1986).

Head injury is two to three times more frequent in males than in females. Rates also vary with race and economic levels, with nonwhites and lower socioeconomic groups being at higher risk (Cooper et al. 1983; Kraus 1987; Rivara and Mueller 1986). Most studies of pediatric head injury suggest that more than 80% of hospital admissions are mild injuries (e.g., unconsciousness not exceeding 1 hour; initial Glasgow Coma Scale score of 12 or greater), with the remainder being moderate or severe. Including all degrees of severity of injury, falls account for a majority of injuries in young children, while the automobile is involved in a majority of adolescent cases. Considering only severe injuries, the motor vehicle is involved in a majority of cases in all age groups, with the exception of infants, whose injuries are associated in large numbers with abuse.

Age and Outcome

Until recently, there has been widespread acceptance of the hypothesis that age is inversely related to outcome (i.e., the younger the individual at the time of injury, the better the outcome). This plasticity principle was originally based on studies of outcome after surgically induced unilateral lesions in experimental animals (Finger 1991). The conclusion was supported by relatively good language development in children with brain injury early in life (Lenneberg 1967) and by optimistic early reports of general outcome following head injury in children (Bruce et al. 1978, 1979).

Unfortunately, this positive prognosis for children with TBI has been seriously challenged in recent years. Several investigators have reported that infants as a group are at greatest risk for serious long-term sequelae after severe head injury (Mahoney et al. 1983; Raimondi and Hirschauer 1984). Beyond infancy, Ewing-Cobbs et al. (1989) found that younger preschoolers were more severely impaired than older preschoolers (cut-off = 30 months) on intellectual, motor, and expressive language measures when tested at least 6 months after severe CHI. Furthermore, investigators who have compared young school-aged children with adolescents with grossly similar injuries have found outcome to be either comparable in the two age groups or relatively depressed in the younger group (Brink et al. 1970; Chadwick et al. 1981; Ewing-Cobbs et al. 1987; Klonoff et al. 1977; Levin et al. 1982).

Finally, recent studies of prefrontal injury in children have revived the concern, expressed earlier by Kennard and Fulton (1942), that early frontal lobe lesions may have delayed consequences—possibly years after the injury—and that these consequences may have their primary impact on social interactive competence and general control over cognitive processes (Dennis 1991; Grattan and Eslinger 1991; Kolb 1989; Mateer and Williams 1991). The prediction of increasing behavioral and psychosocial problems during the months and years after the injury in children is ominously supported by longitudinal data (G. Brown et al. 1981; Eslinger et al. 1992; Fletcher et al. 1990; Grattan and Eslinger 1992; Marlowe 1992; Williams and Mateer 1992). Furthermore, the cumulative effect of new learning problems is likely to result in increasing developmental lags over time in academic and other areas.

Stages of Cognitive Recovery

Use of the word *recovery* may misleadingly suggest to parents and others that return to preinjury levels of functioning is anticipated. *Stages of improvement* would be a better choice of terms; nevertheless, we will follow standard practice in using the word recovery. Because outcome and rehabilitative needs after head injury are often dominated by cognitive and psychosocial issues, recovery scales tend to highlight these variables. For example, the Rancho Los Amigos (RLA) Levels of Cognitive Functioning (Hagen 1981), presented in Table 10–1, is commonly used to track recovery in adolescents and adults with head injury. With modifications, it can be used with younger children as well, although stages of normal cognitive development in infants and toddlers also are useful in tracking cognitive recovery in very young children.

Cognitive improvement after severe CHI is often slow and varies from individual to individual. However, there is a pattern to recovery that scales are designed to capture. We have found it useful to group the many qualitatively distinct levels of cognitive recovery into three general stages that are associated with different types of rehabilitative intervention. The early stage of cognitive recovery (roughly RLA II and III) generally takes place in a hospital or rehabilitation facility and encompasses the period from medical stabilization to beginning purposeful interaction with the environment. Following eye opening and resumption of sleep-wake cycles, individuals may show recognition of objects or people and have at best generalized responses to stimulation (e.g., flexion of the arms in response to any type of stimulation). Responses gradually become more specific to the stimulus as alertness improves (e.g., turning to sound; recognizing familiar faces). This period is often characterized as the *stimulation* phase of rehabilitation, a term that should not be taken to imply the absence of attempts to enable the child to have effects on the environment and in other ways to be an agent and not just a passive recipient of stimulation.

The middle stage of cognitive recovery (roughly RLA IV through VI) is characterized by overall alertness and recognition of objects, people, and events in the environment, but also some degree of confusion, disorientation, impulsiveness, severely impaired attention, and shallow processing of information. At this stage, the child may remain hospitalized, may be receiving home-bound educational services, or may have returned to school. Superficial academic skills (e.g., spelling, word recognition, basic calculation) may return quickly, but comprehension, organized thinking, abstract thinking, problem solving, new learning, and general self-regulation tend to lag far behind. Cognitive rehabilitation during this phase includes selecting meaningful and functional tasks that challenge specific components of cognition with progressively greater demands, promoting reacquisition of familiar organizational schemes that guided thought processes and behavior before the injury, and preventing maladaptive behavior through environmental structuring and careful modulation of task demands.

During the late stage of recovery (roughly RLA VII, VIII, and beyond), behavior is generally goal directed and appropriate (relative to age expectations), but specific constellations of cognitive deficits may emerge related to

Table 10–1.   Rancho Los Amigos levels of cognitive functioning

Early stages of recovery

Level I—*No response*
Patient appears to be in deep sleep and is completely unresponsive to any stimuli presented (coma).

Level II—*Generalized response*
Patient reacts inconsistently and nonpurposefully to stimuli.

Level III—*Localized response*
Patient reacts specifically but inconsistently to stimuli; may turn head toward sound or extend hand upon request.

Middle stages of recovery

Level IV—*Confused-agitated*
Patient is in a heightened state of activity; may show aggressive behavior and excessive irritation disproportionate to stimuli; exhibits significantly decreased ability to process information. Short-term memory and selective attention are nonexistent. Patient is unable to perform self-care.

Level V—*Confused, inappropriate, nonagitated*
Patient is alert and able to respond to simple commands in a fairly consistent manner; highly distractible; lacks ability to focus and sustain attention; makes inappropriate verbalizations (when motoric speech is not impaired); exhibits severe problems with short-term memory; unable to learn new information. Patient can perform self-help activities with assistance.

Level VI—*Confused-appropriate*
Patient shows goal-directed behavior and carryover for old skills that have been relearned (toothbrushing, feeding, etc.); continued short-term memory deficits. Long-term memory (recall) is improving. Patient may show inconsistent orientation to time and place; recognizes caretakers and shows some awareness of basic needs.

Late stages of recovery

Level VII—*Automatic-appropriate*
Patient shows increased awareness of self and environment; able to follow a routine schedule with prompts; lacks insight into condition; demonstrates poor judgment and problem-solving skills; unrealistic about future; independent in self-care with supervision; unable to drive a car.

Level VIII—*Purposeful and appropriate*
Alert and oriented; able to recall and integrate past with recent events; shows carryover for new learning; requires little supervision in carrying out relearned tasks; may continue to show an overall decrease in ability to reason, tolerate stress, and make emergency decisions. Vocational rehabilitation may be indicated.

Source.   Reprinted from Hagen C, Malkmus D, Durham P: *Rancho Los Amigos: Levels of Cognitive Functioning.* Downey, CA, Rancho Los Amigos Medical Center, Adult Brain Injury Service, 1981. Used with permission.

the nature of the child's injury as well as his or her preinjury status. After CHI, residual deficits often include generally impaired executive functions (including reduced control over behavior and emotions and cognitive processes such as attention and memory), impaired organizational skills (negatively affecting reading, writing, speaking, and other complex tasks), slow and inefficient processing of information in any modality, concrete and inflexible thinking, and reduced social perception. Unlike adults, children continue to change over time not simply as a result of neurologic recovery and rehabilitative services, but also because of normal developmental forces. However, children also are more likely than adults to experience delayed onset of deficits as brain injury interacts with developmental challenges over the years after the injury.

Cognitive Rehabilitation With Children

The purpose of cognitive rehabilitation is to enable individuals to achieve goals that may be impeded by cognitive impairment. That is, the goal is to promote successful performance of real-world tasks, not necessarily to improve "cognition." In ways that are analogous to the modalities of physical rehabilitation, cognitive rehabilitation may include interventions designed to do the following:

- Promote restoration of cognitive processes or systems that were impaired by the injury
- Promote development of cognitive processes or systems that may be delayed by the injury
- Facilitate acquisition of new knowledge that increasingly facilitates effective information processing
- Help individuals become increasingly strategic and equip them with strategic procedures that enable them to accomplish goals despite ongoing cognitive impairment
- Identify ways in which academic, social, and vocational environments can be modified to promote success despite ongoing cognitive impairment
- Identify instructional strategies that are consistent with the child's profile of cognitive strengths and weaknesses and that can be used with greatest effectiveness in school
- Heighten children's understanding of their needs and adjustment to their disability so that they are increasingly active participants in the process of solving the many problems caused by the injury and consequent cognitive deficits

Cognitive Rehabilitation as Restoration of Function Through Process-Specific Remedial Exercises

In the early years of intense program development in adult head injury rehabilitation, there was a tendency to associate cognitive rehabilitation or "retraining" with a hierarchically organized set of exercises designed to restore or at least improve impaired components of cognition considered in isolation (Diller 1976). This "building-block" approach often began with precisely targeted attentional and perceptual exercises (e.g., reaction time with and without distractors [for improved alertness, maintenance of response set, and selective attention]; continuous performance tasks; alternating performance tasks [for attentional shifts]; tracking and scanning tasks; and memory tasks, beginning with immediate recall of simple, nonmeaningful stimuli and gradually adding complexity to the stimuli and increasing delays between presentation and recall). Initially, exercises were conducted as paper-and-pencil activities or with customized electronic retraining devices. Subsequently, exercises of this sort were computerized, and cognitive retraining came to be associated with computer activities. The attractiveness of this approach lay in its orderliness (i.e., clinicians created sequenced programs of exercises based on purported cognitive hierarchies and therefore knew at any time what to do and where to go next), the relative ease with which progress (or lack of it) could be measured, and the prospect for the patient of genuinely regaining lost function.

Enthusiasm for this approach to cognitive rehabilitation for adults has waned in recent years (Ben Yishay and Prigatano 1990; Berrol 1990; Lynch 1992). Skepticism has resulted from evidence that certain cognitive processes either do not respond to remedial exercises or the improvements in function are insufficient to support meaningful change in real-world performance of meaningful tasks (Schacter and Glisky 1986). Moreover, concern with the ecological validity of cognitive retraining exercises has grown with the observation that improvements in cognitive functioning do not readily transfer from highly contrived retraining tasks to real-world tasks and settings (Lynch 1992). The latter concern is strongly supported by systematic investigations of transfer of cognitive skill in individuals with normal cognitive functioning, investigations that have led cognitive scientists in recent years to emphasize the domain specificity of many cognitive skills and procedures that would appear to be highly generalizable (Singley and Anderson 1989). Applied to cognitive rehabilitation, these considerations at the least recommend the use of ecologically valid tasks for retraining purposes. In the case of students, academic tasks should be the context of rehabilitation, even if the goals are better control of attention, faster processing of information, better organized perceptual searches, and the like.

Skepticism about the effectiveness of restorative cognitive retraining, using a hierarchy of decontextualized exercises designed to engage component cognitive processes, should come as no surprise to those familiar with the past three decades of research in educational psychology and special education. The building block approach to cognitive retraining bears a strong resemblance to the specific abilities approach to cognitive and academic remediation proposed in the 1950s and 1960s by Kirk, Frostig, Getman, Kephart, Strauss, and others. In a recent review of historical approaches to cognitive dysfunction in students with learning disabilities, Hresko and Reid (1988) concluded that the specific cognitive abilities remedial approach was the only one of five approaches under consideration that has been shown to be "incapable" of supporting effective educational planning for students with learning disabilities. A similarly negative conclusion was drawn by Kavale and Mattson (1983) who completed a meta-analysis of 181 studies of the effectiveness of perceptual and perceptual-motor exercises in relation to cognitive and academic improvement in special education students. In a book on the history of process-specific cognitive training, Mann (1979) traced remedial proposals through 2,500 years of Western educational theory and practices and derived similar pessimistic conclusions about the potential of this approach.

Restoration Versus Compensation: A False Dichotomy

It may seem natural to opt for a purely compensatory model of cognitive rehabilitation in the face of pessimism regarding process-specific remedial approaches. Perhaps one reason for the resilience of the debate between restorative and compensatory approaches to cognitive rehabilitation is that they present a false dichotomy. For example, teaching or reteaching children specific organizational schemata (discussed below) that they then use in processing information more efficiently is not (or need not be) compensatory. Still this approach is quite different from simply exercising a process to make it work better. Similarly, teaching children strategic procedures is often included under the general heading "compensation," but may be better understood as promoting normal cognitive development, that is, acquisition of helpful procedures (e.g., outlining strategies, review strategies, monitoring strategies) that also are acquired by normally developing students. Many strategic procedures are part of normal cognition and therefore not compensatory in the sense that they would not be needed but for the brain injury. Indeed, some cognitive processes are by their very nature strategic (e.g., problem-solving processes).

The restoration versus compensation dichotomy also is inapplicable to children because they are a work in progress (Lehr 1990). Intervention for children with cognitive deficits after brain injury is, at least in part, an attempt to encourage development of cognitive skills and content knowledge not possessed before the injury. Given the well-documented positive relation between knowledge and processing efficiency, there is an important sense in which all attempts to teach general knowledge and specific curricular content to children are aspects of cognitive rehabilitation.

Cognitive Assessment for Planning Rehabilitation and Education

Cognitive assessment of children with TBI is at the same time particularly important and particularly challenging. Its importance lies in the pervasiveness of cognitive deficits after severe TBI; in their profound implications for academic, social, and vocational success; and in the extent to which important decisions about educational services and supports hang in the balance. For the following reasons, cognitive assessment is especially challenging for children with TBI:

Misleading Profiles Based on Recovery of Knowledge and Skill

Following moderate or even apparently severe TBI, children may recover much of the knowledge and academic skill that they had acquired before the injury. This pattern of recovery often results in the decision to provide no special support for the student when he or she returns to school. However, these students may have organizational and learning problems that easily lead to academic failure and associated behavior problems if undetected.

The solution to this problem is not to assume that all children with TBI will have serious learning problems and therefore need intensive services and supports. Rather, assessments should include teaching new information and skills, with careful documentation of learning rate and style, as part of the school reentry cognitive assessment. Professionals should monitor children who appear not to have special educational needs, so that early signs of unexpected difficulty with the curriculum will be noted. Frequent reassessment should be prescribed in the Individualized Educational Plan (IEP) for children who are judged to need support.

Misleading Profiles Based on Gaps in the Knowledge Base

It is not uncommon for students with TBI to have preserved knowledge and skill at relatively high levels along with significant gaps at relatively low levels. Indeed, this can occur in content domains that are hierarchical in nature. For example, a 15-year-old student may remember much of ninth-grade algebra despite having lost most of the third-grade multiplication tables. If the low-level gaps are not recognized, the student is likely to experience failure and frustration. If the preserved high-level strengths are not identified, instruction will likely be at a uniformly low level, the student may feel infantilized, and the teacher will fail to capitalize on important skills that can be used in motivating the student and compensating for weaknesses. The solutions to this assessment challenge include proceeding above ceilings and below basals in standardized tests and vigilantly searching for both gaps and preserved ability during diagnostic instruction.

Misleading Profiles Based on Executive System Weakness

Prefrontal injury and associated executive system weakness (among the most common types of injury and deficit in CHI) have been tied to a set of assessment challenges in both adult and pediatric neuropsychological literatures (e.g., Lezak 1982). Unfortunately, most psychological tests yield high false-negative rates when assessing executive functions (Benton 1991; Bigler 1988; Dennis 1991; Eslinger and Damasio 1985; Grattan and Eslinger 1991; Mateer and Williams 1991; Stelling et al. 1986; Stuss and Benson 1986; Welsh et al. 1991). Consistent with this theme, Perrott et al. (1991), Fletcher et al. (1990), and Petterson (1991) all found that the high rates of behavioral adjustment difficulties in children and adolescents with severe TBI were not predicted by their relatively satisfactory performance on standardized tests of cognitive ability.

There are many features of the testing situation and commonly used tests of intellectual, academic, and language ability that easily generate misleadingly successful performance in children whose ability to control and organize their cognitive processes is relatively impaired as a result of prefrontal injury. For example, controlled and distraction-free testing environments may compensate for poorly regulated attention. Use of clear test instructions may compensate for weak task orientation and impaired flexibility in shifting from task to task. Use of highly structured tasks and clear instructions may compensate for weak initiation, inhibition, and problem solving. Tasks that do not include real-life quantities of information to be organized may compensate for difficulty imposing organizing schemes on incoming information or tasks. Tests that do not require storage and retrieval of information from day to day may compensate for an inability to use encoding and retrieval strategies. The supportive and encouraging manner of the evaluator may compensate for the child's inability to read social cues in context and to cope with interpersonal stress. Each of these themes has been associated with prefrontal injury and should guide clinicians in developing valid assessment procedures for children suspected of such injury.

The general solution to this complex assessment challenge is to ensure that cognitive assessment includes ecologically valid tasks. Ecologically valid assessment of children includes mobilizing planned classroom observations and diagnostic teaching as part of cognitive assessment. Planned observations should also be conducted in natural social environments as part of communication and psychosocial assessment. Elsewhere we have listed procedures that can be used to guide this detective work and have outlined a dialectical model of cognitive assessment that includes structured interaction among school psychologists, classroom teachers, and others (Ylvisaker et al. 1990, 1994a). Procedures are presented within a framework that includes cognitive processes and subprocesses (attentional, perceptual, memory/learning, organizing, and reasoning/problem-solving processes), cognitive systems (working memory, knowledge base, executive system, and response system), and variables that define functional-integrative performance (scope, manner, efficiency, and level of performance).

Case Example

P.N. had multiple head injuries as a preschooler as a result of abuse. At age eight he was integrated into a general education first-grade class for a small part of his school day but spent most of the day in a self-contained special education class and in one-to-one therapy and tutorial instruction. Behavioral outbursts, including screaming, throwing materials, and hitting himself, occurred several times every day. No academic progress had been observed over the past year, despite IQ estimates that suggested reasonable learning potential. Academic instruction occurred in a quiet environment, because of a high level of distractibility, and was based on the principles of direct instruction, because of P.N.'s apparent need for clear learning tasks and many learning trials.

Because of the lack of progress and deteriorating behavior, the school psychologist suggested to the teaching and therapy staff that they systematically explore what effects alternative contexts and task orientations might have on P.N.'s learning. For several weeks, staff attempted to teach various types of content under systematically varying conditions, carefully documenting P.N.'s performance. Contrary to expectations, it emerged that P.N. learned more effectively in a small group than when he received one-to-one attention and that he learned more effectively under incidental or involuntary conditions than under deliberate learning conditions of direct instruction (i.e., when he was oriented to a concrete task that was intrinsically meaningful for him rather than being oriented to the task of learning the lesson for the day). In addition, the psychologist recommended giving P.N. the right to choose some aspect of each lesson. As expected, this reduced his manipulative behavior. Instruction in groups and the use of involuntary learning procedures had not been indicated by the psychologist's earlier testing but were revealed by real-world assessment experiments to be critical modifications of P.N.'s educational program.

Cognitive Intervention: Illustrations

Given the broad understanding of cognitive rehabilitation, virtually every text-book on educational intervention would fall under this umbrella. Although approaches to teaching specific curricular content may not seem to be cognitive rehabilitation, they belong in this arena because growth in content knowledge has an important secondary benefit of increasing efficiency with which information can be processed. Furthermore, "curricular content" is not always easy to distinguish from "cognitive process." For example, middle-school English teachers routinely teach reading comprehension strategies (e.g., actively searching texts for answers to Wh- questions) and writing strategies (e.g., outlining procedures). This strategy instruction is just as much a part of the curricular content as regrouping strategies (i.e., borrowing and carrying) are part of the grade school arithmetic curriculum. Under other circumstances, teaching of this sort would be considered strategic cognitive rehabilitation.

Organization and memory are critical aspects of cognitive development, contribute heavily to academic success, and are frequently impaired in TBI. Equally important to academic success and equally vulnerable in TBI is executive control over cognitive functions or strategic behavior. In the sections that follow, we use these two areas of intervention to illustrate an approach to cognitive rehabilitation.

Organization and Memory

Important aspects of development: memory.   In their review of research on memory development in children, Schneider and Pressley (1989) summarized major aspects of development under four interconnected headings: 1) short-term memory, 2) memory strategies, 3) metamemory, and 4) knowledge base. *Short-term,* or *working memory* (the temporary "holding space" in which information is attended to and operated on) is believed to develop largely in its functional rather than structural capacity. That is, as individuals become increasingly able to organize information, the "chunks" of information that can be held in working memory become increasingly large, thereby increasing its functional capacity. For example, when a number of separate units of information are brought together under one heading (e.g., battles of the Civil War), they can be held in memory as one large "chunk." Increased speed and automaticity of information processing as well as increased use of organizing schema contribute to this growth in functional capacity.

The use of encoding and retrieval *strategies* (procedures that are potentially deliberate and that are used to increase the likelihood that information will be stored and subsequently retrieved) is closely tied to the gradual development of *metamemory*, which includes knowledge of memory as an activity (e.g., that learning and remembering are identifiable covert activities that one can do well or poorly), of tasks (e.g., that some memory tasks are more difficult than others), and of strategies (e.g., that there are things that can be done to make remembering easier). Young children and many individuals with TBI are poorly aware of the limits on their ability to remember, fail to identify tasks that require special effort, and have little understanding of what procedures to use to enhance successful performance.

The *knowledge base* includes information, concepts, organizational schemes, and words along with their interrelations. With increases in the organization of this knowledge comes an increase in the ease with which new information can be processed (attended to, understood, encoded, stored, and retrieved). Particularly as children gain conscious control over their organization of information (i.e., deliberately use organizing strategies), it is easier for them to integrate and elaborate new information, and therefore make it more memorable (Bjorklund 1985; Chi 1978).

Because young children lack understanding of and deliberate control over cognitive activity, learning is largely a by-product of active engagement in personally meaningful activities (Smirnov 1973). That is, their goal is intrinsic to the activity as opposed to the abstract goal of learning or remembering something. Efficiency of *involuntary* or *incidental* learning in this sense (Postman 1964) is a function of features of the task relative to the child's interests and prior knowledge. The goal of the teacher within this framework of learning is to engage students in personally meaningful tasks and focus their attention on relevant aspects of the activity so that the new information is processed as deeply as possible within the student's base of knowledge, increasing the likelihood of encoding, storage, and future recall.

For example, a preschool teacher might teach the word "wider" by having the children move zoo animals into their new cages through gates that are too narrow. The children's goal is simply to get the animals into the cages, which requires overcoming the gate problem by asking that it be made wider. The teacher's goal is to teach "wider." For the children, the concept and corresponding word are processed as a means of accomplishing their primary and concrete goal. This processing is an important feature of preschool learning tasks and may be equally important for older children and adolescents whose injuries have resulted in their being nonstrategic in relation to the abstract goal of learning.

Deliberate or *voluntary* learning is characterized by an intent to remember something (A. L. Brown 1975, 1979). Effectiveness of deliberate learning assumes that the learner understands the abstract goal of learning and has voluntary access to procedures (strategies) that will facilitate achievement of this abstract goal. For this reason, memory or learning performance of preschoolers is understandably impeded by explicitly or implicitly making it their goal to learn or remember (Schneider and Pressley 1989). Using the example from the previous paragraph, if the children had been told that their job was simply to remember that "wider" means that the opening is bigger, their retention would predictably deteriorate. There is gradual development of deliberate learning over the school years, leading ultimately to the facility with which college students use varied strategies to study for exams. Unfortunately, it is common for teachers and therapists to orient "impaired" learners to the abstract task of learning (e.g., "You've got to work real hard to remember this"), even though there is reason to believe that this orientation interferes with learning. Orienting tasks that promote deeper semantic processing and make the learning involuntary will likely be more effective.

Important aspects of development: organization.   As mentioned earlier, children with TBI often show disorders of organizational functioning, manifested by disorganized activities of daily living, poorly organized expressive language (e.g., disjointed conversations and narratives), inefficient word retrieval, weak language comprehension because of difficulty integrating a text, and weak retention of new information because it was not adequately integrated with existing knowledge at the time of encoding. The problem may be temporary but often persists. Furthermore, it may have its basis in loss of organizing schemes and principles or in failure to use organizing schemes that survived the injury. The latter phenomenon is frequently observed in older children and adults with frontal lobe injury.

Well-organized information is learned more easily and remembered longer than poorly organized information, but only if the information is organized in a way that can be appreciated by the learner (Bower 1972; A. L. Brown 1975, 1979; Hagen et al. 1975). Investigations of the effects of different types of organization (e.g., perceptual versus categorical versus thematic organization) on recall have suggested that young children, although capable of a variety of types of organizational thinking, may prefer thematic organization (Ceci and Howe 1978; Szekeres 1988). That is, information is remembered more effectively if it is presented in the context of meaningful real-life functional relationships, scripts, or stories. For example, children remember more target words when they are incorporated into an interesting narrative than when they are presented in categories. Furthermore, because young children cannot be expected to actively organize information to fit their organizational schemata, they profit from organization in the material imposed by and highlighted by an adult (Baumeister and Smith 1979; Ceci 1980; Horowitz et al. 1969; Moely 1977). These developmental themes have interesting implications for teaching organizational schemata to young and cognitively impaired children and, more generally, for structuring any learning task.

Intervention

Although normal cognitive development is not an infallible guide in designing programs of cognitive rehabilitation (Ylvisaker et al. 1992), the general aspects of development that have been outlined do yield important insights for intervention. For example, as recovery progresses from significant confusion and severely compromised cognition to progressively higher levels of functioning, learning tasks can reasonably progress from involuntary to deliberate learning paradigms. The context of presentation of information also moves from personalized thematic activities to more abstract forms of organization. The organizing schemata that are taught or retaught change from concrete routines to more general, but still personally relevant scripts, to more abstract schemata. Metacognitive awareness should gradually be encouraged. Finally, deliberate use of organizing schemata as strategies for effective learning, speaking, writing, and comprehending are gradually introduced.

Table 10–2 lists eight types of organizing schema and activities that can be used to promote the acquisition of that type of schemata and its use in everyday activities. The tasks are designed in such a way that learning occurs incidentally (i.e., the tasks should be personally meaningful and the teacher should highlight the organizational component of the task so that its importance in getting the job done is appreciated by the child). The reflection questions listed in the fourth column are designed to gradually encourage metacognitive appreciation of organizing schemata and their role in accomplishing important tasks effectively. Metacognitive awareness evolves slowly in normal cognitive development. Therefore, it would be unreasonable to expect sudden reacquisition of this understanding in children with TBI.

Young children are capable of a variety of types of organizing. Furthermore, the types of organizational thinking described in Table 10–2 probably develop simultaneously, and they all can be made sufficiently concrete that they are relevant to preschoolers. Nevertheless, there is reason to focus on organization by function (e.g., items needed to make a sandwich or wash a car) and by specific event scripts (e.g., going out to eat or going to the doctor) first in rehabilitation. These types of organizing appear to be most natural to cognitively immature children (e.g., preschoolers), and they are critical for reestablishing organized behavior and general orientation to everyday sequences of events.

Furthermore, parents can be actively involved in helping their children to reacquire *routines* (specific, concrete sequences of behavior, such as getting ready for bed sequences) as well as more general *scripts* (less specific sequences such as playing with toys, visiting relatives, and going to a restaurant). As parents and others promote reacquisition of such real-event scripts, teachers and speech-language pathologists can use the same scripts to promote increasingly well-organized expressive language. Routines and scripts that are important for the child should be recorded in a home-school journal so that a variety of organizational activities can be centered around the same relevant themes. We frequently take photographs of children engaged in sequences of routine events at school or at home. These photos can be used by staff and parents in facilitating the child's real-event narratives and also can be used by the children to guide themselves through sequences of activities that would otherwise require external assistance because of the organizational demands of the task.

At a somewhat more abstract level, highly organized procedures can be used to promote reestablishment of organized networks of concepts in semantic memory. Exploration of semantic features is a common activity for young grade-school children, resulting in "word webs" and other interesting visual representations of connections among word meanings. Often these activities are used by regular education teachers to promote divergent and creative thinking in their students. However, it is critical to impose a consistent structure on semantic feature analysis for students with organizational impairment. We use a feature analysis guide or graphic organizer (Figure 10–1) that includes a center box in which the word (i.e., concept) to be analyzed is placed. Fanning out in clockwise fashion are boxes for the semantic features category, action, use, location, parts, attributes, and other associations.

Initially, highly familiar words are chosen for this organizing activity, with the goals of the activity being to focus the child's attention, encourage a systematic search of his or her knowledge base, and reestablish organization among the pieces of semantic knowledge possessed by the child. Increased organization of conceptual content and words in semantic memory facilitates word and information retrieval and coherence of descriptions. To give feature analysis a meaningful goal, the information gathered during the analysis can subsequently be used to write a description or a story, to complete a similarities and differences exercise, or to complete a problem-solving exercise. If word retrieval problems persist, the feature analysis procedure may be internalized and used as a strategy to search for words or to circumlocute systematically.

Executive Functions and Strategies

Executive functions include self-regulatory or control functions that direct and organize behavior. More specifically, executive functions include awareness of one's strengths and weaknesses; ability to set reasonable goals based on that awareness; planning, organizing, and initiating behavior in pursuit of those

Table 10–2.   Procedures for promoting acquisition of organizational schemata in children

Organizational schemata (means for attaining goal)	Task and goal	Activity	Reflection*
Specific event scripts (e.g., going to a restaurant, going to the dentist)	"Let's play dentist." Let's take turns being the dentist and the patient.	Select items from a large box of appropriate items and foils. Arrange items for dramatic play of the sequence. Play out the event assuming first the role of the patient, then the role of the dentist.	What things do we always see in the dentist's office? What different things (variations) might we see? What events always happen when we go to the dentist? How do they help us to remember? What events might happen only some of the time when we go to the dentist? (e.g., dentist is late, get a shot)
General life scripts (abstracted common life events)	"Let's do a 'This is Your Life' for either Grandma or Grandpa." Talk about all the special things that happened to them.	Use pictures to represent each important category of event: birth, school, marriage, job, and special events. Using the pictures as a guide, make a storybook for the grandparents or older significant other person in the child's life. Then have each child tell the "life story" on the radio show.	How did the pictures help you to remember all the important events? How did we organize all the information about grandma/ grandpa? How did the "books" help you with your radio show?

(continued)

Table 10–2. Procedures for promoting acquisition of organizational schemata in children (*continued*)

Organizational schemata (means for attaining goal)	Task and goal	Activity	Reflection*
Function (use)	"Let's clean the doll house and arrange all the furniture for the play family." "Now let's rearrange some of the furniture for a birthday party for one of the children."	Take all the furniture out of the doll house. Clean the rooms. Then place the furniture back into the house. Have the child rearrange furniture for a party.	How did we arrange all of the furniture and why did we do it that way? Is that the way that the store shows the furniture? How did we change things for the birthday party? Why did we change them?
Perceptual similarity (e.g., color, shape, size, texture, rhyme)	"The art teacher asked us to organize these crayons so that the children can easily and quickly find the ones they want. Let's find a good way to do this."	Label small boxes for different colors. Sort the pieces according to color and put them into the labeled boxes. Call out the colors and time how quickly they can be found, compared with those in a container with a variety of colors.	How did we sort? Why this way? How did it help you find what you wanted? In what other situations might we sort by color? Would we ever want to sort by size (e.g., when we are deciding which crayons to throw away)?

| Semantic similarity (e.g., superordinate category, opposites) | "We are going to set up a grocery store so we can play store." "First, we will make our plan of where we want to put all the items." "Let's make it easy for people to find things." | Make a floor plan showing where the items will be placed. Place play items in the play store as indicated in the plan (e.g., all the fruits in one area). | How did we arrange the store? Why did we arrange it that way? When would this not be a helpful way to arrange the items? How could this arrangement help you to remember where to find things in the store? |
| Main idea and topic (discourse structure) | "Let's do a radio program (or write a letter to a special friend) about a favorite person, place, or thing." | Let the child select a favorite or special person, place, or thing. Use pictures on a chart to cue the child to focus on a main idea about the "topic" (e.g., focus on the main idea, "my dog is lots of fun."). Place representation (e.g., pictures) of main idea in the center of the chart with boxes surrounding it for supporting details. Cue the child to add details to support the main idea (e.g., "he chases a stick; he plays with me," etc.). Use pictures as cues. Record the program (or write the letter). | How did the chart help you to think of details about the special person, place, or thing? How did the chart help you to stay organized when you were talking on the radio show or writing your letter? How did the chart help you to remember what you wanted to say? |

(continued)

Table 10–2. Procedures for promoting acquisition of organizational schemata in children *(continued)*

Organizational schemata (means for attaining goal)	Task and goal	Activity	Reflection*
Story schema	"Let's make a movie about (_____) and show it to your classmates (or to another class)."	Give the child a set of props that are potential elements of a story: —characters (dolls or animals); —settings (e.g., house, barn, fence); —potential problems or goals (e.g., container of water, mud); —potential resolutions for problems (e.g., long stick or ladder, towels). Present a concrete story guide or cues to help the child create a story from the props (e.g., "face" to indicate "who" is in the story or a "large blank square" to indicate "place" or "?" to indicate a "problem," "light bulb" for "solution," "happy face" for "reaction"). Videotape the child's story. Watch the video. Use cues to help the child tell the story.	How did the story guide help to think up your story? How did the story guide help you to tell your story so well? (coherent and organized) How did the story guide help to make your story more interesting? How could the story guide help you to remember the story?

| Integration of scripts | "Let's play going grocery shopping; you be the checker and I'll be the shopper." Use check-out play set with small lunch bags. (Store items have been previously arranged according to semantic similarity.) | Play going to the store and selecting items. Play check-out including scanning items, paying, and packing items into the bags. Pack items according to: size, shape, and weight of items (perceptual) or functional (all refrigerator items together). Shift roles of buyer and checker. | What different things could happen at the store? (variations of the script) How would your Mom want you to pack the bags? How could this help you to remember what you bought? |

*Possible probe question to develop metacognition, understanding, and awareness.

Source. Adapted from Ylvisaker M, Szekeres S, Henry K, et al.: "Topics in Cognitive Rehabilitation Therapy," in *Community Reentry for Head Injured Adults.* Edited by Ylvisaker M, Gobble EMR. Austin, TX, Pro-Ed, 1987, pp. 165–168. Used with permission.

goals; inhibiting behavior that is incompatible with the goals; monitoring and evaluating behavior in relation to the goals; and flexibly solving problems in the event of obstacles. Commonly, executive functions operate automatically; for example, when one makes strategic decisions in a familiar game without special thought. However, executive processes can operate deliberately; for example, when people use strategies such as making note of a telephone number because they might otherwise forget it.

The development of executive functions in relation to cognition includes increasingly accurate judgments of task difficulty and increasingly strategic solutions to cognitive problems (Flavell 1979, 1985). A cognitive strategy is a procedure that one uses in a potentially deliberate, but possibly automatic, manner to enhance performance on cognitively demanding tasks. Strategies may involve the use of external aids (e.g., written reminder, printed schedule, memory book), overt behavior (e.g., asking for information to be repeated or simplified, counting on fingers), or covert behavior (e.g., mentally rehearsing, elaborating, or organizing information; guiding oneself through a task with covert instructions). In normal child development and in recovery from brain injury, strategic behavior progresses from externally prompted use of simple external aids (e.g., reminding preschoolers to put their materials in their boxes

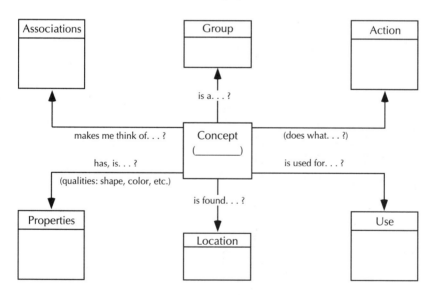

Figure 10–1.   Feature analysis guide. *Source.*   Reprinted from Ylvisaker M, Szekeres S, Henry K, et al.: "Topics in Cognitive Rehabilitation Therapy," in *Community Reentry for Head Injured Adults.*   Edited by Ylvisaker M, Gobble EMR. Austin, TX, Pro-Ed, 1987, pp. 137–220. Used with permission.

so that they will have them when it is time to go home) to internally prompted use of elaborate internal procedures.

Planning.   Planning is an aspect of executive functioning that is important in itself but also can be used to illustrate the concept of preventive or anticipatory cognitive rehabilitation in young children. It is often important to target planning and related executive functions in young children with TBI, even though they would not be expected to possess mature skills at their age in the absence of brain injury. Children who have specific prefrontal injury may need years of targeted intervention in school and at home before they have minimally adequate levels of executive skills. Therefore, it is important for these children to start young. Furthermore, children with cognitive weakness but intact prefrontal areas may need to be more planful and more deliberate in the use of cognitive skills than their intact peers. Therefore, these children also may benefit from an early focus on executive skills, such as planning. Tragically, in the absence of executive system intervention, teachers and parents often become the child's "prosthetic frontal lobes," assuming responsibility for problem identification, problem solving, planning, monitoring, evaluating, and other executive functions. As a result, children who may need more learning trials than their normally developing peers to acquire executive functions actually receive little practice in this area (Meichenbaum 1993).

Ecologically valid approaches to executive system intervention are centered around real-world activities and settings. Ideally, all staff as well as parents deliver the intervention. In the case of planning, this means involving the child in planning meaningful events to whatever extent he or she is capable and with whatever support is necessary. For example, kindergartners may have Velcro boards on which they sequentially place symbols for all of the day's activities. This board is referred to as "The Plan." As activities are completed, the children remove the symbol for that activity. Individual therapy or instructional periods may begin with the teacher indicating a set of alternatives from which the children might choose. Having chosen the activities and their order, the "plan" is somehow represented on paper and the children are frequently reminded that it is their job to stick to the plan. The same procedures should be used at home.

An important aspect of this intervention is the use by adults of consistent terms to stand for the cognitive activity being promoted. These terms might include "your plan," "organize your plan," "stick to your plan," "decide," "reason for deciding," "think," "remember," and the like. Early development of executive functions includes both vocabulary and routines that will later evolve into more mature self-regulatory behavior. There are many advantages of a planning system of this sort, among them the following:

- It promotes predictability and orderliness, which are important for children who may not be well oriented to routines and upcoming events.
- It gives children a sense of control that they might otherwise gain through oppositional and manipulative behavior.
- It promotes goal setting and control of impulsivity.
- It promotes decision-making and thought processes that are needed for thoughtful decision making.
- It creates a system for planning that may yield effective independent planning years after this modest beginning (Ylvisaker and Feeney 1994).

This approach to the early development of planning skill can be used as a model for targeting other aspects of executive functioning in young children, including self-awareness, goal setting, monitoring and evaluating, and problem solving. Elsewhere, we have listed procedures that may be useful in promoting improvements in a variety of executive functions in both children and adults (Ylvisaker and Szekeres 1989).

Strategy intervention.   Many cognitive and academic challenges persist after TBI, despite well-conceived cognitive intervention and academic instruction. Indeed, cognitive disability may worsen over time as impaired new learning has its cumulative effect and as increasingly challenging academic and developmental obstacles are encountered. Therefore, the need to be strategic in overcoming obstacles may be particularly great for these children. The irony is that the parts of the brain associated with strategic thinking are often injured in TBI, generating a need for even more creative intervention.

Table 10–3 includes a set of intervention procedures that are useful in promoting increasingly strategic behavior in general as well as specific cognitive strategies. These procedures highlight the active role of the student in strategy intervention. In our view, there is something deeply contradictory in the common practice of teaching strategies according to the traditional teaching model:

1. The teacher identifies the student's needs.
2. The teacher selects a strategic procedure capable of overcoming the obstacle.
3. The teacher has the student practice the strategy.
4. The teacher monitors performance, evaluates the outcome, and makes modifications if needed.

The contradiction implicit in this approach is that in attempting to promote strategic behavior in the student, the teacher has assumed responsibility for all aspects of strategic behavior. Although the student might benefit from the specific procedure that is taught, it is unlikely that this intervention will result in the student becoming more strategic in a generalizable way.

Table 10–3. Teaching compensatory strategies

Phase I: General strategic thinking

A. Metacognitive-awareness

Goals: Students will discriminate effective from ineffective performance; become aware of their strengths and weaknesses; recognize implications of their deficits.

Rationale: Given the frequency of frontolimbic and right hemisphere damage in TBI, self-awareness is frequently compromised. Individuals are unlikely to acquire and use procedures designed to compensate for problems that they do not recognize as problems.

Procedures:

1. *Objective:* Improve the student's perception of successful versus unsuccessful task performance. Illustrate successful and unsuccessful performance of a functional task through role play or on videotape. With the student, analyze the performances in sufficient detail that the student can identify the features that account for successful versus unsuccessful performance.

2. *Objective:* Improve the student's ability to perceive functional impairments. Individually, request that the student make note of specific deficits of other students in the program or of individuals observed on tape. Discuss these observations. Planned peer teaching is useful. Discuss the effects of TBI on cognitive and social functioning. If appropriate, read and discuss literature on the effects of TBI.

3. *Objective:* Improve the student's awareness of his or her own strengths and weaknesses. Use everyday opportunities to help the student distinguish between easy and difficult tasks. Videotape the student in activities designed to reveal strong and weak areas of functioning. (Alternatively, use role play.) Review the tapes (beginning with strong performance), first without commentary, subsequently inviting comments about what was done well and what needs improvement. Gradually turn over to the student the responsibility for stopping the tape when problems are noted. Note: Considerable desensitizing may be needed before video self-viewing is possible.

4. *Objective:* Improve the student's understanding of the relation between deficits and long-term goals. Discuss in concrete detail the individual's long-term goals and expectations. Jointly create a list of specific skills and resources needed to achieve these goals. Jointly identify the skills that are present and those that are weak relative to this goal.

Note: These metacognitive discoveries are facilitated if the activities are personally meaningful and intimately connected to the student's goals.

(continued)

Table 10–3.   Teaching compensatory strategies *(continued)*

B.   Value of being strategic

    Goal: Students will recognize the importance of being strategic and will identify the characteristics of strategic people.

    Rationale: Because the ultimate goal of this intervention is to promote strategic thinking and strategic behavior in general—not simply to teach specific strategic behaviors as routines—it is important that the student understand what it is to be strategic and that these are valuable attributes.

    Procedures:

    1.   *Objective:* Improve the student's understanding of strategy. Using games, sports, or other relevant models, clarify the concept of strategy as something clever that one does to achieve goals when there are obstacles.

    2.   *Objective:* Heighten the student's appreciation of strategic behavior. Together with the student, identify several individuals who are known to be very strategic (e.g., sports heroes, military heroes). Discuss why they are considered heroic. Clinicians also should clearly model their own strategic behavior and discuss the value of their own strategies.

    3.   *Objective:* Improve the student's understanding of the behaviors that are part of being strategic. Using models relevant to the student (e.g., military, sports, or business analogies), brainstorm about the characteristics of people who are known to be very strategic. Include high level of motivation and initiative, ability to identify and clarify obstacles to goals; ability to plan procedures to overcome obstacles; ability to monitor and evaluate performance; and willingness to engage in ongoing problem solving.

Phase II: **Selecting specific strategic procedures**

    Goal: Students will identify specific procedures useful in overcoming important personal obstacles.

    Rationale: It is important that students participate in the selection of strategic procedures that they will use and that the procedures be truly useful in achieving the goals.

    Procedures:

    1.   Use group brainstorming procedures to identify possible strategies.

    2.   Use "product monitoring" tasks to test the value of strategies: Have the student perform a task with and without the strategy or with a variety of different strategies. Objectively compare the results. (Video analysis may be useful here.)

    3.   Have advanced students demonstrate the value of certain procedures or offer testimonials.

    4.   Discuss the widespread use of compensatory procedures (lists, memos, tape recorders, and so forth) by people who do not have brain injury.

Phase III: Teaching specific strategies
Note: If the discovery procedures in Phase II (e.g., brainstorming and product monitoring) are effective, there may be little need for specific teaching procedures.
Procedures:
A. *Modeling*: The steps in the strategy can be modeled by the therapist or by a peer, or by means of videotape or other media. Modeling is initially accompanied by overt verbalization of the strategy by the model. The student then rehearses the strategy with gradually decreasing cues and self-talk.
B. *Direct instruction*: The carefully programmed behavioral teaching procedures of direct instruction can be used to teach strategies. However, if this is the only approach used, it is likely that the best result will be the acquisition of a learned sequence of behaviors (which may be a desirable outcome), without positive movement in the direction of becoming a strategic person.
C. *Functional practice*: However the strategy is acquired, it must be frequently rehearsed in natural settings using functional activities. The ultimate goal is to make strategic behavior routine.

Phase IV: Generalization and maintenance
Generalization of strategic behavior beyond the context of training is a combined consequence of the perceived utility of the strategy for the individual, the inherent generalizability and utility of the strategy, widespread environmental support for strategic behavior and thinking, and specific teaching procedures designed to enhance generalization.
Note 1: Generalization includes generalized use of specific strategies as well as strategic behavior in general.
Note 2: Generalization may not be a separate phase if the acquisition stage takes place in the context of functional activities and natural settings. This is particularly important for very concrete people.
Note 3: Generalization may be a relatively unimportant phase of intervention if the individual has acquired a strategic attitude and actively seeks occasions for transfer.
Note 4: Some individuals may need environmental reminders indefinitely to use their strategic procedures.
1. *Objective*: Improve the student's discrimination of situations that require or do not require a given strategy.
    a. Use videotaped scenes or role-playing to illustrate the correct use of a strategy in an appropriate situation, inappropriate use of the strategy, and failure to use the strategy when appropriate. Discuss the conditions that require the strategy.

(continued)

Table 10–3.   Teaching compensatory strategies *(continued)*

    b.   Use short videotaped scenes to train the student in efficient and accurate judgments as to whether a strategy is appropriate in a context.

2.   *Objective*: Increase the student's spontaneous use of strategies in varied situations.

    a.   Include family members, work supervisors, and teachers in strategy intervention to (1) provide varied opportunities for the use of specific strategies and of strategic behavior in general, (2) reinforce the student's use of strategies, and (3) model strategic behavior themselves.

    b.   Ask students to keep a log in which they record their successes and failures in strategy use. Make generalization an explicit goal.

3.   *Objective*: Increase the student's acceptance of strategic behavior.

    a.   Ensure that the student is successful using strategies.

    b.   Promote emotional acceptance of strategic behavior by using whatever motivating procedures work: e.g., personal images or metaphors, testimonials, and the like.

Note.   These phases of intervention are not necessarily hierarchical or mutually exclusive.   *Source.*   Adapted from Haarbauer-Krupa J, Henry K, Szekeres S, et al.: "Cognitive Rehabilitation Therapy: Late Stages of Recovery," in *Head Injury Rehabilitation: Children and Adolescents.* Edited by Ylvisaker M. Austin, TX, Pro-Ed, 1985, pp. 318–319. Used with permission.

Promoting active involvement of students in strategy acquisition has many components:

- Relating strategy instruction explicitly to students' interests and goals
- Ensuring that the student understands that performance needs to be enhanced, that strategies enhance performance, that success is a result of effort, not luck or fate, and that he or she is capable of this effort
- Using brainstorming and negotiating procedures in deciding which strategies to pursue
- Ensuring that the student pays attention to the positive consequences of strategic behavior
- Using effective promotional techniques to overcome resistance
- Ensuring that significant people at home and at school are supportive of strategic behavior

Pressley (1993) has attempted to summarize and apply two decades of strategy research in educational psychology to the related field of cognitive rehabilitation after head injury. Among the many important lessons that have been learned by educational psychologists is that strategy instruction must be intensive, comprehensive, and long term. This insight, combined with what is known about transfer of cognitive training, supports the recommendation that strategy intervention be organized as much as possible around classroom activities and supported by practice in other everyday contexts, as opposed to being understood as an isolated therapeutic intervention. This recommendation is discussed in greater detail by Ylvisaker et al. (1994b).

Efficacy of Intervention

In one important respect, the question of effectiveness of cognitive intervention is less critical for children than for adults; children inevitably receive some attention to cognitive skills in school, whereas cognitive intervention for adults is not a standard service and therefore requires special justification. However, it is critical for both children and adults that the service they receive be maximally effective, therefore requiring careful examination of the relative effectiveness of alternative approaches. Unfortunately, there are few reports of efficacy studies in the pediatric TBI literature. Clearly the question, "Does cognitive rehabilitation work for children with TBI?" is far too general. (Compare: "Does surgery work for children with TBI?") Investigators must specify the type and duration of intervention, the nature of the children receiving the intervention (age, type of injury, type and severity of deficits, length of time after injury), cognitive targets, and measures of success.

The only TBI group study that we are familiar with and that meets reasonable methodological standards is that reported by Light et al. (1987). They found that the children with TBI served by their Neurocognitive Education Project demonstrated very slight superiority over an untreated comparison group on standardized cognitive measures but more substantial superiority on measures of adaptive functioning. Although promising, these findings are at best preliminary. For the present, rehabilitation and education professionals who serve students with TBI are best advised to look to the large body of literature dealing with effectiveness of intervention with other groups of children with cognitive impairment, with appropriate cautions in making cross-population inferences.

References

Annegers JF, Grabow JD, Kurland LT, et al: The incidence, causes and secular trends in head trauma in Olmsted County, Minnesota, 1935–1974. Neurology 30:912–919, 1980

Baumeister A, Smith S: Thematic elaboration and proximity in children's recall, organization, and long-term retention of sectorial materials. Journal of Child Psychology 28:231–248, 1979

Benton A: Prefrontal injury and behavior in children. Developmental Neuropsychology 7:275–281, 1991

Ben Yishay Y, Prigatano G: Cognitive remediation, in Rehabilitation of the Adult and Child with Traumatic Brain Injury, 3rd Edition. Edited by Griffith ER, Bond MR, Miller JD. Philadelphia, PA, FA Davis, 1990, pp 393–409

Berrol S: Issues in cognitive rehabilitation. Arch Neurol 47:219–220, 1990

Bigler ED: Frontal lobe damage and neuropsychological assessment. Archives of Clinical Neuropsychology 3:279–297, 1988

Bjorklund D: The role of conceptual knowledge in the development of organization in children's memory, in Basic Processes in Memory Development. Edited by Pressley M, Brainerd C. New York, Springer-Verlag, 1985, pp 103–134

Bower G: A selective review of organizational factors in memory, in Organization of Memory. Edited by Tulving E, Donaldson W. New York, Academic Press, 1972, pp 93–137

Brink JD, Garrett AL, Hale WR, et al: Recovery of motor and intellectual function in children sustaining severe injuries. Dev Med Child Neurol 12: 565–571, 1970

Brown AL: The development of memory: knowing, knowing about knowing, and knowing how to know, in Advances in Child Development and Behavior, Vol 10. Edited by Reese HW. New York, Academic Press, 1975, pp 103–152

Brown AL: Theories of memory and problems of development, activity, growth, and knowledge, in Levels of Processing and Memory. Edited by Craik FIM, Cermak L. Hillsdale, NJ, Lawrence Erlbaum, 1979, pp 225–258

Brown G, Chadwick O, Shaffer D, et al: A prospective study of children with head injuries, III: psychiatric sequelae. Psychol Med 11:63–78, 1981

Bruce DA, Schut L, Bruno LA, et al: Outcome following severe head injuries in children. J Neurosurg 48:679–688, 1978

Bruce DA, Raphaely RC, Goldberg AI, et al: Pathophysiology, treatment, and outcome following severe head injury in children. Child's Brain 5: 174–191, 1979

Ceci SJ: A developmental study of multiple encoding and its relationship to age-related changes in free recall. Child Dev 51:892–895, 1980

Ceci SJ, Howe JA: Age-related differences in free recall as a function of retrieval flexibility. J Exp Child Psychol 26:432–442, 1978

Chadwick O, Rutter M, Shaffer D, et al: A prospective study of children with head injuries, IV: specific cognitive deficits. J Clin Neuropsychol 3: 101–120, 1981

Chi MTH: Knowledge structures and memory development, in Children's Thinking: What Develops? Edited by Siegler RS. Hillsdale, NJ, Lawrence Erlbaum, 1978

Cooper JD, Tabaddor K, Hauser WA: The epidemiology of head injury in the Bronx. Neuroepidemiology 2:70–88, 1983

Dennis M: Frontal lobe function in childhood and adolescence: a heuristic for assessing attention regulation, executive control, and the intentional states important for social discourse. Developmental Neuropsychology 7: 327–358, 1991

Diller L: A model for cognitive retraining in rehabilitation. Clinical Psychology 29:13–15, 1976

Eiben CF, Anderson TP, Lockman L, et al: Functional outcome of closed head injury in children and young adults. Arch Phys Med Rehabil 65:168–170, 1984

Eslinger PJ, Damasio AR: Severe disturbance of higher cognition following bilateral frontal lobe oblation: patient EVR. Neurology 35:1731–1741, 1985

Eslinger PJ, Grattan LM, Damasio H, et al: Developmental consequences of childhood frontal lobe damage. Arch Neurol 49:764–769, 1992

Ewing-Cobbs L, Levin HS, Eisenberg HM, et al: Language functions following closed head injury in children and adolescents. J Clin Exp Neuropsychol 9:575–592, 1987

Ewing-Cobbs L, Miner M, Fletcher JM, et al: Intellectual, motor, and language sequelae following closed head injury in infants and preschoolers. J Pediatr Psychol 14:531–544, 1989

Finger S: Brain damage, development, and behavior: early findings. Developmental Neuropsychology 7:261–274, 1991

Flavell J: Metacognition and cognitive monitoring: a new era of cognitive-developmental inquiry. Am Psychol 34:907–911, 1979

Flavell J: Cognitive development, 2nd Edition. Englewood Cliffs, NJ, Prentice-Hall, 1985

Fletcher JM, Ewing-Cobbs L, Miner M, et al: Behavioral changes after closed head injury in children. J Consult Clin Psychol 58:93–98, 1990

Grattan LM, Eslinger PJ: Frontal lobe damage in children and adults: a comparative review. Developmental Neuropsychology 7:283–326, 1991

Grattan LM, Eslinger PJ: Long-term psychological consequences of childhood frontal lobe lesions in patient DT. Brain Cogn 20:185–195, 1992

Haarbauer-Krupa J, Henry K, Szekeres S, et al: Cognitive rehabilitation therapy: late stages of recovery, in Head Injury Rehabilitation: Children and Adolescents. Edited by Ylvisker. Austin, TX, Pro-Ed, 1985, pp 311–343

Hagen C: Language disorders secondary to closed head injury: diagnosis and treatment. Topics in Language Disorders 1:73–87, 1981

Hagen J, Jongeward R, Jr, Kail R, et al: Cognitive perspectives in the development of memory, Vol 10. Edited by Reese HW. New York, Academic Press, 1975

Horowitz L, Lampel A, Takanishi R: The child's memory of unitized scenes. J Psychol 8:365–386, 1969

Hresko WP, Reid DK: Five faces of cognition: theoretical influences on approaches to learning disabilities. Learning Disability Quarterly 4:211–216, 1988

Kavale K, Mattson P: One jumped off the balance beam: meta-analysis of perceptual-motor training. J Learn Disabil 16:165–173, 1983

Kennard MA, Fulton JF: Age and reorganization of central nervous system. Mt Sinai J Med 9:594–606, 1942

Klonoff H, Low MD, Clark C: Head injuries in children: a prospective five year follow-up. J Neurol Neurosurg Psychiatry 40:1211–1219, 1977

Kolb B: Brain development, plasticity, and behavior. Am Psychol 44:1203–1212, 1989

Kraus JF: Epidemiology of head injury, in Head Injury. Edited by Cooper PR. Baltimore, MD, Williams & Wilkins, 1987, pp 1–19

Kraus JF, Fife D, Conroy C: Pediatric brain injuries: the nature, clinical course, and early outcomes in a defined United States population. Pediatrics 79:501–507, 1987

Lehr E: Psychological Management of Traumatic Brain Injuries in Children and Adolescents. Rockville, MD, Aspen Publishers, 1990

Lenneberg E: The Biological Foundations of Language. New York, Wiley, 1967

Levin HS, Eisenberg HM, Wigg NR, et al: Memory and intellectual ability after head injury in children and adolescents. Neurosurgery 11:668–673, 1982

Lezak MD: The problem of assessing executive functions. International Journal of Psychology 17:281–297, 1982

Light R, Neumann E, Lewis R, et al: An evaluation of a neuropsychologically based reeducation project for the head-injured child. Journal of Head Trauma Rehabilitation 2:11–25, 1987

Lynch WJ: Ecological validity of cognitive rehabilitation software. Journal of Head Trauma Rehabilitation 7:36–45, 1992

Mahoney WJ, D'Souza BJ, Haller JA, et al: Long-term outcome of children with severe head trauma and prolonged coma. Pediatrics 71:756–761, 1983

Mann L: On the Trail of Process: A Historical Perspective on Cognitive Processes and Their Training. New York, Grune & Stratton, 1979

Marlowe WB: The impact of a right prefrontal lesion on a developing brain. Brain Cogn 20:205–213, 1992

Mateer CA, Williams D: Effects of frontal lobe injury in childhood. Developmental Neuropsychology 7:359–376, 1991

Meichenbaum D: The "potential" contributions of cognitive behavior modification to the rehabilitation of individuals with traumatic brain injury. Seminars in Speech and Language 14:18–30, 1993

Moely B: Organization of memory, in Perspectives on the Development of Memory and Cognition. Edited by Kail R, Hagen J. Hillsdale, NJ, Lawrence Erlbaum, 1977, pp 203–236

Perrott SB, Taylor HG, Montes JL: Neuropsychological sequelae, familial stress, and environmental adaptation following pediatric head injury. Developmental Neuropsychology 7:69–86, 1991

Petterson L: Sensitivity to emotional cues and social behavior in children and adolescents after head injury. Percept Mot Skills 73:1139–1150, 1991

Postman L: Short-term memory and incidental learning, in Categories of Human Learning. Edited by Nelson AW. New York, Academic Press, 1964, pp 145–201

Pressley M: Teaching cognitive strategies to brain-injured clients: the good information processing perspective. Seminars in Speech and Language 14:1–16, 1993

Raimondi AJ, Hirschauer J: Head injury in the infant and toddler. Child's Brain 11:12–35, 1984

Raphael RC, Swedlow DB, Downes JJ, et al: Management of severe pediatric head trauma. Pediatr Clin North Am 27:715–727, 1980

Rivara FP, Mueller BA: The epidemiology and prevention of pediatric head injury. Journal of Head Trauma Rehabilitation 1:7–15, 1986

Rosenthal M, Griffith ER, Bond MR, et al: Rehabilitation of the Adult and Child with Traumatic Brain Injury, 2nd Edition. Philadelphia, PA, FA Davis, 1990

Schacter DL, Glisky EL: Memory remediation: restoration, alleviation, and the acquisition of domain-specific knowledge, in Clinical Neuropsychology of Intervention. Edited by Uzzell B, Gross Y. Boston, MA, Martinus Nijhoff, 1986, pp 257–282

Schneider W, Pressley M: Memory Development Between 2 and 20. New York, Springer-Verlag, 1989

Singley MK, Anderson JR: The Transfer of Cognitive Skill. Cambridge, MA, Harvard University Press, 1989

Smirnov A: Problems in the Psychology of Memory. New York, Plenum, 1973

Stelling MW, McKay SE, Carr WA, et al: Frontal lobe lesions and cognitive function in craniopharyngioma survivors. American Journal of Diseases of Childhood 140:710–714, 1986

Stuss DT, Benson DF: The Frontal Lobes. New York, Raven, 1986

Szekeres S: Organization and recall in the young language-impaired child. Unpublished doctoral dissertation. University of Pittsburgh, Pittsburgh, PA, 1988

Welsh MC, Pennington BF, Groisser DB: A normative-developmental study of executive function: a window on prefrontal function in children. Developmental Neuropsychology 7:131–149, 1991

Williams D, Mateer CA: Developmental impact of frontal lobe injury in middle childhood. Brain Cogn 20:196–204, 1992

Ylvisaker M, Feeney T: Communication and behavior: collaboration between speech-language pathologists and behavioral psychologists. Topics in Language Disorders 15:37–53, 1994

Ylvisaker M, Szekeres SF: Metacognitive and executive impairments in head injured children and adults. Topics in Language Disorders 9:34–49, 1989

Ylvisaker M, Chorazy AJL, Cohen SB, et al: Rehabilitative assessment following head injury in children, in Rehabilitation of the Adult and Child with Traumatic Brain Injury, 2nd Edition. Edited by Rosenthal M, Griffith ER, Bond MR, et al. Philadelphia, PA, FA Davis, 1990, pp 393–409

Ylvisaker M, Szekeres SF, Hartwick P: Cognitive rehabilitation following traumatic brain injury in children, in Advances in Child Neuropsychology, Vol 1. Edited by Tramontana MG, Hooper SR. New York, Springer-Verlag, 1992, pp 168–218

Ylvisaker M, Hartwick P, Ross B, et al: Cognitive assessment, in Educational Dimensions of Acquired Brain Injury. Edited by Savage R, Wolcott G. Austin, TX, Pro-Ed, 1994a, pp 69–119

Ylvisaker M, Szekeres SF, Hartwick P, et al: Cognitive intervention, in Educational Dimensions of Acquired Brain Injury. Edited by Savage R, Wolcott G. Austin, TX, Pro-Ed, 1994b, pp 121–184

Part III

Interventions for Severe Psychiatric Disorders

Chapter 11

Cognitive Rehabilitation for Schizophrenia

Daniel M. Storzbach, Ph.D., and Patrick W. Corrigan, Psy.D.

D isturbances of thought have been considered characteristic of schizophrenia since the syndrome was first described (Bleuler 1911/1950; Kraepelin 1902). Treatments for schizophrenia frequently have been judged by their effects on cognitive functions. Although psychopharmacological interventions currently dominate treatment for schizophrenia, research suggests that for many patients cognitive effects of antipsychotic medication are limited. As a consequence, clinical researchers have increasingly sought rehabilitation strategies that ameliorate or compensate for abnormal cognition. In this chapter, we review empirical investigations of cognitive interventions for persons diagnosed with schizophrenia. The review is framed in a theoretical model intended to facilitate both practical clinical application and further research. The chapter also addresses some pragmatic considerations that are relevant to effective cognitive rehabilitation.

Theoretical Considerations

Research on cognitive rehabilitation for schizophrenia has for the most part proceeded unsystematically, lacking coherent goals or unifying concepts. There have been few published attempts to replicate or follow through on previous findings. As a result, research efforts have often been haphazard and apparently uninformed by previous studies. Moreover, the bulk of cognitive rehabilitation studies predate many important recent research advances. These problems have led some researchers to suggest that attempts to develop cognitive rehabilitation interventions for schizophrenia are scientifically premature (Bellack 1992).

Some of the problems with cognitive rehabilitation research may best be addressed by framing research in a network of systematically interrelated and empirically based, theoretical constructs (Cronbach and Meehl 1955). Such a "nomological network" is richly suggestive of predictions regarding the phenomena of interest and helps focus research by suggesting convergent experimental operations and empirical tests of theoretical constructs. Schizophrenia researchers have generated several explanatory models of potential heuristic value for design and evaluation of cognitive rehabilitation strategies. For this chapter, the *limited information processing capacity* model of cognitive functioning in schizophrenia has been chosen as being especially relevant to cognitive rehabilitation.

Experimental data on cognitive abnormalities in schizophrenia have been credibly framed using the limited information processing capacity model (Callaway and Naghdi 1982; Knight and Russell 1978; Nuechterlein and Asarnow 1989; Nuechterlein and Dawson 1984a; Nuechterlein et al. 1990). According to this model, information processing is mediated by a limited pool of processing resources (Kahneman 1973). Individuals flexibly allocate these resources, either focusing them on a single task or sharing them among multiple cognitive processes. For example, the chess master attends closely to the game while being relatively oblivious to his or her surroundings. Conversely, the chess neophyte, distracted by yet unfamiliar rules, is less able to attend closely to the board. Resource allocation is controlled both volitionally and by "automatic" responses.

Specific task characteristics and task difficulty determine the demands placed on processing capacity, with higher-level mental operations incurring greater demands than more elementary functions. Mental operations differ as to where they fall on an automaticity/effortfulness continuum, with more effortful performance demanding greater capacity and more automatized performance requiring less (Hasher and Zacks 1979; Posner and Snyder 1975; Schneider et al. 1984; Shiffrin and Schneider 1977). The individual's total processing capacity also varies with level of psychophysiological arousal and other organismic factors.

In schizophrenia, availability of processing resources is hypothesized to be more limited than in healthy subjects, thereby impairing cognitive function. The limited capacity model has been used to conceptualize the full range of cognitive impairments found in schizophrenia, most especially those of attention, memory, executive functioning, and response selection (Nuechterlein and Dawson 1984b). For example, performance on vigilance tasks has been shown to diminish disproportionately compared with healthy subjects when stimulus items are degraded, thereby requiring greater capacity to attend to task (Nuechterlein 1983). Diminishing task demand or increasing available capacity should therefore improve the schizophrenic individual's cognitive performance. Three cognitive processes have been identified that might account for greater capacity limitations in schizophrenia and explain the effects of cognitive interventions:

1. *Inefficient allocation policy: Allocation policy* is the hypothetical executive function that divides capacity among various cognitive processes in response to perceived environmental contingencies (Kahneman 1973). Schizophrenic patients do not distribute information capacity optimally. Perhaps because schizophrenia is associated with impaired integration of perceptual and cognitive processes (Magaro 1980), internal and external cues necessary for appropriate capacity allocation are ignored. A potential cognitive intervention strategy is to improve allocation policy by making salient the internal goals and environmental cues that control the distribution of capacity.

2. *Impaired modulation of arousal:* The relationship between arousal and capacity is described by a Yerkes-Dodson inverted U curve such that during periods of underarousal or overarousal healthy individuals experience diminished capacity (Gjerde 1983). Available capacity in schizophrenic patients is limited by maladaptive arousal levels. Research suggests that some individuals with schizophrenia experience prolonged or permanent hyperarousal (Broen 1968; Gjerde 1983; Venables 1964; Zahn 1975) or fluctuations between hypo- and hyperaroused states (Dawson and Nuechterlein 1984; Gruzelier 1978). A cognitive intervention strategy would be to improve information processing through optimization of levels of arousal. Hyperaroused patients might be taught relaxation strategies and hypoaroused patients might be shown the benefits of physical exercise.

3. *Impaired automaticity:* Because effortful processes require relatively greater capacity than more automatic processes, delayed or absent automatization would lead to excessive demands on available capacity than in healthy individuals. Individuals with schizophrenia demonstrate an abnormal transition from effortful to automatic processes (Magaro 1984). Moreover, learning might be impaired because performance requires more effort during initial learning. Because effortful processes become more automatic through use of intrinsic mnemonics and repeated practice (Bandura 1986; Fitts and Posner 1967), a potential intervention strategy would use such techniques to facilitate automatization, ultimately reducing capacity load and improving information processing.

Application of the limited capacity model to schizophrenia results in improved description of impaired cognitive processes and suggests possible interrelationships of these impairments with other constructs (e.g., arousal level and psychotic symptoms). The model also appears to have heuristic value for explaining outcome in cognitive rehabilitation. For this reason, it has been chosen to provide an integrative framework for understanding the disparate collection of published studies of cognitive interventions. The model also will be used to generate prescriptions for future research and development of cognitive rehabilitation. Our discussion follows recent reviews (Corrigan, in press; Green 1993) in dividing these investigations into studies targeting more basic information processes and those targeting more "macro" levels of cognitive processing. By *basic information processes*, we mean such cognitive functions as memory and attention that are components of integrated cognitive functioning. Macro-level processes are complex cognitive functions that require integration of multiple basic information processes. Studies of macro-level interventions target such disturbances as conceptual disorganization and delusions.

The limited capacity model is not sufficient to explain all deficits and therapeutic effects. Other models may be valuable for cognitive rehabilitation, including stress-diathesis (Nuechterlein and Dawson 1984a; Zubin and Spring 1977) and lower thresholds for disorganization (Broen and Storms 1966). Rehabilitation researchers are encouraged to be conversant with these and other theories so that the effects of competing rehabilitation hypotheses, and the divergent treatment strategies they entail, might be examined and contrasted.

Cognitive Rehabilitation Approaches to Information Processing Deficits

Investigators of information processing abnormalities associated with schizophrenia have frequently used various laboratory-based cognitive measurement paradigms borrowed from cognitive psychology. Among these are reaction time, dichotic listening, card sorting, backward masking, span of apprehension, and continuous performance (for a brief review, see Spaulding et al., Chapter 5). Most empirically investigated cognitive interventions were derived from these measurement paradigms to ameliorate deficits in attention, memory, or conceptual flexibility.

Attentional Deficits

Operant contingencies have been used to focus attention and improve reaction time in several studies. Framed within the limited capacity model, operant contingencies help regulate capacity allocation such that the schizophrenic patient more optimally assigns cognitive capacity to the processing of appropriate external stimuli. Without the incentive of reinforcing contingencies, patients are more readily distracted by irrelevant external and internal stimuli, capacity dedicated to the attention or reaction time task is diminished, and concentration or processing speed is lower than normal. Several studies have tested operant effects on attentional tasks (Karras 1962, 1968; Meiselman 1973; Rosenbaum et al. 1957; Wagner 1968).

As an example, Wagner (1968) randomly assigned schizophrenic subjects to either an attention task (in which subjects were instructed to match a target stimulus with its replica embedded in a stimulus array) or an abstraction task (one of the three stimuli in the subsequent array shared a common physical or semantic attribute with the target stimulus). Correct performance was reinforced on fixed ratio schedules; mistakes resulted in a mild response cost. Results showed that subjects in the attention training group demonstrated improved scores on the attention task, whereas subjects in the abstract training group did not show significant improvement. No crossover effects were found (i.e., subjects in the attention training group did not improve abstract test scores). These findings suggest that monetary contingencies improve primary attentional function but have little impact on more abstract encoding functions.

To improve reaction times in dual modality tasks, Meiselman (1973) compared the effects of feedback (contingent reinforcement) with repeated practice. During the prototypical single modality task, subjects are instructed to respond to the offset of a light or tone by lifting their finger from a telegraph key. During Meiselman's dual-modality task, one-half of the trials were tone off and one-half of the trials were light off, in random sequence. After pretests, subjects in the feedback group were told a bell would ring after each response in which reaction time was 10 ms shorter than the mean reaction time demonstrated during the pretest, and a buzzer would be heard for any responses slower than the mean. Subjects received 5¢ for each bell and lost 5¢ for each buzzer. Subjects in the repeated practice control group completed the pretest reaction time trials again. Results showed that all 10 subjects in the feedback plus reinforcement condition improved reaction time to dual-modality stimuli; however, six subjects in the control condition were quicker as well. The decrement in reaction times of the feedback group was significantly greater than the repeated practice group.

A more behavioral perspective might view attention and reaction time as not different from other operant behaviors. This alternative to the limited capacity model suggests that reinforcement only strengthens the disturbed patients' responses to specifically reinforced stimuli. The limited capacity model suggests that reinforcing contingencies not only improve attention specific to target stimuli, but also more globally expand information capacity, thus enhancing other cognitive functions such as encoding, consolidation, and retrieval. Future research might profitably test these competing hypotheses.

Memory Deficits

Koh (1978) found that although schizophrenic patient's recognition memory is relatively intact, scores on recall tasks are significantly below normal. This distinction may be explained by limited capacity, because greater cognitive capacity is needed for recall than recognition tasks. Koh concluded that patients lacked basic organizational skills that normally facilitate acquisition and retrieval processes essential to recall memory, thereby making recollection more effortful. Similarly, other investigators have attributed memory deficits in schizophrenia to poor encoding of information into meaningful constructs (Calev et al. 1983). Hence, strategies that compensate for insufficient organization may improve recollection of information.

Koh and colleagues (1976, 1981) found that patients who rated words on a memory task (and thereby aided encoding) in terms of pleasantness were able to increase recall to levels almost those of healthy subjects. Using a similar method, Larsen and Fromholt (1976) instructed schizophrenic subjects to sort a word list into idiosyncratically meaningful categories. After patients had sorted the list into the same categories in two consecutive sorting trials, subjects were asked to recall as many words as possible. Subjects in this group were able to recall words as well as healthy subjects. Improvements in recall memory have been shown in nonverbal domains as well. Patients who rated a series of faces on a pleasantness continuum were able to recall those faces as accurately as a control group (Koh et al. 1981).

Findings from studies in this area are particularly noteworthy because a cognitive function improved to near-normal levels in schizophrenic patients following an information processing intervention. Unlike attentional deficits, which were ameliorated by manipulating the contingencies governing existing cognitive functions, short-term recall was facilitated by an adjunctive information processing strategy. Encoding and organization strategies provide a prosthesis with which patients are able to increase the automaticity of an otherwise highly demanding cognitive task. As a result, the capacity subsequently required to recall well-encoded information is greatly diminished.

Conceptual Flexibility

People normally are able to identify commonalities across stimulus categories and to recognize rules that govern relationships between these categories or concepts. Moreover, healthy individuals are able to adapt rules as changes occur in the task. Conceptual flexibility has been measured using the Wisconsin Card Sorting Task (WCST; Heaton 1981) in which subjects are asked to match stimulus cards to one of four key cards. Subjects must determine the rule by which stimulus cards are matched to key cards (match by color, number, or shape) and sort accordingly. The matching rule is changed after 10 consecutive correct matches without any cues to the subject. Perseverative errors result when individuals continue to incorrectly match stimulus cards to key cards according to the previously operative rule. Schizophrenic patients tend to have significantly more perseverative errors than healthy subjects, suggesting inflexibility in modifying conceptual processing to accommodate environmental feedback (Heaton 1981).

Deficiencies in executive control are especially relevant within the limited-capacity model. Persons with impaired executive functions (e.g., in this case, who are conceptually inflexible) may less effectively allocate cognitive capacity appropriate to environmental demands. Thus, rehabilitation interventions that enhance executive cognitive functions would be expected to improve overall ability to manage processing capacity according to changing environmental information.

In one of the first attempts to directly intervene with patients' conceptual impairments, Goldberg and colleagues (1987) provided instructions on the WCST to schizophrenic patients. Although patients who received instructions had significantly fewer perseverative errors during training, subsequent testing showed that the number of perseverative errors for subjects *returned to baseline* when instructions were no longer provided. Goldberg and his colleagues concluded that impaired conceptual functioning in schizophrenia cannot be ameliorated through cognitive rehabilitation.

Subsequent studies have investigated the effects of combining operant methods with instruction (Bellack et al. 1990; Green et al. 1990; VanderDoes and VandenBosch 1992). Using monetary reinforcement in addition to instruction, Green and colleagues found results similar to those of Goldberg et al. (1987). However, they also found that continuing reinforcement after instructional training enabled half of their subjects to sustain their improved performance. Bellack and colleagues (1990) found that although contingent or noncontingent monetary reward did not improve performance, patients who received both contingent reward and card-by-card instructions significantly increased performance during training *and* during a subsequent testing session.

These studies suggest that motivation plays an important role in modifying WCST performance. A recent study found that combining relatively large monetary reinforcement with response cost for errors resulted in reduced perseverative errors *without* instruction (Summerfelt et al. 1991). However, as these authors point out, differences in clinical state and more enduring population differences such as chronicity or severity of global impairment may account for some of the disparity in findings. This hypothesis is supported by more recent work suggesting that less dysfunctional patients are able to benefit from instruction (Goldman et al. 1992).

Viewed within the limited capacity model, providing instructions and feedback may serve as external organizers that decrease capacity demand or facilitate capacity allocation. However, findings suggest that, for at least some patients, repeated practice or instructions alone are ineffective for improving cognitive flexibility. Adding reinforcement contingencies appears to significantly enhance the effects of these interventions. Within the limited capacity model, reinforcers provide salient stimuli that help patients more effectively allocate cognitive capacity. However, less cognitive motivational explanations also appear to be consistent with the data.

Value of the Limited Capacity Model

The limited capacity model has some value in providing post hoc explanations of positive outcomes found in cognitive intervention studies. Concepts such as allocation policy and automatization appear to shed light on deficient cognitive processes in schizophrenia. However, greater value would be obtained if *predictive* limited capacity hypotheses were supported experimentally. The greatest benefits would be obtained if the model was used prescriptively to develop rehabilitation strategies that diminish these deficiencies. For example, the curvilinear relationship hypothesized between arousal and capacity suggests that strategies teaching patients how to control their anxiety should lead to modulated arousal and improved cognitive functioning. Positive findings would support the heuristic value of the model and suggest further directions for research.

Strategies That Target Psychotic Symptoms

The limited capacity model suggests that psychotic symptoms such as conceptual disorganization may arise when a patient's attempt to perform a task overloads cognitive capacity. For example, as the agitation frequently found in schizophrenia escalates, increasing arousal may reduce capacity, resulting in disorganization and disorientation. This premise predicts that a psychophysiological measure of capacity would covary with psychotic symptoms, and both should normalize with appropriate cognitive rehabilitation. Investigators have found that the experience and subsequent report of delusions and hallucinations, as well as manifestations of conceptual disorganization, can be diminished by using cognitive methods.

Reducing Hallucinations

Investigators have developed a psychophysiological technique, electromyography (EMG), that enables objective investigation of the otherwise subjective experience of hallucinations. Patients' report of auditory hallucinations and EMG activity recorded from chin and lips have been found to be highly correlated (Gould 1948; McGuigan 1966) and thus serve as an empirical marker for the symptom. EMG may be useful in the development of new rehabilitation interventions and measures for objectively testing intervention outcome independent of self-reports.

Clinical investigators have reasoned that, if subvocal activity is somehow causally related to auditory hallucinations, then procedures that interfere with subvocal activity might reduce the frequency of hallucinations. Bick and

Kinsbourne (1987) tested this hypothesis by instructing schizophrenic subjects to perform various muscle movement exercises when experiencing auditory hallucinations. Subjects in the subvocal-specific exercise group were instructed to open their mouth widely, and those subjects in the control condition were told to close their eyes tightly or clench their fist. Patients completing the subvocal-specific exercises reported fewer auditory hallucinations than subjects using the control exercises. Green and Kinsbourne (1990) replicated these findings with humming as the subvocal-specific behavior and opening mouth, biting tongue, and lifting eyebrows as control conditions. Humming increased subvocal EMG activity above baseline, suggesting that this subvocal-specific exercise interfered with EMG activity related to auditory hallucinations.

Green and Kinsbourne also reviewed competing hypotheses that might explain reduced reports of auditory hallucinations. A distraction hypothesis (Margo et al. 1981) suggests that capacity was redirected from attending to hallucinations to attending to the humming. This hypothesis, however, was not supported by Alpert's (1985) survey of patients that found reports of *more* hallucinations at louder noise levels than lower levels. Furthermore, to directly test the distraction hypothesis Green and Kinsbourne's subjects were instructed to hum quietly; significant results were still found.

Perhaps humming required greater effort (and thus cognitive capacity) than control tasks, thereby diminishing attention to hallucinations. However, subjects in Green and Kinsbourne's study reported that the control condition (raising eyebrows) was more effortful than humming. Similarly, highly effortful tasks such as educational or psychotherapy groups do not seem to diminish hallucinations.

An alternative hypothesis is that hallucinations are exacerbated by hyperaroused states that coincided with stressful stimuli. Perhaps during these episodes patients have less available cognitive capacity and thus are more likely to misconstrue environmental stimuli as hallucinations. If so, relaxation and desensitization techniques may diminish stress and secondarily reduce the frequency of hallucinations. Relaxation strategies also may have a prophylactic effect, reducing patients' general reactivity to stress. However, results from the only three studies of the use of relaxation for this purpose were equivocal (Nydegger 1972; Serber and Nelson 1971; Slade 1972). These studies were hampered by serious methodological problems such as lack of baseline data, medication confounds, diagnostic uncertainty, and poor experimental controls. Conclusions regarding the efficacy of relaxation interventions await future studies that more effectively test competing hypotheses.

Operant Strategies for Delusional Speech and Hallucinations

Investigators have studied the effects of punishing contingencies on the frequency of hallucinatory speech (Bucher and Fabricatore 1970; Weingaertner 1971). In one study, 45 patients were randomly assigned to one of three conditions (Weingaertner 1971). Patients in a self-shock condition wore a low-voltage metal box on their belt and were told to deliver a small shock to their hand each time they hallucinated. Patients in a placebo condition wore a similar box that did not deliver a shock and were given the same instructions. These subjects also were told that although they might not feel the shock, it was still effective. Subjects in a third group received no intervention. After 2 weeks of treatment, subjects in *all three* conditions reported significantly reduced hallucinations with no differences between groups. Although equal improvement in both intervention conditions suggests a placebo effect, similar effects in the control group suggest some confounding effect. Because more than half of the potential subjects refused to participate, one possible confound was selection bias. Perhaps subjects who were willing to join in a self-punishment study were highly motivated to decrease hallucinatory speech.

The effects of operant contingencies on "sick talk" also have been examined in various studies (Liberman et al. 1973; Patterson and Teigen 1973). For example, Wincze et al. (1972) compared the efficacy of token contingencies with verbal feedback in decreasing the frequency of delusional speech in 10 paranoid schizophrenic patients. During the token-based intervention, subjects received tokens on a fixed interval schedule for not voicing delusional statements. Feedback consisted of correcting delusional statements by pointing out the falsity in the statement. For example, the therapist would tell a patient who had said he was Jesus Christ, "Your answer is incorrect, Jesus Christ lived almost two thousand years ago. Your name is Mr. M and you are forty years old" (p. 251). Results of the study showed that the rate of delusional statements both within the training sessions and on the ward decreased for seven of the 10 subjects after token contingencies were implemented. Conversely, five of the subjects showed no effects after receiving feedback, and three subjects actually *increased* delusional speech after feedback.

The effects of reinforcing and punishing contingencies on delusional speech and hallucinations may be viewed in two ways. From a strict operant interpretation, these contingencies directly diminish the frequency of symptom report. Given that most people are likely to construe reports about visions and voices as bizarre, patients benefit when they discriminate appropriate versus inappropriate situations for verbalizing their hallucinations. In addition, operant contingencies increase the frequency of competing prosocial behaviors, thereby reducing the likelihood of hallucinations. This explanation contrasts with the limited capacity view that reinforcing contingencies provide the individual with informational feedback that facilitates allocation of cognitive capacity to appropriate external sources. The limited capacity model predicts that psychophysiological measures of capacity will covary with reports of hallucinations and delusions both before and after successful operant interventions; experimentally testing this prediction may support the limited capacity model.

The operant viewpoint of managing psychotic symptoms is limited by its disregard for the subjective experience of psychotic symptoms. Even though patients are taught to display hallucinatory and delusional behaviors less frequently, they may still experience intense psychological discomfort concomitant with symptoms no longer apparent to others. Furthermore, given the growing clinical importance of patients' self-monitoring of symptoms, clinicians should be mindful of the possible deleterious consequences of teaching patients not to share relevant symptoms. Perhaps the best use of operant techniques is for stimulus discrimination training that teaches which social settings are more or less appropriate for verbalization of psychotic symptoms.

Reducing Conceptual Disorganization

Persons diagnosed with schizophrenia often demonstrate disorganized speech marked by tangential associations, autistic logic, and neologisms. Meichenbaum (1966, 1969) used social reinforcement to diminish the rate of "sick talk" and increase the frequency of "healthy talk" in thought-disordered patients. In a followup, Meichenbaum and Cameron (1973) used a mixture of reinforcement, instructions, and self-talk to improve cognitive functioning in several domains. The investigators used confederates as models who "talked aloud" mnemonic strategies governing a digit span task, a second span task with distractors, a proverbs task, a Holzman ink blot test, and an interview. After observing a model, subjects were encouraged to self-instruct similar rules and received positive feedback for correct rehearsals. Subjects who participated in the self-instruction group increased performance on a proverbs test and on an inkblot test at a greater rate than subjects who participated in a practice control group. Hypothetically, teaching patients to self-instruct augments executive capacity allocation. Patients consequently focus on the specific task for which they are instructing themselves instead of attending to irrelevant internal or external stimuli.

Evidence from subsequent studies that investigated self-talk effects on conceptual disorganization was mixed. Although some studies supported and extended Meichenbaum's findings (Bentall et al. 1987; Shuart 1985), other studies failed to replicate his results (Gresen 1974; Margolis and Shemberg 1976). Using a yoked control group, Margolis and Shemberg were unable to find differences between subjects who participated in the self-monitoring treatment and subjects in the no-treatment control group. After the study, these subjects reported that self-reward strategies seemed "silly and babyish" (p. 671). Bentall et al. (1987) concluded that generic self-statements may be ineffective when they are prescribed programmatically, suggesting a need for the goals and content of self-instruction to be highly individualized.

Research by Harrow and his colleagues (1989) regarding impaired perspective and thought disorder challenges some of the assumptions underlying a self-talk approach to conceptual disorganization. In this study, 83 acutely ill patients were asked to rate the "typicality" of their own and of other patients' responses to proverbs on the Gorham Proverbs Test (Gorham 1956). Results indicated that psychotic subjects ratings of other patients' responses were similar to those of independently trained judges. However, *self*-ratings by psychotic patients were markedly disparate from ratings by judges. Although discordance rates were more pronounced for patients who were more thought disordered, even relatively asymptomatic patients were unable to recognize atypicality in their responses. How can patients guide thought processes with self-talk if they cannot reliably recognize their disorganized cognitions? Perhaps judgments requiring self-perspective are more demanding and patients' cognitive capacity is readily exceeded. If so, self-instruction may be more reliably effective if accompanied by adjunctive cognitive interventions that further increase information processing capacity.

Clinical Considerations Relevant to Cognitive Rehabilitation

Multiple factors affect the course of schizophrenia (Spaulding 1986) and require rehabilitation programs to be broadly comprehensive and multimodal (Anthony and Liberman 1992). This finding suggests that cognitive rehabilitation is less likely to be effective as an isolated intervention strategy, but rather ought to be integrated within a comprehensive, multidisciplinary process. Cognitive rehabilitation thus needs to take into account diverse "extraneous" factors usually investigated within other domains of inquiry. The following sections will briefly discuss three such topics: effects of psychotropic medications, assessment of heterogeneous deficits, and effects of the treatment environment.

Interactions Between Psychopharmacological and Cognitive Interventions

Pharmacological intervention is currently the predominant treatment for schizophrenia. Although psychotropic medications frequently reduce or alleviate disruptive positive symptoms such as delusions and hallucinations, their effects on specific information processes are less clear. The results of research on the relationship of antipsychotic and antiparkinsonian medication with cognitive functioning are complex. Based on these results, some hypothetical models of psychotropic drug effects on cognition are illustrated in Figure 11–1.

Numerous studies have found that some of the basic cognitive functions of schizophrenic patients benefit from pharmacological intervention. In particular, antipsychotic medication seems to enhance such early processing functions as readiness to respond, attention, and iconic memory. For example, medicated patients performed better on a backward masking task than an unmedicated comparison group (Braff and Saccuzzo 1982). Similar results have been found for iconic memory (Marder et al. 1984; Spohn et al. 1977). Moreover, improvements in early processing functions correlate with significant reductions in psychotic symptoms (Orzack et al. 1967; Spohn et al. 1977). Several studies also have demonstrated improvements in sustained attention (Orzack et al. 1967; Spohn et al. 1977). Medication appears to improve selective attention as well, possibly by reducing the effects of external distractors (Oltmanns et al. 1978; Strauss et al. 1985; Wahba et al. 1981).

However, not all studies have found basic cognitive functions to improve with drug treatment. For instance, Serafetinides and colleagues (1972) failed to show that neuroleptic medication improved performance on attention tasks. Neither simple reaction time (Held et al. 1970; Spohn et al. 1988) nor the reaction time crossover effect (Spohn et al. 1977, 1988) were found to be responsive

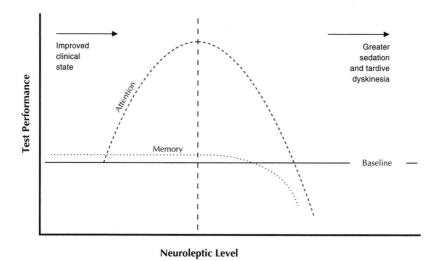

Figure 11–1. Hypothetical relationships between neuroleptic drug dose and cognitive functions.

to medication. Similarly, neuroleptic treatment has not been found to reduce verbal (Koh and Kayton 1974; Koh et al. 1973, 1981; Pearl 1962; Small et al. 1972; Whitehead and Thune 1958) and nonverbal (Castner et al. 1958; Koh et al. 1981; Lloyd and Newbrough 1964; Pearl 1962; Perlick et al. 1986) memory deficits. Three of four studies failed to show improved ability to learn number-symbol pairs on the WAIS Digit Symbol subtest with medication (Killian et al. 1984; Orzack et al. 1967; Serafetinides and Clark 1973), with only one study (Datson 1959) indicating positive effects.

Cognitive effects of neuroleptic medications may vary with dose level. In general, research suggests that optimal clinical effects for neuroleptic medication are achieved at moderate dose levels (500–700 mg chlorpromazine equivalents) with increased risk of side effects and diminished clinical outcome associated with higher dosages (Baldessarini et al. 1988). This principle appears to apply to cognitive functioning as well. One study found a significant negative correlation between neuroleptic dosage level and attention with doses ranging from very low (100 mg chlorpromazine equivalents) to very high (3,500 mg chlorpromazine equivalents; Sweeney et al. 1991). Other research has shown that high doses of neuroleptic medication significantly reduced attention (Pearl 1962) and increased reaction time (Spohn et al. 1985). An inverse relationship between dose of haloperidol and performance on a number-symbol substitution task was demonstrated in healthy subjects (Magliozzi et al. 1989). These findings suggest a threshold for neuroleptic dosage at which improvement in attention plateaus and perhaps declines.

Some antiparkinsonian medications prescribed to diminish the side effects of neuroleptics may impair cognitive functions. These drugs include anticholinergic medications that antagonize neuroleptic effects and dopamine agonists that enhance receptivity of monoaminergic synapses. These two classes of drugs have significantly different cognitive effects. Patients prescribed either of the anticholinergics benztropine (Cogentin) or trihexyphenidyl (Artane) have shown impaired short-term recall (Baker et al. 1983; Hitri et al. 1987; Perlick et al. 1986; Sweeney et al. 1991; Tune et al. 1982; Van Putten et al. 1987). These effects appear to depend on the severity of symptoms and are less apparent in more severely disturbed individuals (Calev et al. 1987). It is possible that anticholinergic effects may account for some of the diminished cognitive functions found at higher doses of neuroleptics. However, dopamine agonists such as amantadine (Symmetrel) have not been found to impair memory (Fayen et al. 1988; Gelenberg et al. 1989; Hitri et al. 1987; Van Putten et al. 1987).

Analysis of both therapeutic and undesirable medication effects suggests curvilinear relationships between medication levels and cognitive functions. The suggested biphasic relationship between dose level and attentional functioning also has been found for dose level and psychotic symptoms (cf. Baldessarini et al. 1988). Thus, although a linear relationship exists as medication dosage approaches optimal levels, attentional functioning appears to decline at higher dosages as sedation and/or movement disorders become more influential. This "inverted U" relationship (shown in Figure 11–1) does not apply to memory function, however. Moderate doses of antipsychotic medication have negligible effects on memory, but with higher doses impairments may occur. These decrements in memory may be related to the addition of anticholinergic drugs to the medication regimen.

Changes in cognitive functioning associated with psychotropic drug treatment need to be assessed when applying rehabilitation strategies. If, as is often the case, drugs and rehabilitation interventions are applied simultaneously, then their relative contributions to outcomes are difficult to discern. Medication changes during a rehabilitation intervention may either enhance or impair the effect of the intervention, whereas the stress that accompanies some interventions may modulate drug responses. Thus, continuing assessment and careful consideration of benefits, costs, and interactions are necessary in attaining an optimal mix of rehabilitation and pharmacological interventions.

Heterogeneity in Schizophrenia: Assessment and Treatment Implications

Uniformity of rehabilitation needs and intervention responses across all persons diagnosed with schizophrenia are contradicted by empirical evidence. Rather, population heterogeneity universally characterizes research findings on cognitive functioning in schizophrenia. Moreover, no specific cognitive deficit has invariably been associated with the disorder. For instance, only 40%–50% of schizophrenic patients are impaired on conventional versions of the Continuous Performance Test (Nuechterlein 1991), approximately 40% are impaired on span of apprehension (Asarnow et al. 1991), and some schizophrenic patients demonstrate normal performance on backward masking (Braff et al. 1991). Similarly, a significant minority of schizophrenic patients demonstrate normal performance on standard neuropsychological batteries (G. Goldstein 1991). Moreover, cognitive functioning varies within individuals across time. For instance, backward masking performance of some schizophrenic patients normalizes with symptom improvement (Braff et al. 1991).

Although research may someday define systems of classification that reliably predict treatment response, current nosology and assessment technology are not yet adequate for this purpose. Because of these limitations, the most effective rehabilitation strategy may be to individualize interventions based on comprehensive idiographic assessment (Spaulding 1986). Within such an approach, cognitive assessment contributes information to a functional analysis of behavior (Ciminero 1977) that defines elements of behavioral sequences for which maladaptive cognitive functioning impairs performance. Highly individual patterns of deficits that interfere with integrated performance may only be discernible through functional analysis of specific task performance (Kaplan 1988). Specification of key deficits facilitates development of individualized treatment programs by identifying the most critical targets for cognitive intervention. Ongoing assessment ideally would accompany intervention to provide feedback on effectiveness and suggest program modifications appropriate to changing clinical status.

However, pragmatic considerations often militate against application of comprehensive idiographic assessment. Detailed idiographic assessment is far too costly in time, money, and professional expertise to be fully implemented in most psychiatric rehabilitation settings. One cost-reduction strategy would be to apply different tiers of assessment dependent on the "difficulty" of a particular case. This stategy could be implemented by initially assessing the patient's capacity to meet the cognitive demands of important rehabilitation activities, followed by increasingly detailed and comprehensive cognitive assessment only to the extent needed to identify and evaluate appropriate interventions. Thus, most patients would receive only the most useful subset of the full assessment armamentarium.

Another approach is to automate significant portions of cognitive assessments. Many cognitive assessment tasks have been adapted for use on relatively inexpensive microcomputer systems. Several of these have been packaged into computerized assessment batteries such as the Ohio Battery (Magaro and Ashbrook 1984) or the COGLAB Battery (Spaulding et al. 1983). As an example of how such a battery can be used in psychiatric rehabilitation, two COGLAB cognitive performance profiles of a patient diagnosed with schizophrenia are shown in Figure 11–2. These profiles cluster COGLAB measures according to whether they evaluate perceptual, preattentional, attentional, or conceptual functions. Note that in this case assessment suggested that the most prominent deficit was conceptual. As the result of this and other data, cognitive treatment to enhance conceptual function was implemented. Subsequent assessment shows conceptual measures falling within normal limits.

It is hoped that further research and development of these and other assessment approaches will result in increased utility and practical availability of cognitive assessment data that enables individualized cognitive intervention. As is sometimes the case with medical treatments that require extremely expensive drugs, even the most powerful interventions are useless if their availability is curtailed by prohibitive cost. However, whatever their general

availability, comprehensive idiographic assessment and treatment may ultimately be a necessity for cognitive rehabilitation research. To the extent that
individual treatment response depends on detailed information of the kind
provided by idiographic assessment, use of generic treatments within traditional group designs may result in misleading group outcomes and erroneous
conclusions as to the general effectiveness of cognitive interventions.

The Environmental Context of Cognitive Rehabilitation

Inadequate consideration may currently be given to the potentially powerful
effects of "nontreatment" environmental variables on psychiatric rehabilitation. Environmental psychology research with healthy subjects has found environmental effects on cognitive processes that are often abnormal in
schizophrenia. Extrapolation of such findings to schizophrenia is further supported by a small number of similar studies that used subjects with schizophrenia or other severe behavioral disorders. Therefore, it is likely that effective
implementation of cognitive interventions requires consideration of

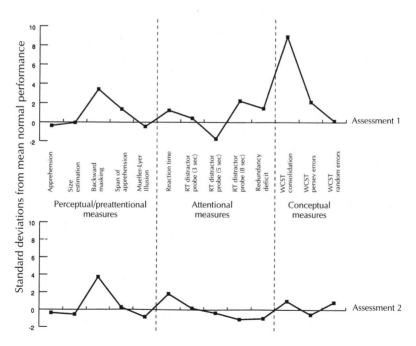

Figure 11–2.   Cognitive assessment profiles obtained with the COGLAB (Spaulding
et al. 1983) computerized assessment battery. Assessments were of the same patient
and occurred more than 1 year apart.

environmental influences on cognition. Because Heinssen (Chapter 15) discusses this issue more fully, only a few key issues are addressed here.

Environmental effects may be most profound in large institutions that often are crowded, noisy, and chaotic. Lack of control over even mildly aversive loud noise has been shown to cause dysphoric mood (Breier et al. 1987). High population densities are associated with increased physiological arousal and negative mood (Epstein et al. 1981). Population density effects are especially adverse in settings where residents have little control and tend not to cooperate with each other (Epstein 1982). Even moderate levels of population density correlate with reduced life satisfaction and more negative forms of behavior (Rohe 1982). Overcrowding in female prisons has been linked to increased rates of disciplinary infractions (Ruback and Carr 1984), whereas increased crowding in a juvenile correctional institution was associated with social disorganization and negative mood (Ray et al. 1982). Within psychiatric settings, lack of privacy has been found to be a significant source of discontent (Sommer and Kroll 1979).

Apparently few studies have directly investigated the effects environmental variables have on cognitive functioning in schizophrenia. Understimulating environments are thought to exacerbate negative symptoms and increase delusional and hallucinatory processes (Falloon et al. 1984). Yet, Alpert's (1985) finding of more frequent hallucinations with louder noise levels suggests that overstimulation also is problematic. Demand-intensive treatment efforts that include high degrees of structure and forced social interaction are associated with symptom exacerbation (Wing 1978). Studies of emotion and communication within families of persons diagnosed with schizophrenia have found high levels of tension and emotionality are associated with increased rates of relapse and exacerbation (M. Goldstein 1987). These effects appear to be at least in part mediated by psychophysiological arousal (Sturgeon et al. 1984; Tarrier and Barrowclough 1987; Tarrier et al. 1979, 1988; Valone et al. 1984).

Environmental psychologists have suggested models of environmental effects on normal functioning that closely correspond with the limited information capacity model (Cohen 1978; Saegert 1978). Environmental stressors are thought by these theorists to result in overload of normal information processing required by social and functional roles. For example, optimal levels of visual environmental complexity exist that, when exceeded for informative or decorative purposes, result in bewilderment or disorientation (Kaplan 1975). Therefore, environmental psychologists recommend designing physical settings such that individuals' cognitive capacities are not adversely affected by them. Analogous concepts and applications may be usefully derived from the limited information processing model of psychotic cognition.

Adverse effects of psychiatric treatment environments have been reduced by environmental modifications. For instance, rearranging dayroom chairs in small groupings oriented to encourage social interaction markedly increased rates of socializing among psychiatric patients (Holohan 1972; Sommer and Ross 1958). Use of color coding and large graphics were followed by increased prosocial and reduced maladaptive behavior of elderly nursing home patients (Lawton et al. 1984). A controlled study of the effects of rearranging a psychiatric ward showed more than a 60% increase in social activity compared with a control ward (Holohan and Saegert 1973). Changes included painting the ward with bright colors, providing attractive and colorful modern furniture and room furnishings, and adding partitions to divide dormitories into two-bed sections. Ittelson et al. (1970) discovered pronounced behavioral differences between psychiatric patients who received either single or multiple occupancy bedrooms, with single occupancy patients exhibiting less withdrawn behavior. Redesign of rooms to provide flexible space options ranging from relatively private to relatively public increased social interactions between patients and staff and reduced maladaptive behavior (C. Whitehead et al., unpublished observations, 1982).

In summary, although few investigations have specifically studied environment-cognition interactions in schizophrenia, principles of environmental psychology regarding vulnerability of normal cognition to environmental effects may be usefully extrapolated to cognitive rehabilitation. As an example, Liberman et al. (1982) recommended keeping rehabilitation training areas uncluttered and posting charts that succinctly summarize learning points so that patients are less likely to be distracted by irrelevant environmental stimuli. However, such extrapolated guidelines need to be more thoroughly validated by empirical evidence. Further research and development in this area would help clinical investigators identify environmental strategies that will facilitate the goals of cognitive rehabilitation.

Conclusion

On the whole, research suggests that the effects of rehabilitation interventions on cognitive functioning in schizophrenia are significant and potentially useful (see Figure 11–3 for a summary of findings). Studies clearly indicate that the outward signs of "cognitive" psychotic symptoms such as delusional thinking and hallucinations are modifiable by psychosocial interventions. Procedures that incorporate positive reinforcement to affect these symptoms are more efficacious than those that do not. Interventions that are most certainly effective for basic information processing deficits are primarily adapted laboratory tasks that incorporate variations and combinations of instruction, repeated

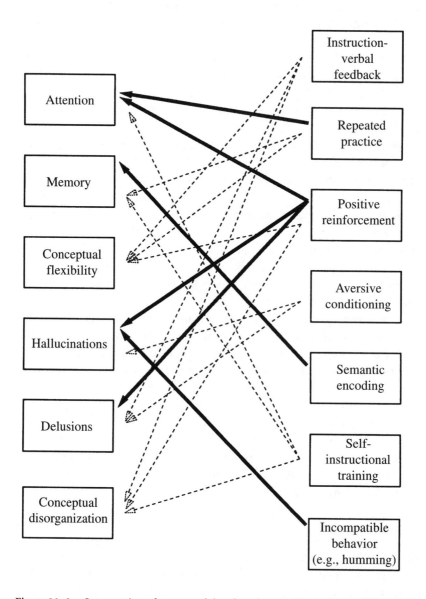

Figure 11–3. Interventions that research has found most effective for specific categories of cognitive deficits. Dark arrows point from classes of interventions to kinds of impairments for which empirical evidence supporting effectiveness is relatively strong. Dotted lines point from classes of interventions to kinds of impairments for which empirical evidence supporting effectiveness is relatively sparse, indirect, or questionable on methodological grounds.

practice, and operant learning procedures. Although such methods demonstrably facilitate the acquisition of task automaticity, there is little evidence that the improved performance generalizes beyond the training task. Thus, clinical utility of these methods may be limited to focal interventions targeting isolated but functionally significant deficits.

There is some evidence of individual differences in responses to cognitive interventions. These findings converge with experimental psychopathology studies demonstrating heterogeneity of cognitive functioning and suggesting that idiographic assessment may be important for effective implementation of cognitive rehabilitation. Unfortunately, cognitive rehabilitation research thus far has been limited by presenting a static, homogeneous picture of cognitive deficits. If treatment response depends on detailed information and individualized treatment, generic treatments within traditional group designs may result in misleading research findings.

The investigated cognitive interventions, although often proximally effective, have not been convincingly demonstrated to result in significant improvement in functioning. For example, it would be important to know whether improvement in elementary cognitive functions facilitates more complex functions as well. The ecological validity of cognitive interventions also is poorly demonstrated (Ellis 1986; Weingaertner 1971). What effects do isolated improvements in cognitive functioning have on complex real-world cognition? Do cognitive interventions significantly affect the impairments of social and instrumental functioning that are the most devastating effects of schizophrenia?

Clinically significant generalization can take several forms. One form of generalization would be transfer from target process to secondary process; for example, improved attentional function might improve working memory. Generalization also may occur as a transfer from target process to broader task. Even if such generalization were limited, clinical utility still might exist if the intervention was strategically applied to obtain temporary cognitive improvement that facilitates learning of specific instrumental or social skills (Spaulding 1992). For example, although global or enduring improvement in working memory might not result, the patient's skills repertoire would still be augmented. Finally, generalization may manifest itself as a nonspecific improvement of life satisfaction (e.g., diminution of troublesome delusions through appropriate reinforcing contingencies yields increased patient statements about quality of life).

Clinical investigators need to account for these varied forms of generalization in developing and testing cognitive interventions that help patients meaningfully improve their perception, comprehension, and utilization of real-world information. It has increasingly become apparent to clinicians that specific procedures may need to be actively incorporated into rehabilitation to facilitate generalization (Stokes and Baer 1977). Such interventions as in vivo role play, independent homework, and natural consequences have been shown to facilitate transfer of newly learned behaviors to other settings (Corrigan et al. 1992). Similar approaches may be necessary to attain clinically significant generalization of cognitive rehabilitation effects as well.

References

Alpert M: The signs and symptoms of schizophrenia. Compr Psychiatry 26: 103–112, 1985

Anthony WA, Liberman RP: Psychiatric rehabilitation, in Handbook of Psychiatric Rehabilitation. Edited by Liberman RP. New York, Macmillan, 1992, pp 95–126

Asarnow RF, Granholm E, Sherman T: Span of apprehension in schizophrenia, in Handbook of Schizophrenia, Vol 5: Neuropsychology, Psychopathology and Information Processing. Edited by Steinhauer SR, Gruzelier JH, Zubin J. Amsterdam, The Netherlands, Elsevier Science, 1991, pp 335–370

Baker LA, Cheng LY, Amara IB: The withdrawal of benztropine mesylate in chronic schizophrenic patients. Br J Psychiatry 143:584–590, 1983

Baldessarini RJ, Cohen MD, Teicher MD: Significance of neuroleptic dose and plasma level in the pharmacological treatment of psychoses. Arch Gen Psychiatry 45:79–91, 1988

Bandura A: The explanatory and predictive scope of self-efficacy. Journal of Social and Clinical Psychology 4:359-373, 1986

Bellack AS: Cognitive rehabilitation for schizophrenia: is it possible? is it necessary? Schizophr Bull 18:43–50, 1992

Bellack A, Mueser K, Morrison R, et al: Remediation of cognitive deficits in schizophrenia: training on the Wisconsin Card Sorting Test. Am J Psychiatry 147:1650–1655, 1990

Bentall R, Higson P, Lowe C: Teaching self-instructions to chronic schizophrenic patients: efficacy and generalization. Behavioral Psychotherapy 15:58–76, 1987

Bick PA, Kinsbourne M: Auditory hallucinations and subvocal speech in schizophrenic patients. Am J Psychiatry 144:222–225, 1987

Bleuler E: Dementia Praecox or the Group of Schizophrenias. New York, International University Press (Original work published 1911), 1950

Braff DL, Saccuzzo DP: The effect of antipsychotic medication on speed of information processing in schizophrenia. Am J Psychiatry 139: 1127, 1982

Braff DL, Sacuzzo DP, Geyer MA: Information processing dysfunctions in schizophrenia: studies of visual backward masking, sensorimotor gating, and habituation, in Handbook of Schizophrenia, Vol 5: Neuropsychology, Psychopathology and Information Processing. Edited by Steinhauer SR, Gruzelier JH, Zubin J. Amsterdam, The Netherlands, Elsevier Science, 1991, pp 303–334

Breier A, Albus M, Pickar D, et al: Controllable and uncontrollable stress in humans. Am J Psychiatry 144:1419, 1987

Broen WE: Schizophrenia: Research and Theory. New York, Academic Press, 1968

Broen W, Storms L: Lawful disorganization: the process underlying a schizophrenic syndrome. Psychol Rev 73:265–279, 1966

Bucher B, Fabricatore J: Use of patient-administered shock to suppress hallucinations. Behavior Therapy 1:382–385, 1970

Calev A, Venables P, Monk A: Evidence for distinct verbal memory pathologies in severely and mildly disturbed schizophrenics. Schizophr Bull 9:247–264, 1983

Calev A, Korin Y, Kugelmass S, et al: Performance of chronic schizophrenics on matched word and design recall tasks. Biol Psychiatry 22:690–709, 1987

Callaway E, Naghdi S: An information processing model for schizophrenia. Arch Gen Psychiatry 39:339–347, 1982

Castner CW, Covington CM, Nickols JE: The effects of a Thorazine-centered treatment program with psychological evaluations. Texas Report of Biological Medicine 16:21–30, 1958

Ciminero A: Behavioral assessment: An overview, in Handbook of Behavioral Assessment. Edited by Ciminero A, Calhoun R, Adams H. New York, Wiley, 1977, pp 3–13

Cohen S: Environmental load and the allocation of attention, in Advances in Environmental Psychology, Vol 1. Edited by Baum A, Singer JE, Valins R. Hillsdale, NJ, Lawrence Erlbaum, 1978

Corrigan PW: Cognitive rehabilitation in schizophrenia, in Schizophrenia. Edited by Brenner H, Perris C. Bern, Switzerland, Springer (in press)

Corrigan PW, Schade ML, Liberman RP: Social skills training, in Handbook of Psychiatric Rehabilitation. Edited by Liberman RP. New York, Macmillan, 1992, pp 95–126

Cronbach LJ, Meehl PE: Construct validity in psychological tests. Psychol Bull 52:281–302, 1955

Datson PG: Effects of two phenothiazine drugs on concentrative attention span of chronic schizophrenics. J Clin Psychol 15: 106–109, 1959

Dawson ME, Nuechterlein KH: Psychophysiological dysfunctions in the developmental course of schizophrenic disorders. Schizophr Bull 10:204–232, 1984

Ellis ES: The role of motivation and pedagogy on the generalization of cognitive strategy training. J Learn Disabil 19: 667–670, 1986

Epstein YM: Crowding stress and human behavior, in Environmental Stress. Edited by Evans GW. Cambridge, England, Cambridge University Press, 1982, pp 133–148

Epstein YM, Woolfolk RL, Lehrer PM: Physiological, cognitive, and nonverbal responses to repeated exposure to crowding. Journal of Applied Social Psychology 11:1–13, 1981

Falloon IRH, Boyd JL, McGill CW: Family Care of Schizophrenia: A Problem-Solving Approach to the Treatment of Mental Illness. New York, Guilford, 1984

Fayen M, Goldman MB, Moulthrop MA, et al: Differential memory function with dopaminergic versus anticholinergic treatment of drug-induced extrapyramidal symptoms. Am J Psychiatry 145: 483–486, 1988

Fitts PM, Posner ML: Human Performance. Belmont, CA, Brooks/Cole, 1967

Gelenberg AJ, Van Putten T, Lavori PW, et al: Anticholinergic effects on memory: benztropine versus amantadine. J Clin Psychopharmacol 9:180–185, 1989

Gjerde PF: Attentional capacity dysfunction and arousal in schizophrenia. Psychol Bull 93:57–72, 1983

Goldberg TE, Weinberger DR, Berman KF, et al: Further evidence for dementia of the prefrontal type in schizophrenia? a controlled study of teaching the Wisconsin Card Sorting Test. Arch Gen Psychiatry 44:1008–1014, 1987

Goldman RS, Axelrod BN, Tompkins LM: Effects of cues on schizophrenic patients' performance on the Wisconsin Card Sorting Test. Am J Psychiatry 149:1718–1722, 1992

Goldstein G: Comprehensive neuropsychological test batteries and research in schizophrenia, in Handbook of Schizophrenia, Vol 5: Neuropsychology, Psychopathology and Information Processing. Edited by Steinhauer SR, Gruzelier JH, Zubin J. Amsterdam, The Netherlands, Elsevier Science, 1991, pp 525–551

Goldstein M: Psychosocial issues. Schizophr Bull 13:157–171, 1987

Gorham DR: A Proverbs Test for Clinical and Experimental Use. Psychological Reports 1:1–12, 1956

Gould LN: Verbal hallucinations and the activity of vocal musculature. Am J Psychiatry 105:367–372, 1948

Green MF: Cognitive remediation in schizophrenia: is it time yet? Am J Psychiatry 150:178–187, 1993

Green MF, Kinsbourne M: Subvocal activity and auditory hallucinations: clues for behavioral treatments. Schizophr Bull 16:617–625, 1990

Green MF, Ganzell S, Satz P, et al: Teaching the Wisconsin Card Sorting test to schizophrenic patients (letter). Arch Gen Psychiatry 47:91–92, 1990

Gresen R: The effects of instruction and reinforcement versus a multifaceted self-control procedure in the modification and generalization of behavior in schizophrenia. Unpublished doctoral dissertation, Bowling Green University, Bowling, OH, 1974

Gruzelier JH: Bimodal states of arousal and lateralized dysfunction in schizophrenia: effects of chlorpromazine, in The Nature of Schizophrenia: New Approaches to Research and Treatment. Edited by Wynne LC, Cromwell RL, Matthysse S. New York, Wiley, 1978, pp 167–187

Harrow M, Lanin-Kettering I, Miller JG: Impaired perspective and thought pathology in schizophrenic and psychotic disorders. Schizophr Bull 15: 605–623, 1989

Hasher L, Zacks RT: Automatic and effortful processes in memory. J Exper Psychol Gen 108:356–388, 1979

Heaton RK: Wisconsin Card Sorting Test Manual. Odessa, FL, Psychological Assessment Resources, 1981

Held JM, Cromwell RL, Frank ET, et al: Effect of phenothiazines on reaction time in schizophrenics. J Psychiatr Res 7:1–5, 1970

Hitri A, Craft RB, Fallon J, et al: Serum neuroleptic and anticholinergic activity in relationship to cognitive toxicity of antiparkinsonian agents in schizophrenic patients. Psychopharmacol Bull 23:33–37, 1987

Holohan CJ: Seating patterns and patient behavior in an experimental dayroom. J Abnorm Psychol 80:1115–1124, 1972

Holohan CJ, Saegert S: Behavioral and attitudinal effects of large-scale variation of the physical environment of psychiatric wards. J Abnorm Psychol 82:454–462, 1973

Ittelson WH, Proshansky HM, Rivlin LG: Bedroom size and social interaction on the psychiatric ward. Environment and Behavior 2: 255–270, 1970

Kahneman D: Attention and Effort. Englewood Cliffs, NJ, Prentice-Hall, 1973

Kaplan E: A process approach to neuropsychological assessment, in Clinical Neuropsychology and Brain Function. Edited by Boll T, Bryant BK. Washington, DC, American Psychological Association, 1988, pp 129–167

Kaplan S: An information model for the prediction of preference, in Landscape Assessment. Edited by Zube EH, Brown RO, Fabos JG. Stroudsburg, PA, Dowden, Hutchinson, & Ross, 1975, pp 129–167

Karras A: The effects of reinforcement and arousal on the psychomotor performance of chronic schizophrenics. Journal of Abnormal and Social Psychology 65: 104–111, 1962

Karras A: Choice reaction time of chronic acute psychiatric patients under primary or secondary aversive stimulation. Br J Soc Clin Psychol 7:270–279, 1968

Killian GA, Holzman PS, Davis JM, et al: Effects of psychotropic medication on selected cognitive and perceptual measures. J Abnorm Psychol 93: 58–70, 1984

Knight RG, Russell PN: Global capacity reduction and schizophrenia. Br J Soc Clin Psychol 17:275–280, 1978

Koh SD: Remembering in schizophrenia, in Language and Cognition in Schizophrenia. Edited by Schwartz S. Hillsdale, NJ, Lawrence Erlbaum, 1978

Koh SD, Kayton L: Memorization of "unrelated" word strings by young nonpsychotic schizophrenics. J Abnorm Psychol 83:14–22, 1974

Koh SD, Kayton L, Berry R: Mnemonic organization in young nonpsychotic schizophrenics. J Abnorm Psychol 81:299–310, 1973

Koh SD, Kayton L, Peterson RA: Affective encoding and consequent remembering in schizophrenic young adults. J Abnorm Psychol 85: 156–166, 1976

Koh SD, Grinker RR Sr, Marusarz TZ, et al: Affective memory and schizophrenic anhedonia. Schizophr Bull 7:292–303, 1981

Kraepelin E: Dementia praecox, in Clinical Psychiatry: A Textbook for Students and Physicians, 6th Edition. Edited by Kraepelin E. Leipzig, Germany, Thieme, 1902

Larsen S, Fromholt P: Mnemonic organization and free recall in schizophrenics. J Abnorm Psychol 85:61–65, 1976

Lawton MP, Fulcomer M, Kieban MH: Architecture for the mentally impaired elderly. Environmental Behavior 16:730–757, 1984

Liberman RP, Teigen J, Patterson R, et al: Reducing delusional speech in chronic paranoid schizophrenics. J Appl Behav Anal 6:57–64, 1973

Liberman RP, Nuechterlein KH, Wallace CJ: Social skills training and the nature of schizophrenia, in Social Skills Training: A Practical Handbook for Assessment and Treatment. Edited by Curran JP, Monti PM. New York, Guilford, 1982

Lloyd DN, Newbrough JR: Sensory changes with phenothiazine medication in schizophrenic patients. J Nerv Ment Dis 139:169–175, 1964

Magaro PA: Cognition in Schizophrenia and Paranoia: The Integration of Cognitive Processes. Hillsdale, NJ, Erlbaum, 1980

Magaro PA: Psychosis and schizophrenia, in The Nebraska Symposium on Motivation. Edited by Spaulding W, Cole JK. Lincoln, University of Nebraska Press, 1984

Magaro PA, Ashbrook R: The application of an information processing model to the diagnosis and treatment of functional disorders through the use of a mini-computer. Fourth International Symposium on Models and Techniques of Cognitive Rehabilitation, Indianapolis, IN, 1984

Magliozzi JR, Mungas D, Laubly JN, et al: Effect of haloperidol on a symbol digit substitution task in normal male adults. Neuropsychopharmacology 29:29–37, 1989

Marder SR, Asarnow RF, Van Putten T: Information processing and neuroleptic response in acute and stabilized schizophrenic patients. Psychiatric Research 13:41–49, 1984

Margo A, Hemsley DR, Slade PD: The effects of varying auditory input on schizophrenic hallucinations. Br J Psychiatry 139:122–127, 1981

Margolis RB, Shemberg KM: Cognitive self-instruction in process and reactive schizophrenia: a failure to replicate. Behavior Therapy 7: 668–671, 1976

McGuigan FJ: Covert oral behavior and auditory hallucinations. Psychophysiology 3:78–80, 1966

Meichenbaum DH: Effects of social reinforcement on the level of abstraction in schizophrenics. J Abnorm Psychol 71:354–362, 1966

Meichenbaum DH: The effects of instructions and reinforcement on thinking and language behavior of schizophrenics. Behav Res Ther 7:101–114, 1969

Meichenbaum DH, Cameron R: Training schizophrenics to talk to themselves: a means of developing attentional controls. Behavior Therapy 4:515–534, 1973

Meiselman KC: Broadening dual modality cue utilization in chronic nonparanoid schizophrenia. J Consult Clin Psychol 41:447–453, 1973

Nuechterlein KH: Signal detection in vigilance tasks and behavioral attributes among offspring of schizophrenic mothers and among hyperactive children. J Abnorm Psychol 92:4–28, 1983

Nuechterlein KH: Vigilance in schizophrenia and related disorders, in Handbook of Schizophrenia, Vol 5: Neuropsychology, Psychopathology and Information Processing. Edited by Steinhauer SR, Gruzelier JH, Zubin J. Amsterdam, The Netherlands, Elsevier Science, 1991, pp 397–433

Nuechterlein KH, Asarnow RF: Cognition and perception, in Comprehensive Textbook of Psychiatry. V. Edited by Kaplan HI, Sadock BJ. Baltimore, MD, Williams & Wilkins, 1989, pp 241–256

Nuechterlein KH, Dawson ME: A heuristic vulnerability/stress model of schizophrenic episodes. Schizophr Bull 10:300–312, 1984a

Nuechterlein KH, Dawson ME: Information processing and attentional functioning in the developmental course of schizophrenic disorders. Schizophr Bull 10:160–202, 1984b

Nuechterlein KH, Dawson ME, Ventura J, et al: Testing vulnerability models: stability of potential vulnerability indicators across clinical state, in Search for the Causes of Schizophrenia, Vol 2. Edited by Hafner H, Gattaz WF. Heidelberg, Germany, Springer-Verlag, 1990

Nydegger R: The elimination of hallucinatory and delusional behavior by verbal conditioning and assertive training: a case study. J Behav Ther Exp Psychiatry 3:225–227, 1972

Oltmanns TF, Neale JM, Ohayon J: The effect of anti-psychotic medication and diagnostic criteria on distractibility in schizophrenia. J Psychiatr Res 14:81–91, 1978

Orzack MH, Kornetsky C, Freeman H: The effects of daily administration of carphenazine on attention in the schizophrenic patient. Psychopharmacologia 11:31–38, 1967

Patterson RL, Teigen JR: Conditioning and post-hospital generalization of nondelusional responses in a chronic psychotic patient. J Appl Behav Anal 6: 65–70, 1973

Pearl D: Phenothiazine effects in chronic schizophrenia. J Clin Psychol 18: 86–89, 1962

Perlick D, Stastny P, Katz I, et al: Memory deficits and anticholinergic levels in chronic schizophrenia. Am J Psychiatry 143:230–232, 1986

Posner MI, Snyder CRR: Attention and cognitive control, in Information Processing and Cognition, The Loyola Symposium. Edited by Solso RL. Hillsdale, NJ, Lawrence Erlbaum, 1975, pp 55–85

Ray DW, Wandersman A, Ellisor J, et al: The effects of high density in a juvenile correctional institution. Basic Applied Social Psychology 3:95–108, 1982

Rohe WM: The response to density in residential settings: the mediating effects of social and personal variables. Journal of Applied Social Psychology 12:292–303, 1982

Rosenbaum G, MacKavey WR, Grisell JL: Effects of biological and social motivation on schizophrenic reaction times. Journal of Applied Social Psychology 54:364–368, 1957

Ruback RB, Carr TS: Crowding in women's prisons: attitudinal and behavioral effects. Journal of Applied Social Psychology 14:57–68, 1984

Saegert S: High density environments: the personal and social consequences, in Human Response to Crowding. Edited by Baum A, Epstein YM. Hillsdale, NJ, Lawrence Erlbaum, 1978, pp 257–281

Schneider W, Dumais ST, Shiffrin RM: Automatic and control processing and attention, in Varieties of Attention. Edited by Parasuraman R, Davies DR. Orlando, FL, Academic Press, 1984, pp 1–27

Serafetinides EA, Clark ML: Psychological effects of single dose antipsychotic medication. Biol Psychiatry 7:263–267, 1973

Serafetinides EA, Collins S, Clark ML: Haloperidol, clopenthixol, and chlorpormazine in chronic schizophrenia. J Nerv Ment Dis 154:31–42, 1972

Serber M, Nelson P: The ineffectiveness of desensitization and assertiveness training in hospitalized schizophrenics. J Behav Ther Exp Psychiatry 2:107–109, 1971

Shiffrin RM, Schneider W: Controlled and automatic human information processing, II: perceptual learning, automatic attending, and general theory. Psychol Rev 84:127–190, 1977

Shuart W: Effects of self-instructional training on performance in a social skills training group. Unpublished doctoral dissertation, University of Nebraska-Lincoln, 1985

Slade P: The effects of systematic desensitization on auditory hallucinations. Behav Res Ther 10:85–91, 1972

Small IF, Small JG, Milstein V, et al: Neuropsychological observations with psychosis and somatic treatment. J Nerv Ment Dis 155:6–13, 1972

Sommer R, Kroll B: Personal privacy in a psychiatric ward setting. Environment and Behavior 11:114–129, 1979

Sommer R, Ross H: Social interaction on a geriatrics ward. Int J Soc Psychiatry 4:128–133, 1958

Spaulding W: Assessment of adult-onset pervasive behavior disorders, in Handbook of Behavior Assessment. Edited by Adams H, Calhoun K. New York, Wiley, 1986, pp 631–669

Spaulding W: Design prerequisites for research on cognitive therapy for schizophrenia. Schizophr Bull 18:39–42, 1992

Spaulding W, Crinean J, Martin T: Microcomputerized clinical and research laboratories in psychiatric inpatient settings. Behavior Research Methods and Instrumentation 15:171–176, 1983

Spaulding W, Crinean J, Martin T: Microcomputerized clinical and research laboratories in psychiatric inpatient settings. Behavior Research Methods and Instrumentation 15:171-176, 1983

Spohn HE, Lacoursiere RB, Thompson R, et al: Phenothiazine effects on psychological and psychophysiological dysfunction in chronic schizophrenics. Arch Gen Psychiatry 34:633–644, 1977

Spohn HE, Coyne L, Lacoursiere R, et al: Relation of neuroleptic dose and tardive dyskinesia to attention, information-processing, and psychophysiology in medicated schizophrenics. Arch Gen Psychiatry 42:849–859, 1985

Spohn HE, Coyne L, Spray J: The effect of neuroleptics and tardive dyskinesia on smooth-pursuit eye movement in chronic schizophrenics. Arch Gen Psychiatry 45:833–840, 1988

Stokes TF, Baer DM: An implicit technology of generalization. J Appl Behav Anal 10:349–367, 1977

Strauss ME, Lew MF, Coyle JT, et al: Psychopharmacologic and clinical correlates of attention in chronic schizophrenia. Am J Psychiatry 142:497–499, 1985

Sturgeon D, Turpin D, Kuipers L, et al: Psychophysiological responses of schizophrenic patients to high and low expressed emotion relatives: a follow-up study. Br J Psychiatry 145:62–69, 1984

Summerfelt AT, Alphs LD, Wagman AMI, et al: Reduction of perseverative errors in patients with schizophrenia using monetary feedback. J Abnorm Psychol 100:613–616, 1991

Sweeney JA, Keilp JG, Haas GL, et al: Relationships between medication treatments and neuropsychological test performance in schizophrenia. Psychiatry Res 37:297–308, 1991

Tarrier N, Barrowclough C: A longitudinal psychophysiological assessment of a schizophrenic patient in relation to the expressed emotion of his relatives. Behavioral Psychotherapy 15: 45–57, 1987

Tarrier N, Vaughn CE, Lader MH, et al: Bodily reactions to people and events in schizophrenics. Arch Gen Psychiatry 36:311–315, 1979

Tarrier N, Barrowclough C, Porceddu K, et al: The assessment of psychophysiological reactivity to the expressed emotion of the relatives of schizophrenic patients. Br J Psychiatry 152: 618–624, 1988

Tune LE, Strauss ME, Lew MF, et al: Serum levels of anticholinergic drugs and impaired recent memory in chronic schizophrenic patients. Am J Psychiatry 139:1460–1462, 1982

Valone K, Goldstein MG, Morton JP: Parental expressed emotion and psychophysiological reactivity in an adolescent sample at risk for schizophrenic spectrum disorders. J Abnorm Psychol 93:448–457, 1984

VanderDoes AJW, VandenBosch RJ: What determines Wisconsin Card Sorting performance in schizophrenia. Clinical Psychology Review 12:567–583, 1992

Van Putten T, Gelenberg AJ, Lavori PW, et al: Anticholinergic effects on memory: benztropine vs. amantadine. Psychopharmacol Bull 23:26–29, 1987

Venables PH: Input dysfunction in schizophrenia, in Progress in Experimental Personality Research. Edited by Maher BA. New York, Academic Press, 1964, pp 1–47

Wagner BR: The training of attending and abstracting responses in chronic schizophrenia. Journal of Experimental Research in Personality 3:77–88, 1968

Wahba M, Donlon PT, Meadow A: Cognitive changes in acute schizophrenia with brief neuroleptic treatment. Am J Psychiatry 138:1307–1310, 1981

Weingaertner AH: Self-administered aversive stimulation with hallucinating hospitalized schizophrenics. J Consult Clin Psychol 36:422–429, 1971

Whitehead WA, Thune LE: The effects of chlorpromazine on learning in chronic psychotics. J Consult Psychol 22:379–383, 1958

Wincze JP, Leitenberg H, Agras WS: The effects of token reinforcement and feedback on delusional verbal behavior of chronic paranoid schizophrenics. J Appl Behav Anal 5:247–262, 1972

Wing JK: Social influences on the course of schizophrenia, in The Nature of Schizophrenia: New Approaches to Research and Treatment. Edited by Wynne LC, Cromwell RL, Matthysse S. New York, Wiley, 1978, pp 599–616

Zahn TP: Psychophysiological concomitants of task performance in schizophrenia, in Experimental Approaches to Psychopathology. Edited by Kietzman ML, Sutton S, Zubin J. New York, Academic Press, 1975, pp 109–131

Zubin J, Spring B: Vulnerability: a new view of schizophrenia. J Abnorm Psychol 86:103–126, 1977

Chapter 12

Integrated Psychological Therapy Program: Training in Cognitive and Social Skills for Schizophrenic Patients

Hans Dieter Brenner, M.D., Ph.D., Anita Hirsbrunner, M.A., and Daniela Heimberg, M.A.

The Integrated Psychological Therapy Program Training in Cognitive and Social Skills for Schizophrenic Patients

Despite 80 years of intensive research on predisposing genetic, biological, developmental, psychosocial, and sociological factors, no researcher or research team has found the one necessary or sufficient factor that causes schizophrenia. Consequently, in recent years researchers have moved away from linear deterministic approaches to multifactorial systemic models of the origin of schizophrenia, claiming that only an interacting combination of hereditary, biochemical, social, and psychological variables are responsible for the outbreak of this mental disorder (e.g., the Vulnerability Stress Model for schizophrenia by Zubin and Spring 1977).

Although treatment with neuroleptic medication has proved to be effective in treating acute psychotic episodes and in preventing relapses, it does not help the patient to gain greater insight into his or her personal problems and, perhaps more importantly, does not enable him or her to acquire appropriate coping strategies when faced with stress. Consequently, under the influence of integrative views of schizophrenia, therapy for schizophrenic patients has been extended to supplement neuroleptic medication with various other intervention modes. The latter can be subsumed under four headings: token economy programs (e.g., Cohen et al. 1972), social skills training programs (e.g., Wallace et al. 1980), therapy that focuses on the fostering of problem-solving skills (e.g., Liberman 1982), and therapy that incorporates the situative/emotional context as described in expressed emotion theories (overview in Olbrich 1983).

A growing number of experts agree that it is essential to provide combined therapy packages, including biological, social-learning, and psychosocial interventions, when treating schizophrenic patients. Nevertheless, even these combined packages have not shown the expected impact. Recent longitudinal studies (e.g., Schubart et al. 1986; Möller and Zerssen 1986; World Health Organization 1979) have proved that, in spite of multimodal efforts, the treatment of schizophrenic patients has been ineffective in influencing major behavioral consequences of schizophrenia, such as social withdrawal, lack of role orientation, deficient role fulfillment, negative symptoms, and low levels of stress resistance. In our opinion this is partly because combined therapy approaches have little regard for those processes in therapy that mediate between specific components of information processing and specific symptoms or symptom complexes. Strangely enough, although clinicians claim that cognitive disorders are a key indicator of schizophrenia and the basis of its characteristic symptomatology, therapy programs have paid little attention to cognitive processes.

One of the reasons why cognition has been neglected may be that experimental research on information processes (and therefore its application to therapy with schizophrenic patients) has been hampered by a multitude of divergent theoretical concepts with different operational terms. The situation improved toward the end of the 1970s when various authors (Hemsley and Zawada 1976; Koh et al. 1977; Kukla 1980; Magaro 1980; Schwartz 1978) began to apply the research and methods developed by cognitive psychologists concerned with "normal" information processing to schizophrenia.

Two models of information processing have emerged, one known as the bottom-up approach (e.g., Broga and Neufeld 1981) and the other as the top-down approach (e.g., Marousarz and Koch 1980). The former claims that schizophrenic symptoms emerge because of the impairment of basic cognitive functions (e.g., psychotic symptoms result from attentional deficits). The latter model suggests that the breakdown of more complex cognitive functions is responsible for the impairment of basic cognitive functions and simultaneously for the emergence of the symptoms. Magaro (1980) attempted to synthesize these discrepancies, proposing a model of dynamic interaction between elementary cognitive functions and higher-level controlling functions.

Unfortunately the interrelationship between information processing and cognitive, emotional, and behavioral factors has only been described in general terms. Lack of integrative theories may explain why therapy programs for schizophrenic patients have neglected the treatment of cognitive dysfunctions. The main question remains: where are the roots of schizophrenic cognitive dysfunctions to be localized and, therefore, where should the point of action for therapy be?

Another reason for this neglect probably lies in the unverified but widespread hypothesis that cognitive disorders are normalized by neuroleptic medication, leading clinicians to believe that specific treatment is unnecessary. Although certain elementary cognitive disorders seem to improve after psychophysiological arousal is normalized, neuroleptical medication has little or no effect on less elementary levels of mental functioning. Selective attention, for example, can be improved, but not the ability to modulate concepts to changing demands from the environment. This may explain why the combined treatment packages are not as efficient as they could be. Neuroleptic medication does not have a sufficient impact on disorders of abstraction capacity, concept formation, or concept modulation. Alternatively, therapy programs that focus exclusively on overt behavior or indirectly on cognitive dysfunctions are not sufficiently effective; although these programs produce short-lived improvements, generalization of learned skills into everyday life usually is not achieved. Numerous authors attribute the relative insufficiency of combined treatment to the persistence of elementary cognitive dysfunctions that may interfere with the patient's ability to profit from social-learning and psychosocial treatment.

Some efforts have been undertaken to develop therapy forms that specifically target isolated cognitive functions (e.g., Larsen and Fromholt 1979; Wishner and Wahl 1974). In the opinion of Magaro (1980) and Spaulding et al. (1986), the findings of these studies prove that specific cognitive dysfunctions can be normalized. Also, cognitive therapy programs of a more systematic nature have been developed and undergone evaluation under controlled conditions (Liberman 1988; Meichenbaum and Cameron 1973). However, relationships between different levels of functioning have not been expressedly taken into consideration. Whether a transfer to other levels of functioning (such as overt behavior) is possible and whether the effects of treatment are durable is open to speculation. Several questions must be answered to address this shortfall: Does faulty information processing play a mediating role in schizophrenia? How do cognitive disturbances mediate between neurochemical dysfunctions, clinical symptoms, and maladjusted behavior? Which consequences should be drawn for a more effective therapy?

An Integrative Model of Cognitive and Social Dysfunctions in Schizophrenia: Vicious Circles and Pervasiveness

The relationship between basic and more complex cognitive dysfunctions in schizophrenia and between cognitive deficits and social dysfunction can be seen as two vicious circles (Figure 12–1). In the first vicious circle, deficits in elementary cognitive functioning diminish higher order cognitive processes at the same time preventing coordination of elementary processes. This positive feedback loop causes continuous dysfunction, where complex and elementary functions exacerbate one another. The second vicious circle describes how cognitive deficits prevent sufficient acquisition of interpersonal coping skills. Insufficient interpersonal coping causes exposure to social stress, leaving the schizophrenic patient in a state of heightened arousal, wherein his or her intellectual capacity is further limited. The positive feedback loop to the first vicious circle is thus completed (Brenner et al. 1992b).

Based on an understanding of cognitive dysfunctions as moderating variables within a Vulnerability Stress Model rather than as structural characteristics, a "Model of Pervasiveness" was proposed (Brenner 1987; Brenner et al. 1992a; Spaulding 1986). According to this model, the relationship between cognitive systems and symptomatology is explained in terms of the effect impaired information processing has on the development and organization of behavior.

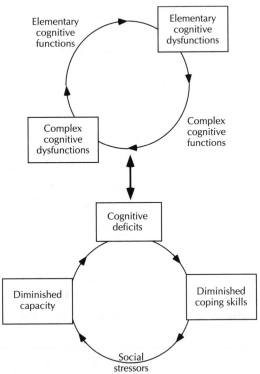

Figure 12–1.   The model of vicious circles: schematic representation of the positive feedback loops that define the interaction of cognitive and social variables.

This assumption implies that all levels of behavior are related to each other hierarchically. Considering this hierarchy, it was assumed that relatively molecular functions would be progressively combined with more complex molar behavior. The "Model of Pervasiveness" (Figure 12–2) was based on three hypotheses: 1) Schizophrenic patients have deficits at various levels of behavioral organization; 2) Deficits at one level have a detrimental effect on functions at other levels; and 3) The various levels of behavioral organization are related to each other in ordinal hierarchy. Disorders at more molecular levels result in impaired functioning at more molar levels, implying that deficits have a pervasive effect on all levels of behavioral organization.

The various levels of functioning (as depicted in Figure 12–2), with respect to schizophrenic deficits, were described as follows: 1) Attention/perceptual level: impairment in attention span, selective focus of attention, accuracy of perception, etc.; 2) Cognitive level: impairment in concept acquirement and modulation, inadequate or inappropriate prelinguistic associative processes or attributions, etc.; 3) Microsocial level: directly observable inadequacy of so-called social skills or overt behavior that is manifested in a given social context; 4) Macrosocial level: impairment in the fulfillment of complex tasks, i.e., inadequate coping with the assumption of specific social roles.

Brenner (1987) assumed that deficits at lower hierarchical levels impair the ability to function adequately at the next level in a serial progression of behavioral organization. For example, impairment in attentional processes

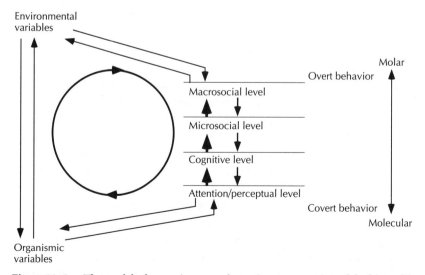

Figure 12–2. The model of pervasiveness: schematic representation of the hierarchical development and organization of deficient behavior in schizophrenia.

prevents adequate attributional processes. These difficulties in turn hinder appropriate behavior in a given social situation. In some instances an inversion of this process may be likely, where relatively molar deficits impair molecular functions at lower hierarchical levels. For example, failure to cope with a stressful social situation may release specific attentional dysfunctions.

Since the variability of maladjusted behavior could not be explained solely by referring to molecular deficits, the model included environmental and organismic variables that were thought to interact with each described level of functioning. Organismic variables were seen as specific psychophysiological phenomena (level of arousal, etc.) that influence covert mental functioning and overt behavior. In the same way, specific environmental variables (e.g., critical life events) were seen as responsible for variations of overt behavior and, therefore, covert mental functioning.

The Integrated Psychological Therapy Program for Schizophrenic Patients: A Therapeutic Approach Based on the Model of Pervasiveness

Two important conclusions for cognitive therapy with schizophrenic patients were drawn from the considerations mentioned previously: 1) An important aim of therapy with schizophrenic patients should be the reduction of disorders of attention, perception, and cognition; and 2) Therapy also must aim to break the vicious circles between attentional and more complex cognitive functioning and between cognition and behavior. It should focus on the connections between impaired attentional/perceptual and conceptual processes and their integrating organizations, as well as on positive feedbacks between cognitive dysfunctions and psychosocial stressors.

Based on the previously mentioned hypotheses, Brenner and co-workers initiated a group therapy program for schizophrenic patients at the Central Institute for Mental Health in Mannheim, Germany (Brenner et al. 1980). The program has been continually elaborated and has found widespread recognition under the name of "Integrated Psychological Therapy" (IPT). The term "integrated" refers to a main feature of the program, the demand that cognitive therapy for schizophrenic patients should occur within a social setting and under application of meaningful therapy materials. "Integrated" also means that therapy is implemented in such a way that dysfunctions in attention, perception, and cognition are reduced together with the development of adequate social and problem-solving skills, rather than under laboratory conditions where isolated dysfunctions are the target. IPT aims to provide therapy for both dysfunctions of cognitive processes (covert behavior in the Model of Pervasiveness) and for specific deficiencies in overt social behavior. A short description of the general structure of the IPT is provided with the specific aims of each subprogram. A comprehensive description of the program, its practical application, and its theoretical background can be found in Roder et al. (1992), or in an English version in Brenner et al. (1994).

The General Structure of the IPT

The IPT consists of five subprograms—cognitive differentiation, social perception, verbal communication, social competence, and interpersonal problem solving—that are each designed to meet the specific needs of schizophrenic patients and, in their combination, to form an integral approach to therapy (see Figure 12–3).

Each of the five subprograms can be seen as lying on a continuum of two inseparably linked dimensions—one concerning cognitive functions and the other concerning social competence. Both dimensions are jointly focused on throughout each subprogram, although the former is accentuated at the beginning of a subprogram and the latter toward its end.

This also is true for the entire program. The first two subprograms concentrate on the rebuilding of basic cognitive functions, the last two subprograms foster more complex interactional modes of behavior, with the third subprogram taking an intermediary role. Here again the proceeding prescribes a progression from a more cognitive to a more social dimension.

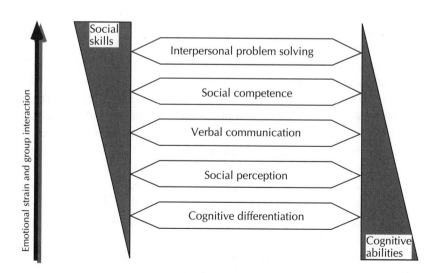

Figure 12–3. The five subprograms of the Integrated Psychological Therapy Program.

Demands of the patients increase as they progress through IPT. Therapy begins with a high level of structure and proceeds toward increasing demands on the patients' spontaneous participation and group interaction. Similarly, tasks at the beginning of therapy focus on relatively "objective" topics, where emotional involvement is kept low and a group consensus can usually be found with ease, and progress toward tasks with more "subjective" topics that evoke a greater degree of emotional involvement and contain issues of ambiguous content.

The Specific Aim of Each of the Five Subprograms

The cognitive differentiation subprogram concerns the improvement of specific basic cognitive functions such as attentional skills (e.g., selective attention, shifting attention, sustaining focused attention) and conceptualization abilities (e.g., stimuli abstraction, concept formation, concept discrimination, concept modulation, and concept recall). Intervention techniques include card sorting exercises and verbal exercises. Patients are required to draw up hierarchies of concepts; find suitable definitions, synonyms, or antonyms for given words; and distinguish between words with different contextual meanings. These skills are subsequently practiced in a game, comparable to 20 questions, where using appropriate search strategies (such as the use of conceptual rather than concrete questions) is required.

The social perception subprogram aims to improve analysis of social information (i.e., it focuses on the improvement of skills pertaining to discrimination between relevant and irrelevant social stimuli). The intervention technique is based on a series of slides that depict social situations. During early stages of this subprogram, the group members are asked to list all the visual information they observed on the slide. Each group member must then give an interpretation of this information. Individual interpretations are discussed and group consensus is sought. The actions and goals of social situations shown in the first slides of this subprogram are unambiguous. Those shown later, however, usually evoke ambiguous interpretations. It is not the reaching of a consensus on interpretation that is central to the training, but rather the contemplation of various interpretation possibilities, on the basis of individual perception and experience. Every interpretation is accepted as long as the reference to actual visual information makes sense and can be accepted by the entire group. Extremely discrepant opinions are gently confronted with contradictory evidence. In a final step, each group member also is asked to give the social situation in question a pertinent headline.

The verbal communication subprogram aims to improve conversational skills. The program starts with simple tasks that elicit skills learned in the previous programs. These may include shifting of attention to a statement made by another group member by listening closely and repeating the statement verbatim. The exercises mentioned earlier facilitate the associative-semantic processes necessary for reciprocal communication that is then practiced with the help of prompts. Patients are encouraged to discuss topics in free communication, without the help of prompts.

The social skills subprogram parallels more conventional behavioral social skills training except that cognitive components of social functioning are specifically focused on. Intervention techniques include a careful definition of the goal of specific social actions, the elaboration of possible dialogues that will be used in subsequent role plays, the naming of a pertinent title for the social action, the analysis of anticipated difficulties in the role play, and the rating of these difficulties on a scale. The role play itself is first modeled by a co-therapist and then enacted by the group member who rated the difficulties of the social situation lowest. After the role play, feedback is given by the observers and the therapist regarding the adequacy of verbal and nonverbal behavior. The group member also is told how he or she may improve on interpersonal difficulties observed during the role play.

The interpersonal problem solving subprogram also is similar to conventional problem-solving techniques, except that its cognitive components are accentuated. Certain steps of problem solving are supplemented with cognitive structuring especially designed for persons with schizophrenic deficits. For example, the identification and analysis of a given problem will include a careful separation of facts from assumptions and the correction of idiosyncratic perspectives. Similarly, the selection of a solution from the pool of generated solution alternatives involves the analysis of the success and failure of this solution in other problem situations, thus promoting a discriminative approach to the assessment of the suitability of specific solutions for various problems.

IPT's Role in Multimodal Treatment

The theoretical considerations discussed earlier suggest a multimodal concept of treatment for schizophrenic patients. Thus, a comprehensive treatment program must include a variety of therapeutic strategies. A treatment program for cognitive functions and social skills based on empirical findings and theoretical models, such as the IPT, only can be optimally effective when applied in a multimodal setting that includes psychopharmacotherapy, milieu therapy, social therapy, and family counseling. IPT should be embedded in a ward where both long- and short-term therapy planning and implementation are performed by a stable team of cooperating medical, psychological, and nursing staff. Ideally, the patient will progress through all of the IPT subprograms that are relevant to his or her special needs, and receive opportunities to practice newly acquired skills within the ward's daily routine. Patients also receive support from the staff in transferring these skills to social situations outside the clinic. Patients are motivated to cooperate with an optimal medication plan. Cooperation of the patient's relatives or other important persons should be established through family therapy sessions.

Recent Studies on the Effectiveness of the IPT

IPT has undergone many controlled experimental investigations and single case studies in different clinics (Brenner et al. 1987, 1989, 1990; Hermanutz and Gestrich 1987; Hodel, in press; Hodel et al. 1990; Kraemer et al. 1987, 1990; Roder 1988, 1990; Roder et al. 1987; Vogel 1987).

Three main studies evaluated the effectiveness of the complete therapy program on experimental versus control groups. The first study (Brenner et al. 1987), conducted in Mannheim, Germany, and Bern, Switzerland, involved 43 hospitalized, moderately chronic schizophrenic patients in a control group design. A second control group study (Brenner et al. 1987), involving 18 patients, happened in Heilbronn, Germany, with schizophrenic outpatients whose illness, again, had developed into moderate chronicity. The third control group study (Roder et al. 1987) was conducted in Münsterlingen, Switzerland, with 12 hospitalized, severely chronic schizophrenic patients. The main characteristics of these studies are shown in Table 12–1.

Because all three studies followed approximately the same design and produced comparable results, a joint description is provided; interested readers should read Brenner et al. (1987), for a more comprehensive report. All patients participating in the studies were selected according to the following criteria: ICD-9 diagnosis of schizophrenia (295.5 and 295.7 were exempted), WAIS IQ (Reduced Wechsler Intelligence Test, cf. Dahl 1972) rating of at least 85 points, minimal hospitalization duration of one year; and age between 20 and 50 years. Patients with neurological dysfunctions and alcohol or drug abuse were not considered. Patients were assigned to either experimental groups (therapy with the IPT) or control groups (standard treatment). In the Mannheim/Bern study, a placebo-attention group was added. (This was not considered necessary in the other two studies because no major differences were found between the two control groups.) In the Mannheim/Bern study, patients were assigned to groups according to their admittance date to the clinic. In the other two studies, groups were stratified according to age, sex, intelligence, duration of hospitalization, and duration of illness.

Table 12–1. The main evaluative studies of the Integrated Psychological Therapy Program

Study	Subjects	Diagnostic criteria	Therapy duration	Control measures	Investigation groups	Treatment effects (pre-post comparison)
Brenner et al. 1989: Study 1	43 chronic schizophrenic patients	ICD-9 (World Health Organization, 1978)	3 months	Benton D2 FCQ MMPI BPRS PSA	Experimental group ($N = 14$) Placebo-attention group ($N = 15$) Empty control group ($N = 14$)	FCQ (F value: 6.04; $P < .01$)[a] D2 (F value: 2.4 ; $P < .01$)[a] BPRS (F value: 6.79; $P < .01$)[a] in follow-up (18 months after therapy end) FCQ (F value: 5.37; $P < .05$)[a] D2 (F value: 9.10; $P < .01$)[a] BPRS (F value: 6.58; $P < .05$)[a] PSA (F value: 5.99; $P < .05$)[a]
Brenner et al. 1987: Study 2	18 chronic schizophrenic patients	ICD-9	4 months	Benton D2 KVT FCQ BPRS PSA AMDP SASKA	Experimental group ($N = 10$) Empty control group ($N = 8$)	BPRS[b]: Anergia (T value: 2.19; $P < .05$) Hostility (T value: 2.67; $P < .05$) SASKA[b]: Word-synonym (T value: 2.07; $P < .01$) Word-antonym (T value: 2.31; $P < .01$) Attribution (T value: 2.19; $P < .01$)

(continued)

Table 12–1. The main evaluative studies of the Integrated Psychological Therapy Program (*continued*)

Study	Subjects	Diagnostic criteria	Therapy duration	Control measures	Investigation groups	Treatment effects (pre-post comparison)
Roder et al. 1987	12 chronic schizo-phrenic patients	ICD-9	5 months	Benton D2 KVT SASKA FCQ BPRS PSA AMDP	Experimental group (N = 6) Empty control group (N = 8)	SASKA[a]: General score (z value: 2.20; $P < .05$) Word-antonym (z value: 2.02; $P < .05$) Word-selection (z value: 2.20; $P < .05$)
Hermanutz and Gestrich 1987	64 chronic schizo-phrenic patients	ICD-9	6–12 weeks	D2 WAIS BPRS GAS NOSIE	Experimental group (N = 32) Empty control group (N = 32)	GAS (F value: 5.07; $P < .05$) BPRS[b]: Activation (F value: 4.99; $P < .05$) Hostility (F value: 4.49; $P < .05$) Depression (deterioration: F value: 6.40; $P < .05$)
Kraemer et al. 1987	30 chronic schizo-phrenic patients	ICD-9	3 months	RPM FCQ BPRS PD-S Bf-S AT DT SW PS SB	Experimental group (N = 17) Empty control group (N = 13)	FCQ[c]: Loss of automatism ($P < .05$) Motoric disorders ($P < .01$) Thought disorders ($P < .05$) Paranoia ($P < .05$) Restlessness ($P < .05$) AT ($P < .01$)(3) DT ($P < .01$)(3) SW ($P < .05$)(3) PL ($P < .01$)(3) SB ($P < .05$)(3)

[a]Results of nonparametric Wilcoxon-tests. Significant results are shown in the table only if they are free of interfering variables such as group-processes or learning-effects.

[b]Results of covariance-analysis with pretest measures as co-variables. Additional analyses of average showed superiority of the experimental groups.

[c]Results of T tests (no further information about T values), only for interference-free significant results (see [b]).

Note. Benton = Benton Test (Benton 1981); D2 = Attention-Encumbrance Test (Brickenkamp 1978); FCQ = Frankfurt Complaint Questionnaire (Süllwold 1991); MMPI = Minnesota Multiphase Personality Inventory (Hathaway & McKinley 1977); BPRS = Brief Psychiatric Rating Scale (CIPS 1981); PSA = Scale of Psychological Adjustment, only in follow-up (PSA 1979); KVT = Test for Performance of Concentration (Abel 1961); SASKA = Verbal Performance Test (Riegel 1967); AMDP = Manual for the Documentation of Psychiatric Findings (Arbeitsgemeinschaft für Methodik und Dokumentation in der Psychiatrie AMDP 1979); GAS = Global Assessment Scale (Endicott et al. 1976); NOSIE = Nurses' Observation Scale for Inpatient Evaluation (CIPS 1981); WAIS = Reduced Wechsler Intelligence Test, only nonverbal part (Dahl 1972); RPM = Repeated Psychological Measurements, only Word Recognition and Crossing Out Numbers (Fahrenberg et al. 1977); PD-S = Paranoid-Depression Scale (CIPS 1981); Bf-S = Individual Condition Scale (CIPS 1981); AT = Abstraction Ability Test, as internal control measure (Kraemer et al. 1987); DT = Verbal Differentiation Test, as internal control measure (Kraemer et al. 1987); SW = Social Perception Test, as internal control measure (Kraemer et al. 1987); PL = Problem-Solving Test, as internal control measure (Kraemer et al. 1987); SB = Stress-Coping Test, as internal control measure (Kraemer et al. 1987).

Source. Reprinted from Brenner HD, Hodel B, Genner R, et al.: "Biological and Cognitive Vulnerability Factors in Schizophrenia: Implications for Treatment." British Journal of Psychiatry 161:154–163, 1992. Used with permission.

The studies followed a pre-post design, with a follow-up period of 18 months in the Mannheim/Bern study. Group comparisons were made with psychological tests for cognitive performance (e.g., Benton-A, Benton 1981; D2 Attention-Encumbrance Test, Brickenkamp 1978), observation and self-rating scales of psychiatric symptoms (e.g., BPRS, CIPS 1981; FBF/FCQ Frankfurt Complaints Questionnaire, Süllwold 1991) and rating scales for social adjustment (e.g., PSA Scale of Psychosocial Adjustment 1979).

Compared with patients in the control groups, patients participating in the experimental groups showed significant improvements in the pre-post comparison and also after 18 months. It was found that rehospitalization rates of the patients who had received IPT training were significantly lower than those of the control group patients during the follow-up period.

In another study, Hermanutz and Gestrich (1987) evaluated the effectiveness of three IPT subprograms: cognitive differentiation, social perception, and verbal communication. The subprograms were implemented in a slightly adapted version; e.g., not only slides but also audiotaped material were used in the social perception subprogram. Therapy and control groups were stratified according to age, sex, and attained level of education. The patients in the experimental group had a higher average hospitalization length than the patients in the control group. Both groups showed improvements in six of the 19 measures (Table 12–1), but the therapy group scored significantly higher in three measures of the Brief Psychiatric Rating Scale (CIPS 1981) and in the Global Assessment Scale (Endicott et al. 1976) (Table 12–1).

Kraemer et al. (1987) combined the cognitive differentiation and social perception subprograms with a program for the promotion of cognitive coping strategies, according to Meichenbaum (Kraemer et al. 1987). Thirty severely chronic schizophrenic patients were randomly referred either to the experimental group or to the control group. The patients in the experimental group showed significant improvements in most of the measures (Table 12–1) and scored significantly higher in some measures concerning self-perception (Frankfurt Complaints Questionnaire, Table 12–1) and all internal criteria for therapy success (abstraction ability, verbal differentiation etc., Table 12–1).

Although the main studies proved the general effectiveness of the IPT, a number of interesting questions remained unanswered. Do IPT interventions show effects on both cognitive and social functions? Where does the main impact of each subprogram lie? Are improvements in cognitive functions automatically followed by improved social behavior, as suggested by the Model of Pervasiveness? After these studies, more were conducted that aimed to clarify the differential effects of the IPT.

One study (Roder 1988, 1990), using an intragroup design, with 4 weeks baseline, 8 weeks therapy, and 4 weeks follow-up, addressed whether therapies that exclusively target basic cognitive dysfunctions show concomitant effects on higher-level functions. The cognitive differentiation subprogram was implemented alone, and effects in cognitive, psychopathological, and social measures were evaluated. The study showed that cognitive functions were significantly improved, though these effects were apparent only after five weeks of therapy. Positive effects were present during the four weeks of follow-up. Significant effects on the psychopathological or social level of functioning, however, could not be found. These results were reproduced in several other studies (Hodel et al. 1990; Kraemer et al. 1990; Vogel 1987), although results concerning social adjustment measures were inconsistent.

These studies suggest that improvements in impaired cognitive functions are not necessarily followed by improvements in social functioning. Thus stable and undisturbed information processing seems to be a necessary, but not a sufficient, condition for adequate social behavior on higher functional levels. Possibly other moderating factors that have not been considered have an inhibiting effect on pervasive processes that should coincide with cognitive improvements. These factors may reside in improvements that occur from participation in the social skills and interpersonal problem solving subprograms. A series of single case studies (Hodel, in press) showed improvements in social and cognitive functions that plateaued toward the end of therapy. These plateaus may reflect persisting deficient metafunctions or controlling processes that were insufficiently influenced by therapy.

Finally, practical experience suggests that emotions and level of arousal play a key role in the transition of improved cognitive abilities to the improvement of overt social behavior.

Further Development of the IPT

Attempts are being made at further development of the IPT subprograms with a greater consideration of emotional factors. The extent to which training of perception and appraisal of emotions can be integrated into IPT subprograms is being evaluated. Efforts are being made to incorporate training of emotional awareness, fostering an understanding of the events concomitant with the appearance of emotions and of the appraisal of consequences of emotions.

Hodel and co-workers have drafted a manual of IPT training steps that take special consideration of respective emotional factors (Brenner and Hodel 1990; Sandner et al. 1991). In this training, slides are shown that depict emotionally "loaded" situations. Patients are asked to describe them, thereby promoting awareness for emotions and understanding of situation stimuli that evoke them. Possible coping strategies to the emotional situation are sought and their application is practiced during role plays.

The interventions of this manual have been evaluated in a pre-post design (Hodel 1992). An experimental group of seven chronic schizophrenic patients was compared with a placebo-attention group of nine patients participating in a physical expression program. Results show significant differences between groups in emotion identification (Brenner and Hodel 1990). Unfortunately, these differences were already in evidence in the pre-test, so a conclusion cannot be drawn. Both groups showed significant improvements in their subjective perception of well-being (FBS/FCS Frankfurt Subjective Condition Scale, Süllwold and Herrlich 1987). However, in accordance with expectations, only the experimental group attained significant reduction of subjectively perceived cognitive disturbances (FCQ, Süllwold 1991) and only the experimental group showed significant improvement in central cognitive skills (Word Recognition Test of the RPM Repeated Psychological Measurement, Fahrenberg et al. 1977). It seems that the patients in the experimental group compensated cognitive disorders with less "interference" from distracting emotions. These findings encourage further research in this direction.

On the social level, independent living skills training (Liberman et al. 1987) is being incorporated into IPT. The social skills subprogram is being extended to include special interventions that focus on certain important areas of social life. In particular, three new programs have been developed by Roder and coworkers that try to improve social skills in the work, housing, and leisure. All subprograms follow IPT's basic principles, proceeding from a focus on cognitive aspects toward a focus on social behavior and the subsequent encouragement of a transfer of skills learned in therapy to real-life situations.

The three programs have undergone evaluation in pilot studies (Heimberg and Hirsbrunner 1991; Jenull 1992; Schwab and Zemp 1991). The pilot studies sought to evaluate whether the interventions were realizable in their conception (i.e., would they be comprehensible to schizophrenic patients), whether they were capable of motivating the therapy group (i.e., would the group members participate actively), and whether the topics discussed would evoke interest (i.e., were they considered of importance by the patients themselves). Results showed that the interventions were largely comprehensible to schizophrenic patients. Participants rated all the topics discussed within the programs of sufficient or immediate importance. A first evaluation of therapy effects also was undertaken, using intragroup designs with a baseline period of 4 weeks, therapy duration of 8 weeks, and a follow-up period of another 4 weeks. Results showed significant short-term improvements in most practiced skills. However, these could not be maintained in the follow-up period. More evaluation studies of the programs' efficacy with intergroup designs are planned.

Plans are being discussed to compare the IPT with other therapy forms. These include cognitive training following constructivist principles (Perris

1989), and a newly developed psychoeducative training program using the coping paradigm (Brenner et al. 1993). Depending on the outcome of these studies, elements of these treatment approaches will be incorporated into the IPT.

References

Abel D: Konzentrations-Verlaufs-Test. Göttingen, Germany, Hogrefe, 1961
Arbeitsgemeinschaft für Methodik und Dokumentation in der Psychiatrie AMDP: Das AMDP-System. Manual zur Dokumentation psychiatrischer Befunde. Berlin, Germany, Springer, 1979
Benton AL: Der Benton Test. Bern, Switzerland, Huber, 1981
Brenner HD: On the importance of cognitive disorders in treatment and rehabilitation, in Psychosocial Treatment of Schizophrenia: Multidimensional Concepts, Psychological, Family and Self-Help Perspectives. Edited by Strauss JS, Böker W, Brenner HD. Toronto, Ontario, Huber, 1987, pp 136–166
Brenner HD, Hodel B: Information processing in schizophrenia: a clinical approach, in Psychiatry: A World Perspective, Vol 1. Edited by Stefanis CN, Rabavilas AD, Soldatos CR. Amsterdam, The Netherlands, Excerpta Medica, 1990, pp 293–298
Brenner HB, Stramke WG, Mewes J, et al: Erfahrungen mit einem spezifischen Therapieprogramm zum Training kognitiver und kommunikativer Fahigkeiten in der Rehabilitation Chronischschizophrener Patienten. Nervenarzt 51:106–112, 1980
Brenner HD, Hodel B, Kube G, et al: Kognitive Therapie bei Schizophrenen: Problemanalyse und empirische Ergebnisse. Nervenarzt 58:72–83, 1987
Brenner HD, Böker W, Hodel B, et al: Cognitive treatment of basic pervasive dysfunctions in schizophrenia, in Schizophrenia: Scientific Progress. Edited by Schulz SC, Tamminga CA. New York, Oxford University Press, 1989, pp 358–367
Brenner HD, Kraemer S, Hermanutz G, et al: Cognitive treatment in schizophrenia, in Schizophrenia: Concepts, Vulnerability and Intervention. Edited by Straube ER, Hahlweg K. Berlin, Germany, Springer, 1990, pp 161–191
Brenner HD, Hodel B, Genner R, et al: Biological and cognitive vulnerability factors in schizophrenia: implications for treatment. Br J Psychiatry 161:154–163, 1992a
Brenner HD, Hodel B, Roder V, et al: Treatment of dysfunctions and behavioral deficits in schizophrenia. Schizophr Bull 18:21–26, 1992b
Brenner HD, Schaub A, Böker W: Umsetzung des Copingparadigmas in therapeutisches Handeln: Evaluation einer bewältigungsorientierten Gruppentherapie. Psychiatrische Universitatsklinik Bern, Switzerland, research grant request to Swiss National Fund, 1993
Brenner HD, Roder V, Hodel B, et al: Integrated Psychological Therapy for Schizophrenic Patients (IPT). Toronto, Ontario, Canada, Hogrefe & Huber, 1994

Brickenkamp R: Test d2, Aufmerksamkeits-Belastungs-Test. Göttingen, Germany, Hogrefe, 1978

Broga MI, Neufeld RWJ: Evaluation of information sequential aspects of schizophrenic performance: framework and current findings. J Nerv Ment Dis 169:558–568, 1981

CIPS Collegium Internationale Psychiatriae Scalarum: Internationale Skalen für Psychiatrie. Weinheim, Germany, Beltz, 1981

Cohen R, Florin I, Grushe A, et al: The introduction of a token economy in a psychiatric ward with extremely withdrawn chronic schizophrenics. Behav Res Ther, 10:69–74, 1972

Dahl G: WIP: Reduzierter Wechsler Intelligenztest. Anwendung - Auswertung, Statistische Analysen, Normwerte. Meisenheim, Germany, Hain, 1972

Endicott J, Spitzer RL, Fleiss JL, et al: The Global Assessment Scale. Arch Gen Psychiatry 33:766–772, 1976

Fahrenberg I, Kuhn M, Kulick B, et al: Repeated psychological measurement. Diagnostica 23:15–36, 1977

Hathaway SR, McKinley JC: MMPI Saarbrücken. Bern, Switzerland, Huber, 1977

Heimberg D, Hirsbrunner A: Entwicklung und Evaluation eines Gruppentherapieprogrammes zur Rehabilitation schizophren Erkrankter im Wohnbereich. Unpublished master's thesis, Universität Bern, Switzerland, 1991

Hemsley DR, Zawada SL: Filtering and the cognitive deficit in schizophrenia. Br J Psychiatry 128:456–461, 1976

Hermanutz M, Gestrich J: Kognitives Training mit Schizophrenen. Nervenarzt 58:91–96, 1987

Hodel B: Das Training von Coping Verhalten bei störenden Emotionen für schizophrene Patienten. Paper presented at the GFTS Symposium, Münsterlingen, Switzerland, October 1992

Hodel B: The Course of Cognitive and Social Interventions in Schizophrenia: Descriptive Results of Two Single Cases. Bern, Switzerland, Huber, in press

Hodel B, Brenner HD, Merlo M: Cognitive and social training for chronic schizophrenic patients: a comparison between two types of therapeutic interventions, in Psychiatry: A World Perspective, Vol 3. Edited by Stefanis C, Rabavilas A, Soldatos CR. Amsterdam, The Netherlands, Excerpta Medica, 1990

Jenull B: Freizeitrehabilitation schizophrener Patienten. Unpublished master's thesis, Universität Wien, Austria, 1992

Koh SD, Szog R, Peterson RA: Short term memory scanning. J Abnorm Psychol 86:415–460, 1977

Kraemer S, Sulz KHD, Schmid R, et al: Kognitive Therapie bei standardversorgten schizophrenen Patienten. Nervenarzt 58:84–90, 1987

Kraemer S, Zinner HJ, Riehl T, et al: Kognitive Therapie und Verhaltenstraining zur Förderung sozialer Kompetenz für chronisch schizophrene Patienten, in Kognitive Therapie bei Schizophrenen. Edited by Kühne GE, Brenner HD, Huber G. Jena, Germany, Fischer, 1990

Kukla F: Zum Konzept der Informationsverarbeitung bei der Untersuchung und Erklärung kognitiver Störungen—ein Überblick unter besonderer Berücksichtigung der Schizophrenie. Probleme und Ergebnisse der Psychologie 73:75–94, 1980

Larsen S, Fromholt P: Mnemonic organization and free recall in schizophrenia. J Abnorm Psychol 85:61–65, 1979

Liberman RP: Assessment of social skills. Schizophr Bull 8:63–83, 1982

Liberman RP (Ed.): Psychiatric Rehabilitation of Chronic Mental Patients. Washington DC, American Psychiatric Press, 1988

Liberman RP, Jacobs HE, Boone SE, et al: Skills training for the community adaption of schizophrenics, in Psychosocial Treatment of Schizophrenia. Edited by Böker W, Brenner HD. Toronto, Ontario, Huber, 1987

Magaro PA: Cognition in Schizophrenia and Paranoia: The Integration Process. Hillsdale NJ, Lawrence Erlbaum, 1980

Marousarz TZ, Koch SD: Contextual effects on short-term memory retrieval of schizophrenic young adults. J Abnorm Psychol 89:683–690, 1980

Meichenbaum D, Cameron R: Training schizophrenics to talk to themselves: a means of developing attentional controls. Behavior Therapy 4:515–534, 1973

Möller HJ, Zerssen D: Der Verlauf schizophrener Psychosen unter gegenwärtigen Behandlungsbedingungen. Berlin, Germany, Springer, 1986

Olbrich R: Expressed Emotion (EE) und die Auslösung schizophrener Episoden: Eine Literaturübersicht. Nervenarzt 54:113–121, 1983

Perris C: Cognitive Therapy with Schizophrenic Patients. London, Cassell, 1989

PSA: Skala der psychosozialen Kompetenz. Internes Papier der Arbeitsgruppe für Evaluative Forschung der psychiatrischen Klinik am Zentralinstitut für Seelische Gesundheit. Mannheim, Germany, 1979

Riegel KF: Der sprachliche leistungstest SASKA. Gottingen, Germany, Hogrefe, 1967

Roder V: Untersuchungen zur Effektivität kognitiver Therapieinterventionen mit schizophrenen Patienten. Unpublished dissertation, Universität Bern, Switzerland, 1988

Roder V: Evaluation einer kognitiven Schizophrenietherapie, in Kognitive Therapie bei Schizophrenen. Edited by Kühne GE, Brenner HD, Huber G. Jena, Germany, Fischer, 1990

Roder V, Studer K, Brenner HD: Erfahrungen mit einem integrierten psychologischen Therapieprogramm zum Training kommunikativer und kognitiver Fähigkeiten in der Rehabilitation schwer chronisch schizophrener Patienten. Schweizer Archiv für Neurologie und Psychiatrie 138:31–44, 1987

Roder V, Brenner HD, Kienzle N, et al: Integriertes Psychologisches Therapieprogramm für schizophrene Patienten (IPT). Weinheim, Germany, Psychologie Verlags Union, 1992

Sandner M, Hodel B, Brenner HD: Treatment of emotional and cognitive vulnerability of schizophrenic patients [Abstract]. Abstracts Book: International Congress on Schizophrenia and Affective Psychoses, Geneva, Switzerland, Institution Universitaires de Psychiatrie Geneva (IUPG)-WHO, September 1991

Schubart C, Schwarz R, Krumm B, et al: Schizophrenie und Soziale Anpassung. Berlin, Germany, Springer, 1986

Schwab T, Zemp A: Therapiemanual zur Arbeitsrehabilitation schizophrener Patienten. Unpublished manual, Psychiatrische Universitätsklinik Bern, Switzerland, 1991

Schwartz S (ed): Language and Cognition in Schizophrenia. Hillsdale, NJ, Lawrence Erlbaum, 1978

Spaulding W: Assessment of adult-onset pervasive behavior disorders, in Handbook of Behavior Assessment. Edited by Cummero A, Adams H, Calhoun K. New York, Wiley, 1986

Spaulding W, Storms L, Goodrich B, et al: Applications of experimental psychopathology in psychiatric rehabilitation. Schizophr Bull 12:560–577, 1986

Süllwold L: Manual zum Frankfurter Beschwerde-Fragebogen FBF. Berlin, Germany, Springer, 1991

Süllwold L, Herrlich J: Frankfurter Befindlichkeits-Skala (FBS) für schizophren Erkrankte. Berlin, Germany, Springer, 1987

Vogel B: Empirischer Vergleich und Evaluation der Auswirkungen zweier Therapiestufen eines Therapieprogrammes zum Training kognitiver und sozialer Fertigkeiten in der Rehabilitation chronisch schizophrener Patienten. Unpublished master's thesis, Universität Konstanz, Germany, 1987

Wallace CJ, Nelson CJ, Liberman RP, et al: A review and critique of social skills training with schizophrenic patients. Schizophr Bull 6:42–63, 1980

Wishner J, Wahl O: Dichotic listening in schizophrenia. J Consult Clin Psychol 42:538–546, 1974

World Health Organization: Schizophrenia: An International Follow-up Study. Chichester, England, Wiley, 1979

Zubin J, Spring BJ: Vulnerability—a new view of schizophrenia. J Abnorm Psychol 86:103–126, 1977

Chapter 13

Cognitive Rehabilitation for Negative Symptoms

Joel O. Goldberg, Ph.D., and Peter E. Cook, M.D.

When rehabilitation practitioners ask people to describe the most frequent and most difficult problems they encounter in family members with schizophrenia, they accurately report the debilitating impact of negative symptoms on daily living. More than 85% of one sample of families cited troublesome issues such as "few friends," "few hobbies," and "few interests" (Runions and Prudo 1983); only one of the 10 most common problems pertained to acute psychosis. Experimental follow-up studies have confirmed these observations by families and community caregivers.

Negative symptoms of schizophrenia, not positive symptoms, are the most robust predictors of long-term outcome (Fenton and McGlashan 1991). Yet a conceptual and heuristic framework from which clinicians might formulate and test interventions has remained elusive. As a result, psychiatric rehabilitation practitioners have not developed effective therapeutic approaches to alleviate negative symptoms in schizophrenic patients.

To date, clinicians have neglected the role of cognitive elements in psychiatric rehabilitation. Textbooks on the topic of rehabilitation with psychiatric patients are not explicit about the neuropsychological impairments these individuals face, nor do they acknowledge cognitive mediators in interventions. We believe that the recognition of an association between negative symptoms and cognitive impairments challenges the pessimistic view that negative symptoms may represent a "core deficit" of schizophrenic illness, or an immutable trait phenomenon.

In this chapter, we highlight the cognitive elements that are relevant to patients' functional adaptation to the community and their ability to benefit from psychosocial rehabilitation strategies. First, we describe the significance of negative symptoms in relation to neuropsychological dysfunction. We then review psychiatric rehabilitation principles and methods that address negative symptoms and cognitive impairments. Finally, we outline three approaches to the cognitive rehabilitation of negative symptoms.

Negative Symptoms and Cognitive Impairment

Diminution or loss of normal function is the hallmark of negative symptoms in schizophrenia (Greden and Tandon 1991). Common negative symptoms include poverty of speech, apathy or amotivation, blunted or restricted affect, and attention troubles (Andreason and Olsen 1982; Carpenter et al. 1991; Kay et al. 1987). Although most clinicians are familiar with negative symptom terminology, they do not always recognize that negative symptoms are associated with multiple significant neuropsychological dysfunctions.

Converging evidence from investigators in different centers, using a variety of methodologies, points to a link between negative symptoms and cognitive impairments (e.g., Braff et al. 1991; Buchanon et al. 1994). Although the pathophysiology of underlying brain dysfunction remains uncertain, researchers now suspect that cognitive impairments are causally associated with negative symptoms (Levin 1984; Liddle 1992; Wolkin et al. 1992). To address the question of how cognitive dysfunction might be associated with negative symptoms, we review conceptual issues in four symptom categories that are important in clinical practice.

Poverty of Speech and Language Dysfunction

Researchers traditionally categorize language disturbances in schizophrenia as positive symptoms of thought disorder. An alternative explanation, which we describe later, is that impairments in speech processing are related to verbal memory deficits and verbal learning dysfunctions. Furthermore, at least some of the speech difficulties found in patients with schizophrenia may relate to primary cognitive deficits such as those observed in aphasia.

Hoffman et al. (1986) proposed a cognitive model of schizophrenic language dysfunction that posits underlying deficits in the coherent organization of language output. According to this view, some schizophrenic patients demonstrate subtle mistakes in organizing their words into meaningful verbal narratives.

Hoffman and Satel (1993) applied language rehabilitation technologies adapted from work with adult aphasic patients to address these verbal organization deficiencies. They used audiotape replay to provide immediate feedback on speaking performance. Success on these language exercises was associated with improved speech coherence.

For other patients, language planning difficulties lead to an inability to generate spontaneous communication, which produces the negative symptoms of poverty of speech. Gruzelier et al. (1988) found significantly diminished word fluency in patients with negative symptoms, compared with those who had positive symptoms or affective disorders.

One reason that clinicians may fail to appreciate speech processing difficulties is that basic language functions remain intact (Levin et al. 1989). For example, Dalby and Williams (1986) determined that, as with organic dementias, word pronunciation and spelling are preserved in schizophrenia. Instead, schizophrenic patients show an inability to plan multi-sentence communication, which results in impaired language production.

Apathy, Amotivation, and Drive Dysfunction

Unfortunately, many individuals with cognitive impairments are unable to initiate responses and formulate goals, leading therapists to mislabel them as lazy, resistant, or personality-disordered. Failure to initiate, organize, and maintain a set of goals, which researchers believe are primarily frontal lobe functions (Weinberger 1987), may lead to the negative symptoms of amotivation and anhedonia.

Evidence in support of this perspective is indirect. Some research indicates that schizophrenic patients perform adequately on tasks that require automatic responses but are impaired when mental effort is required (e.g., Callaway and Naghdi 1982). Thus, apparent poor motivation actually is caused by an inability to meet the effortful processing demands that some problems present. Likewise, poor drive, which stigmatizes a patient as lazy, actually may reflect mental fatigue, as shown on tasks that require cognitive persistence or vigilance (Everett et al. 1989).

Brain imaging research, for example, has begun to show that schizophrenic patients may have subtle impairments in crucial pathways between the prefrontal and hippocampal brain regions (T. E. Goldberg et al. 1990). Thus, the negative symptoms of amotivation may reflect a deficit in a schizophrenic patient's ability to initiate action (Frith and Done 1988). Findings of reduced speed in carrying out spontaneous actions corroborate this model. Nelson et al. (1990) and Pantelis et al. (1992) found that cognitive slowness in patients with negative symptoms correlated with their failure to show initiative—findings that could not be explained by medication effects or extrapyramidal symptoms.

Embarking on a course of action or setting a personal goal requires intact brain links between the prefrontal cortex and the hippocampus (Benson and Stuss 1990; Stuss and Benson 1986). Neuroimaging and cognitive studies suggest that deficits in higher-order mental activities may underlie the negative symptoms of drive dysfunction and amotivation.

Restricted Emotion and Affect Dysfunction

Researchers have developed growing interest in the relationship between schizophrenic patients' inability to recognize and express emotions and impaired cognitive abilities (Feinberg et al. 1986; Walker et al. 1984). Levin et al. (1985) found that patients with negative symptoms were less accurate in producing vocal affect and were particularly poor in differentiating sad and angry emotions. A study by Blanchard et al. (1994), however, failed to support an association between affective expression and neuropsychological impairment found in earlier work (Borod et al. 1989).

Morrison et al. (1988) confirmed evidence of marked impairments in social perception related to patients' inability to accurately identify negative emotions displayed by others. Role-play testing shows that schizophrenic patients have difficulty managing social interactions, even when they exhibit mild negative affect, because of their faulty perception of emotions. Patients with attentional deficits on negative symptom rating scales exhibit the most severely impaired social perceptual processes (Bellack et al. 1992).

These results suggest that cognitively based perceptual deficits and impaired processing of affective information are significant factors in the social deficits of schizophrenic patients. These deficits appear to persist despite the alleviation of acute symptoms of schizophrenia (positive symptoms); they also are associated with poor long-term community adjustment.

Attention Dysfunction and Memory Deficits

The most significant source of impairment for schizophrenic patients is attention dysfunction, which clinicians and family members alike frequently neglect and misunderstand. Despite decades of empirical findings of serious attention and memory deficits on a diverse range of tests in people with schizophrenia (Levin et al. 1989), rehabilitation practitioners have not integrated the results into hospital and community practice. Impaired attention is not simply an epiphenomenon of psychosis; Neuchterlein and Dawson (1984) showed that it is an unrelenting deficit that remains despite the remission of positive symptoms.

One reason that therapists may overlook attention dysfunction and memory deficits is that basic alertness and simple recognition skills remain intact in schizophrenic patients (Gjerde 1983). Rather, individuals with chronic mental illness may have serious but subtle attentional impairments that disrupt many common daily activities (Green 1996). Table 13–1 lists four kinds of common attention impairments, with definitions and examples of each difficulty.

As an example of these different attention demands, reading requires not only comprehension skills but also *sustained attention*: the ability to concentrate so that the reader can absorb the information. Reading in a noisy cafeteria demands the increased skill of *selective attention*. Switching between reading and talking requires *alternating attention*. Most difficult of all, reading and eating at the same time involves *divided attention*.

Recognizing the characteristics of sustained, selective, alternating, and divided attention can be useful in pinpointing subtle dysfunctions that arise in various contexts with schizophrenic patients. For example, when a clinician changes topics during a session, the patient may fail to recognize the switch. Even more commonly, some therapy or social skills groups can become disrupted because the length of the session demands significant sustained attention by group members. Liberman and Green (1992) and Kern et al. (1992) confirmed experimentally that the ability to sustain vigilance is an important predictor of the extent to which group members benefit from treatment programs.

Memory impairments also have been associated with schizophrenia. Recent advances in neuroimaging have shown that cognitive impairments correlate with dysfunction in brain regions associated with memory (T. E. Goldberg et al. 1990). Like other cognitive deficits, memory problems in schizophrenia may be neglected because of their subtlety rather than their insignificance. Most patients exhibit impairments when they are called upon to recall information and not simply recognize facts (T. E. Goldberg et al. 1989; Larsen and Fromholt 1976). For example, asking a patient whether the phrase "sustained attention" appeared in the previous paragraph would involve a relatively easy "recognition" demand; on the other hand, having a patient recite, without looking back, the names of the four kinds of attention would entail more effortful "recall."

Table 13–1. Common attention impairments in schizophrenia

Kind of attention	Definition	Examples
Sustained attention	Maintaining focus over time	Trouble listening on the phone
Selective attention	Responding to relevant information despite distractions	Trouble listening when background noise is high
Alternative attention	Disengaging and redirecting focus	Cannot switch topics easily in conversation
Divided attention	Performing multiple tasks	Cannot do two things at once

Source. Reprinted from Goldberg JO, Triano-Antidormi L: "Cognitive Rehabilitation," in *What Works! Innovation in Community Mental Health and Addiction Programs.* Edited by Duplessis G. Toronto, Ontario, Canadian Scholars Press, 1993, p 139. Used with permission.

Some caregivers find themselves frustrated when they must repeatedly remind patients about appointment times, recent decisions, or facts they have just discussed. Failure to recall such information is a major source of impairment for some schizophrenic patients (Gold et al. 1992; Saykin et al. 1991). When clinicians are sensitive to the recall demands that they impose and the difficulties that these demands engender for their patients, they can take steps to reduce the memory requirements of some situations. For example, regular appointment times are easier to recall than irregular or frequently shifted sessions.

The cognitive model suggests that schizophrenic patients may have subtle but significant memory impairments. This paradigm offers an alternative to the psychodynamic interpretation that attributes an appointment no-show, for example, to patient "resistance."

Psychiatric Rehabilitation and Cognitive Dysfunction

Two conceptual frameworks guide interventions with chronic psychiatric patients: the traditional medical model and the newer rehabilitation model. The comprehensive medical model (Engel 1980) embeds individuals in a biopsychosocial matrix and directs providers to consider interventions at various levels, as illustrated in Figure 13–1. The medical model is limited, however, in that it traditionally has led practitioners to focus on the presence or absence of illness, rather than on functional outcomes in community adaptation and quality of life that are of primary interest to patients and families.

In contrast, the rehabilitation model was developed from a World Health Organization paradigm (Anthony and Liberman 1986) describing health as the ability to be successful in major family, community, and society roles. From this point of view, the overall goal of psychiatric rehabilitation is to ensure that patients can perform the physical, emotional, social, and intellectual tasks they need to live, learn, and work in the community with minimum support from the helping professions (Anthony et al. 1990).

Conventional pharmacotherapy using neuroleptics has been relatively ineffective in treating the negative symptoms of schizophrenia and associated

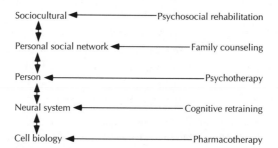

Figure 13–1. Medical model of interventions and their targets

cognitive deficits. Even newer drugs such as clozapine do not alter enduring neuropsychological dysfunctions (T. E. Goldberg et al. 1993). Rehabilitation alternatives to the traditional medical approach are receiving increased consideration because of their focus on the patient's functional disabilities. As Carpenter and Conley (1991) outlined, psychiatric rehabilitation interventions build social, vocational, and other skills of daily living. Rehabilitation strategies also suggest the need to engineer supportive environments to minimize the deleterious impact of negative symptoms and cognitive deficits on the patient's adaptive roles.

Although psychologists usually describe rehabilitation practices for the chronic mentally ill patients in psychosocial terms, the most critical ingredients implicitly incorporate cognitive rehabilitation strategies in their implementation. Consider three key psychiatric rehabilitation methods: case management, long-term planning, and skills training. In case management, the clinician usually is characterized as a support worker but often serves as an "alternative problem solver" for patients who are experiencing problem-solving impairments. Long-term planning assists patients in setting goals; this type of intervention attempts to compensate for patients' reduced drive and initiative. Finally, skills-training approaches often target cognitive disabilities such as poor organization of daily activities; in developing instructional techniques, therapists also must consider the patient's information processing limitations.

Rehabilitation Case Management

In his overview of brain development in schizophrenia, Weinberger (1987) reflected on the need for a "lend/lease" of another's ego as the equivalent of a patient's surrogate dorsolateral prefrontal cortex. In fact, for many patients with chronic mental disorders, the availability of a case manager is as crucial for problem solving as an attendant can be for someone with a physical handicap. Unfortunately, psychiatrists often pejoratively label the use of long-term support by the mentally ill patient to assist in solving problems as "dependency."

One prospective 6-year follow-up study (Wykes and Dunn 1992) confirmed significant correlations between cognitive impairments and increased staffing and services in community housing and rehabilitation, illustrating the need for community support. In fact, no patient with information-processing deficits was able to move to more independent residential care. Fenton and McGlashan (1991) showed in their long-term follow-up study that the negative symptoms of schizophrenia are associated most significantly with poor outcomes.

Goal-Setting in Rehabilitation Planning

Rehabilitation professionals have made many attempts to target the planning and goal-setting impairments found in schizophrenic patients. For example, Zec and Meisler (1986) developed an "executive board system" (EBS) designed to compensate for impaired initiative and defective ability to shift mental set.

Rehabilitation practitioners have used the EBS in hospital and community settings. In this system, therapists provide patients with explicit information on cue cards about the timing and sequencing of tasks. Patients receive instruction and practice writing out cards for each job they plan to do. The EBS essentially is a prosthesis for organizing and monitoring discrete task steps. Patients can make plans for the "day in preview," "week in preview," or even "year in preview." Besides providing salient cues to direct action, the EBS approach makes concrete the "hidden" cognitive functions of anticipatory thinking and foresight.

The psychiatric rehabilitation model developed at Boston University is the most comprehensive approach to the remediation of goal-setting impairments (Anthony et al. 1990). This technique helps patients choose goals following an orderly process that involves evaluating necessary skills and supports, identifying alternatives, and planning interventions (Cohen et al. 1990). Having patients choose their own goals is important: Brown et al. (1991) showed that patients who chose their community housing options had significantly lower rehospitalization rates than patients who were assigned or placed in residences.

Rehabilitation workers face a dilemma regarding how to assist patients in making their own choices. Clinicians frequently hear patients respond perseveratively, i.e., saying they want the same residential setting even when it has not been a satisfactory living arrangement in the past. Anthony et al. (1990) described a rehabilitation technique, which they termed Researching Alternative Environments, that mitigates perseverative decision making. With housing decisions, for example, this method identifies the three or four best choices from a pool of alternatives. Patients work with rehabilitation practitioners to collect information about the most pertinent characteristics of each setting and depict it in chart form (see, e.g., Table 13–2) to provide meaningful comparisons and make decision making explicit. This method facilitates the best match between the patient's personal criteria and the available alternatives. This process contrasts sharply with traditional methods of clinician-directed housing placements.

Case Example

Sue is a 36-year-old single woman diagnosed with schizophrenia and treated with chlorpromazine. Neuropsychological evaluation revealed low intelligence, impaired mental flexibility, and problem-solving abilities. Sue's negative symptom ratings also were significant. Test results showed that she had difficulties generating alternatives and articulating choices. Nevertheless, Sue worked with her case manager in a rehabilitation process over 6 months to move from a boarding home to her own residence. She used the chart displayed in Table 13–2 to record her research about three alternative environments (Anthony et al. 1990) and then selected the group home based on the best "fit" with her own personal criteria.

Skills Training

Researchers have showed that social skills training is effective in remediating impairments in emotional perception and expression, social withdrawal, and lack of initiative (Liberman et al. 1989; Penn 1991). In our own rehabilitation work, we address our patients' information processing limitations by designing lesson plans that do not overload them with performance demands. For example, breaking down lesson plans into manageable "chunks" of information is an important cognitively based teaching strategy.

Table 13–3 illustrates the skills training approach: One of our patients describes in her own words the orderly skills training steps of instruction, modeling, role play, feedback, and homework. To help this patient generalize her newly

Table 13–2. Potential alternative environments for Sue

Personal criteria	Group home	YWCA	Subsidized apartment
Affordable rent	1	1	1
Social activities	1	0	0
Near my friends	1	0	0
Close to bus stop	0	1	1
Want authority figures	1	1	0
Jobs to do	1	0	1
Writing desk in room	1	0	0
People to talk to about many topics	1	0	0
Things to keep busy	1	0	1
Windows	0	0	1
Total score	8*	3	5

*Sue's choice based on the best match with her personal criteria.

Source. Adapted from Anthony W, Cohen M, Farkas M: *Psychiatric Rehabilitation.* Boston, MA, Boston University Center for Psychiatric Rehabilitation, 1990. Used with permission.

acquired skills, we presented this "patient's view" as a poster at our annual department of psychiatry research day (J. O. Goldberg et al. 1991), with the patient participating as a coauthor and answering questions. Her account highlights how she has memorized the individual learning points; such capacity is a crucial cognitive mediator of success.

Skills training with an emphasis on generalization appears to have been effective for our group members. Ratings of their social skills (Goldstein and Gershaw 1976) indicated important pre-group versus post-group improvements. One of our graduates has been hired at competitive wages as a role-play instructor in our entry-phase group, and the visible success of a fellow patient has inspired other patients with negative symptoms, increasing their enthusiasm and motivation.

Table 13–3.   Patient's view of social skills training

"The group started in December and finishes in June. The group is very helpful because it is very well organized and very structured: nothing wishy-washy about it. This group deals with people's communication, e.g., problems with listening, problems with maintaining a conversation.

The group in general initiates with each person identifying his or her communication problems from a very long list. (This list does not leave out too much.) For each problem, there is a step-by-step procedure to look after the problem, e.g., to start a conversation, the procedure is:
1) Choose right place and time
2) Greet each other
3) Decide if other person is listening
4) Small talk
5) Present main topic

We all have partners to whom we work on our problems. The partners compliment each other, e.g., a partner who is working on maintaining a conversation with a partner who's working on listening to a conversation. The partners work on their problems by role playing, trying to go through the procedure of steps for their particular problem. The rest of the group play an active role by telling the two actors their strengths and weaknesses according to the steps of the procedure. After we become professional in our areas of problem, we go out and practice this on a person whom we agreed on in the group—this is our homework.

The group is important so that we can communicate well with friends and maintain them and lead a more meaningful life. So as you can see, this is a very helpful group."

As an alternative to structured group training approaches, individual skills teaching is distinguished by an emphasis on individualized planning and limits on the size of lesson plans (Nemec et al. 1992). Individual teaching avoids the discouraging redundancy of teaching skills that a patient already has acquired; lessons address impairments relevant to the patient's stated goals. This approach, however, involves increased staff time and therefore additional cost.

The "real world" benefits of classroom teaching are important. For individuals with impairments, the inability to make mental shifts and the lack of mental flexibility reflect compromised cognitive components of generalization that lead to failures in skill transfer to a new environment. A systematic approach to analyzing and overcoming the barriers inhibiting generalization is needed. Anthony et al. (1990) developed "skills programming" techniques, which identify barriers to skill utilization in the patient's own environment and help the patient develop steps for actually performing the skill where it is needed, not just in the classroom. When rehabilitation workers target generalization problems, they assist patients in overcoming the neuropsychological dysfunctions that inhibit skill transfer.

Case Example

Steve is a 38-year-old man diagnosed with paranoid schizophrenia who is treated pharmacologically with long-acting haloperidol. He shows predominantly negative symptoms, according to the Positive and Negative Syndrome Scale (PANSS) (Kay et al. 1987). Steve's verbal IQ scores have declined 10 points, correlating with increased negative symptoms compared with evaluations conducted more than a decade ago with the onset of schizophrenia.

Steve described his difficulty as "not being able to give my opinion in a straightforward way." Although he learned the skill of "saying no" in the social skills classroom group, he used this ability only intermittently in community settings. Steve developed a skills programming plan with his therapist in which the goal was to generalize the use of "saying no" outside the class. The plan specified discrete steps, beginning with "saying no" in a case management session and proceeding to "saying no" to a cigarette request and to a telephone solicitation. Steve monitored his own success on a chart listing "percentage of times when requests are denied"; his plan specified a "praise system" of rewards for behavioral reinforcement. Despite Steve's reduced verbal skills and negative symptoms, the plan was effective in helping him practice assertiveness skills outside the classroom.

Practical Strategies for Cognitive Rehabilitation in the Community

In this section, we consider three approaches to cognitive rehabilitation in the community: adjustment, compensation, and retraining (cf. J. O. Goldberg 1994).

Adjustment Approaches

The adjustment approach to cognitive rehabilitation represents a shift from the differential diagnostic use of neuropsychological tests of two decades ago. In the adjustment approach, rehabilitation practitioners formulate individualized descriptions of the patient's impaired functions and intact capacities in a comprehensive neuropsychological report, then tailor treatment plans to circumvent areas of major loss and capitalize on the patient's skill strengths.

Neuropsychological evaluations can help clinicians face the confusing task of deciphering the pattern of patients' cognitive impairments and preserved skills. Psychologists identify distinct and meaningful profiles using neuropsychological parameters to define subtypes (Heinrichs 1993; Heinrichs and Awad 1993). The assessment of cognitive functions for rehabilitation purposes emphasizes the patient's current adaptive abilities, such as attention, learning, memory, and problem-solving skills. These neurocognitive abilities are most relevant to a patient's capacity to adapt to the demands of living in the community; they also are particularly vulnerable to the effects of chronic mental illness.

Comparison with "overlearned" or *crystallized* abilities provides a contrasting reference point for estimating the patient's level of premorbid functioning. Overlearned behaviors such as reading, vocabulary, and fund of information are least affected by psychiatric illness. These preserved skills can mislead the clinician into overestimating the patient's ability to perform and adapt, causing the therapist to miss cognitive deficits that are subtle, easily overlooked, and subject to misinterpretation (Erickson and Burton 1986). Traditional mental status examinations do not assess such impairments well.

To ensure that the results of neuropsychological testing are meaningful, rehabilitation practitioners must go beyond test scores and diagnosis in drawing conclusions; they also must relate the patient's test performance to premorbid community functioning, relevant living skills, social demands faced by the patient, and available socioenvironmental supports. In addition, qualitative information, obtained from direct observation, that describes how patients succeed or fail provides clues to how they cope with their impairments.

The utility of a neuropsychological assessment depends largely on the questions the evaluation addresses (Erickson and Binder 1986). For example, relevant questions might include the following: How well can the patient direct, sustain, and shift attention? Can the patient easily learn and retain verbal material? How does the patient approach complex problems? Can the patient organize new material and make decisions in the face of increasing task demands? How much support is required for the patient to accurately anticipate, detect, and monitor errors? Framed by these and other questions, assessment results can reveal strengths and weaknesses in the patient's information processing capacities and highlight rehabilitation implications for the clinician.

The adjustment approach also has the advantage of making deficits tangible to the patient (Flesher 1990). Many patients express frustration about their failure to obtain places to live, jobs, and friendships. They are puzzled about the source of their difficulties. To sort out the confusion, test feedback sessions reframe the functional consequences of negative symptoms in terms of common cognitive deficits, such as troubles with attention or difficulties in making plans.

Recommendations about adjustment and coping strategies (see Table 13–4) provide the patient with potential remedies. Such recommendations, learned from experience and gleaned from the cognitive rehabilitation literature, help patients cope more effectively with their cognitive impairments.

Case Example

> Sally is a 26-year-old woman diagnosed with schizophrenia and living in the community. She was having difficulty in her part-time work in a small grocery store; her employer complained that she was "slow." The employer's judgment was perplexing because Sally's initial work skills were good. In response to these difficulties, Sally was referred for a neuropsychological evaluation.
>
> Sally's neurocognitive profile helped clarify the nature of her problems and suggested specific rehabilitation recommendations based on the adjustment approach. The assessment results indicated that Sally's adaptive abilities, such as her capacity to shift set (change tasks quickly), were below average. She demonstrated preserved skills, however, in the area of mental calculations, which she performed at superior levels. The overall profile suggested that Sally would function best performing mainly cashier functions (at which she excels) while avoiding tasks that required her to shift sets frequently.

Strategy-Building or Compensation Approaches

Therapists trained in traditional models learn methods to change the *person*. Alternative rehabilitation approaches seek to alter the patient's *environment* to

Table 13–4.   Coping with cognitive impairments in schizophrenia

Impairment	Adjustment to loss	Strategy-building
Sustained attention	Shorter, more frequent sessions	Self-instruction
	Short breaks at work setting	Recognize when mind wanders
Selective attention	Quiet, uncluttered work or learning environment	Walkman-type radio Build routines
Memory difficulties	Reminder calls	Daily planner
	Try to maintain a daily routine	Posted notes
		Dosette for self-administration of medication
New learning	Present information in simple, brief, step-by-step manner	Read list of steps until routine
	Use prompts to increase generalization	Practice skills in own setting to enhance generalization
Problem solving	Develop a step-by-step problem-solving procedure	Deck of cards to organize and monitor task-related behavior
		Devote sessions to long-term goal setting, not just relief of immediate problems

reduce the disabling impact of impairments. Stuve et al. (1991) distinguished two kinds of environmental approaches: using coping aids or prosthetic devices and adapting the social or physical setting to accommodate deficits.

First-person accounts and naturalistic surveys provide initial clues regarding effective coping aids for patients with chronic mental disorders. Carr (1988) uncovered some valuable coping techniques in a study of 200 patients in the community. One method that patients frequently cited involved listening to music on a Walkman-type personal radio. Some patients described the effect as soothing; for others, the music redirected their attention from internal psychotic processes to external reality. Regardless, the radio became a beneficial coping device.

Cues or aids also can be effective compensatory strategies for making demands less effortful and more routine. Meiselman (1973) found that some chronic schizophrenic patients benefited from visual rather than auditory cues. Putting a note or object in a place where the patient is likely to see it and checking notice boards are common strategies (Harris 1980). Elsewhere in this volume (see Chapter 15), Heinssen describes the use of posters on job sites to remind patients of job routines. Patients can use lists posted in the bathrooms of their apartments for morning hygiene routines. Telephones with speed-dial functions can be programmed with frequently used numbers to minimize the mental effort required to recall the numbers. Microwave ovens can be a less demanding and safer alternative to stove cooking. Case workers or patients can fill medication dosettes on a weekly basis to reduce the demands of remembering when to take daily oral medications.

The use of a diary is the single most common technique for managing memory impairment. Researchers have showed that systematically using a "memory book" is a very effective coping strategy (Miller 1992). Merely handing a notebook to a patient rarely is useful, however; many patients with memory problems need to be taught how to use a diary (Sohlberg and Mateer 1989).

Chunking is a general technique that restricts information demands (Flesher 1990). In transactions with patients, therapists model chunking by making reference to the category being discussed (e.g., "We are talking about housing today"). The treatment environment is geared to categorizing and tagging information so that it does not overload the patient's capacity. Appointments are scheduled as briefer sessions with a single-issue agenda.

Adaptation of physical or social environments has been neglected in community-based work with people who have psychiatric disabilities. The challenge is designing apartment, school, or work environments that minimize the impact of cognitive impairments. Psychogeriatric facilities, for example, use colored lines on the floor so that residents with organic dementias can follow a path to the dining area, thus compensating for spatial confusion. In a similar vein, Liberman and Green (1992) suggested that uncluttered training settings would enable schizophrenic patients to avoid distractions.

Retraining Approaches

Rehabilitation techniques that attempt to directly remediate patients' cognitive deficits through specific training have generated a great deal of controversy. Reviews of cognitive remediation of impairments from traumatic brain injuries (Benedict 1989) have determined that successful outcomes often rely on the performance of attention functions because other brain systems depend on attention for effective cognitive processing (Gummow et al. 1983).

Attention Process Training (APT), designed by Sohlberg and Mateer (1987), is one of the most promising techniques for such remediation. We use this cognitive rehabilitation technology for patients whose neurocognitive profiles show significant attentional dysfunctions (defined by impaired scores on a battery of attention tests).

APT represents a major advance because the training proceeds through graduated steps in increasing attentional demands:

1. *Sustained attention:* Patients initially learn to build vigilance on auditory and visual tasks. In our experience, patients in this phase of APT begin to show awareness of their attentional processing and make meta-cognitive statements ("I notice my mind wandering"). This first phase of training provides an in vivo opportunity for self-instructional training (cf. Meichenbaum and Cameron 1973).
2. *Selective attention:* Auditory exercises appear to be particularly well-suited to remediating schizophrenic impairments. In this phase, patients listen to audiotapes consisting of target numbers or letters with radio broadcast distraction in the background.
3. *Alternating attention:* In this phase, visual and auditory exercises require that patients redirect their attention in response to demands by the trainer to switch their focus. This training may be effective in improving the mental-shift problems noted in some information-processing studies (Everett et al. 1989) and that are prominent in some "deficit" symptom patients (Buchanon et al. 1994).
4. *Divided attention:* The final phase of training requires patients to work simultaneously on tasks with two different demands. This procedure may increase the patient's information-processing capacity, allowing the patient to handle more information at one time.

APT involves at least 6 months of training. We keep the initial sessions brief to accommodate the limited persistence and attention that are characteristic of our patients. In every session, we remind our patients that the goal of their work is to improve their attention skills. By the end of the training, therapists and patients explore generalization issues by listing daily situations that require the different forms of attention.

APT outcome measures consist of tests other than the tasks that patients practice in training, thus providing a measure of generalization. J. O. Goldberg (1994) and Triano-Antidormi and Goldberg (1992) reported successful outcomes in pilot studies on the effectiveness of APT with schizophrenic patients who are living in the community. We currently are conducting controlled case studies concerning the efficacy of APT and examining the impact of APT on negative symptom ratings and quality of life.

Summary

Unlike vegetative signs of depression, clinicians find that the negative symptoms of chronic mental disorders are elusive targets for traditional interventions. In this chapter, we have outlined how neuropsychological measures appear to specify the functional impairments described by accounts of negative symptoms. Cognitive impairments are evident in schizophrenic patients even after acute episodes of psychosis have subsided, yet rehabilitation practitioners often misunderstand and neglect the serious liability of persistent negative symptoms. Clinicians may misinterpret or ignore subtle but disabling information-processing deficits—leading to pejorative interpretations.

Despite a lack of knowledge about the underlying pathophysiology of negative symptoms, rehabilitation practitioners can design effective strategies to diminish the disabling impact of those symptoms. The techniques that appear to be most effective in addressing negative symptoms use cognitive rehabilitation methods either explicitly or implicitly as components of psychiatric rehabilitation plans.

References

Andreason NC, Olsen S: Negative and positive schizophrenia: definition and validation. Arch Gen Psychiatry 39:789–794, 1982

Anthony WA, Liberman RP: The practice of psychiatric rehabilitation: historical, conceptual and research base. Schizophr Bull 12:542–559, 1986

Anthony W, Cohen M, Farkas M: Psychiatric Rehabilitation. Boston, MA, Boston University Center for Psychiatric Rehabilitation, 1990

Bellack AS, Mueser KT, Wade J, et al: The ability of schizophrenics to perceive and cope with negative affect. Br J Psychiatry 160:473–480, 1992

Benedict RHB: The effectiveness of cognitive remediation strategies for victims of traumatic head-injury: a review of the literature. Clinical Psychology Review 9:605–626, 1989

Benson DF, Stuss DT: Frontal lobe influences on delusions: a clinical perspective. Schizophr Bull 16:403–412, 1990

Blanchard JJ, Kring AM, Neale JM: Flat affect in schizophrenia: a test of neuropsychological models. Schizophr Bull 20:311–325, 1994

Borod JC, Alpert M, Brozgold A, et al: A preliminary comparison of flat affect schizophrenics and brain damaged patients on measures of affective processing. J Commun Disord 22:93–104, 1989

Braff DL, Heaton R, Kuck J, et al: The generalized pattern of neuropsychological deficits in outpatients with chronic schizophrenia with heterogeneous Wisconsin Card Sort Test results. Arch Gen Psychiatry 48:891–898, 1991

Brown MA, Ridgeway P, Anthony WA, et al: Comparison of outcomes for clients seeking and assigned to supported housing services. Hosp Community Psychiatry 42:1150–1153, 1991

Buchanon RW, Strauss ME, Kirkpatrick B, et al: Neuropsychological impairments in deficit vs nondeficit forms of schizophrenia. Arch Gen Psychiatry 51:804–811, 1994

Callaway E, Naghdi MA: An information processing model for schizophrenia. Arch Gen Psychiatry 39:339–347, 1982

Carpenter WT, Conley RR: Therapeutic approaches to negative symptoms, in Negative Schizophrenic Symptoms: Pathophysiology and Clinical Implications. Edited by Greden JF, Tandon R. Washington, DC, American Psychiatric Press, 1991, pp 207–214

Carpenter, WT, Buchanan RW, Kirkpatrick B: The concept of the negative symptoms of schizophrenia, in Negative Schizophrenic Symptoms: Pathophysiology and Clinical Implications. Edited by Greden JF, Tadon R. Washington, DC, American Psychiatric Press, 1991, pp 5–20

Carr V: Patients' techniques for coping with schizophrenia: an exploratory study. Br J Med Psychol 61:339–352, 1988

Cohen MR, Farkas MD, Cohen BF, et al: Psychiatric Rehabilitation Technology: Setting an Overall Rehabilitation Goal (trainer package). Boston, MA, Boston University Center for Psychiatric Rehabilitation, 1990

Dalby JT, Williams R: Preserved reading and spelling ability in psychotic disorders. Psychol Med 16:171–175, 1986

Engel GL: The clinical application of the biopsychosocial model. Am J Psychiatry 137:535–544, 1980

Erickson RC, Binder LM: Cognitive deficits among functionally psychotic patients: a rehabilitative perspective. J Clin Exp Neuropsychol 8:257–274, 1986

Erickson RC, Burton MA: Working with psychiatric patients with cognitive deficits. Cognitive Rehabilitation 4:26–31, 1986

Everett J, Laplante L, Thomas J: The selective attention deficit in schizophrenia: limited resources or cognitive fatigue? J Nerv Ment Dis 177:735–738, 1989

Feinberg TE, Rifkin A, Schaffer D, et al: Facial discrimination and emotional recognition in schizophrenia and affective disorders. Arch Gen Psychiatry 43:276–279, 1986

Fenton WS, McGlashan TH: Natural history of schizophrenia subtypes, II: positive and negative symptoms and long-term course. Arch Gen Psychiatry 48:978–986, 1991

Flesher S: Cognitive habilitation and schizophrenia: a theoretical review and model of treatment. Neuropsychology Review 1:223–246, 1990

Frith CD, Done DJ: Towards a neuropsychology of schizophrenia. Br J Psychiatry 153:437–443, 1988

Gjerde PF: Attention capacity dysfunction and arousal in schizophrenia. Psychol Bull 93:57–72, 1983

Gold JM, Randolph C, Carpenter CJ, et al: Forms of memory failure in schizophrenia. J Abnorm Psychol 101:487–494, 1992

Goldberg JO: Cognitive retraining in a community psychiatric rehabilitation program, in Cognitive Technology in Psychiatric Rehabilitation. Edited by Spaulding W. Lincoln, University of Nebraska Press, 1994, pp 67–85

Goldberg JO, Triano-Antidormi L: Cognitive rehabilitation, in What Works! Innovation in Community Mental Health and Addiction Programs. Edited by Duplessis G. Toronto, Ontario, Canadian Scholars Press, 1993, pp 137–144

Goldberg JO, Babiski L, McGurk T, et al: Social skills: beyond the group to the community. Paper presented at the McMaster University annual research day in psychiatry, Hamilton, Ontario, April 1991

Goldberg TE, Weinberger DR, Pliskin NH, et al: Recall memory deficit in schizophrenia: a possible manifestation of prefrontal dysfunction. Schizophr Res 2:251–257, 1989

Goldberg TE, Ragland JD, Torrey EF, et al: Neuropsychological assessment of monozygotic twins discordant for schizophrenia. Arch Gen Psychiatry 47:1066–1072, 1990

Goldberg TE, Greenberg RD, Griffin SJ, et al: The effect of clozapine on cognition and psychiatric symptoms in patients with schizophrenia. Br J Psychiatry 162:43–48, 1993

Goldstein AP, Gershaw NJ: Skills Training for Community Living. Toronto, Ontario, Pergamon, 1976

Greden JF, Tandon R: Negative Schizophrenic Symptoms: Pathophysiology and Clinical Implications. Washington, DC, American Psychiatric Press, 1991

Green MF: What are the functional consequences of neurocognitive deficits in schizophrenia? Am J Psychiatry 153:321–330, 1996

Gruzelier J, Seymour K, Wilson L, et al: Impairment on neuropsychological tests of temperohippocampal and frontohippocampal functions and word fluency in remitting schizophrenia and affective disorders. Arch Gen Psychiatry 45:623–629, 1988

Gummow L, Miller P, Dustman R: Attention and brain injury: a case for cognitive rehabilitation of attentional deficits. Clinical Psychology Review 3: 255–274, 1983

Harris J: Memory aids people use: two interview studies. Memory Cognition 8:31–38, 1980

Heinrichs RW: Schizophrenia and the brain: conditions for a neuropsychology of madness. Am Psychol 48:221–233, 1993

Heinrichs RW, Awad AG: Neurocognitive subtypes of chronic schizophrenia. Schizophr Res 9:49–58, 1993

Hoffman RE, Satel SL: Language therapy for schizophrenic patients with persistent voices. Br J Psychiatry 162:755–758, 1993

Hoffman RE, Stopek S, Andreason N: A discourse analysis comparing manic versus schizophrenic speech organization. Arch Gen Psychiatry 43: 831–838, 1986

Kay SR, Fiszbein A, Opler LA: The positive and negative syndrome scale (PANSS) for schizophrenia. Schizophr Bull 13:261–275, 1987

Kern RS, Green MF, Satz P: Neuropsychological predictors of skills training for chronic psychiatric patients. Psychiatry Res 43:223–230, 1992

Larsen SF, Fromholt P: Mnemonic organization and free recall in schizophrenia. J Abnorm Psychol 85:61–65, 1976

Levin S: Frontal lobe dysfunctions in schizophrenia, II: impairments of psychological and brain functions. J Psychiatr Res 18:57–72, 1984

Levin S, Hall JA, Knight RA, et al: Verbal and nonverbal expressions of affect in speech of schizophrenia and depressed patients. J Abnorm Psychol 94: 487–497, 1985

Levin S, Yurgelun-Todd D, Craft S: Contributions of clinical neuropsychology to the study of schizophrenia. J Abnorm Psychol 98:341–356, 1989

Liberman RP, Green MF: Whither cognitive-behavioral therapy for schizophrenia? Schizophr Bull 18:27–36, 1992

Liberman RP, DeRisi WJ, Mueser KT: Social skills training for psychiatric patients. New York, Pergamon Press, 1989

Liddle PF: PET Scanning and schizophrenia—what progress? Psychol Med 22:557–560, 1992

Meichenbaum D, Cameron R: Training schizophrenics to talk to themselves: a means of developing self-controls. Behavior Therapy 4:515–534, 1973

Meiselman KC: Broadening dual modality cue utilization in chronic non-paranoid schizophrenics. J Consult Clin Psychol 41:447–453, 1973

Miller E: Psychological approaches to the management of memory impairments. Br J Psychiatry 160:1–6, 1992

Morrison RL, Bellack AS, Mueser K: Facial affect recognition deficits and schizophrenia. Schizophr Bull 14:67–83, 1988

Nelson HE, Pantelis C, Carruthers K, et al: Cognitive functioning and symptomatology in chronic schizophrenia. Psychol Med 20:357–365, 1990

Nemec PB, McNamara S, Walsh D: Direct skills teaching. Psychosocial Rehabilitation Journal 16:13–25, 1992

Neuchterlein KH, Dawson ME: Information processing and attentional functioning in the developmental course of schizophrenic disorders. Schizophr Bull 10:160–203, 1984

Pantelis C, Barnes TRE, Nelson HE: Is the concept of frontal-subcortical dementia relevant to schizophrenia? Br J Psychiatry 160:442–460, 1992

Penn D: Cognitive rehabilitation of social deficits in schizophrenia: a direction of promise or following a primrose path? Psychosocial Rehabilitation Journal 15:27–41, 1991

Runions J, Prudo R: Problem behaviors encountered by families living with a schizophrenic member. Can J Psychiatry 28:382–386, 1983

Saykin AJ, Gur RC, Gur RE, et al: Neuropsychological function in schizophrenia: selective impairment in memory and learning. Arch Gen Psychiatry 48:618–624, 1991

Sohlberg MM, Mateer CA: Effectiveness of an attention training program. J Clin Exp Neuropsychol 9:117–130, 1987

Sohlberg MM, Mateer CA: Training use of compensatory memory books: a three-stage behavioral approach. J Clin Exp Neuropsychol 11:871–891, 1989

Stuss DT, Benson DF: The Frontal Lobes. New York, Raven, 1986

Stuve P, Erickson RC, Spaulding W: Cognitive rehabilitation: the next step in psychiatric rehabilitation. Psychosocial Rehabilitation Journal 15:9–26, 1991

Triano-Antidormi L, Goldberg JO: The efficacy of attention training: the case for schizophrenia (abstract). Canadian Psychology 33:433, 1992

Walker E, McGuire M, Bettes B: Recognition and identification of facial stimuli by schizophrenics and patients with affective disorders. British Journal of Clinical Psychiatry 23:37–44, 1984

Weinberger DR: Implications of normal brain development for the pathogenesis of schizophrenia. Arch Gen Psychiatry 44:660–669, 1987

Wolkin A, Sanfilipo M, Wolf AP, et al: Negative symptoms and hypofrontality in chronic schizophrenia. Arch Gen Psychiatry 49:959–965, 1992

Wykes T, Dunn G: Cognitive deficit and the prediction of rehabilitation success in a chronic psychiatric group. Psychol Med 22:389–398, 1992

Zec RF, Meisler N: Executive Board System (EBS): a self-help approach to cognitive-behavior rehabilitation. Paper presented at the annual meeting of the International Association of Psychosocial Rehabilitation Services, Cleveland, Ohio, June 1986

Chapter 14

Cognitive Rehabilitation Interventions for Depressed Patients

John E. Roberts, Ph.D., and Shirley Hartlage, Ph.D.

ognitive therapy, along with interpersonal psychotherapy (Klerman et al. 1984), is one of the most widely used and effective psychological treatments for unipolar depression. Cognitive therapy is a relatively brief, structured intervention that is believed to reduce the cognitive biases and maladaptive thought processes associated with depression. In this chapter we discuss basic assumptions of cognitive therapy, specific therapeutic techniques, and the nature of the therapeutic relationship. Therapeutic implications of environmental adversity, depressive realism, and vulnerable self-esteem also are addressed. Finally, empirical findings concerning the efficacy of cognitive therapy for depression also are reviewed. Although there are many varieties of cognitive therapy (Ellis 1962; Mahoney 1974; Meichenbaum 1977; Rehm 1988), Beck's model (Beck et al. 1979), the most widely used and empirically validated cognitive intervention for depression, will be the focus of this chapter.

After providing a conceptual orientation to cognitive therapy, we will introduce Susan, a fictitious, although not atypical, depressed patient. Aspects of Susan's treatment will demonstrate various issues and techniques in cognitive therapy.

Conceptual Underpinnings of Cognitive Therapy

All cognitive therapies share several basic assumptions. The most important and fundamental of these is cognitive relativism: the idea that one's cognitions or thoughts are simply beliefs and not necessarily accurate accounts of reality. There can be numerous alternative cognitive frames, angles, or perspectives on the same experience. Of particular interest is the hypothesized relationship between cognition and emotion. It is believed that the person's appraisal or construal of the meaning of events shapes the events' emotional consequences (Lazarus 1991). In Epictetus' words, "Men are not moved by things but by the views which they take of them" (quoted in Beck 1976, p. 47). Consequently, there are many possible emotional reactions to an event, each directly related to how that event is construed. Some therapists, social theorists, and philosophers suggest that we construct meaning out of the world based on our belief structures (e.g., Berger and Luckman 1966; Feyerabend 1975; Guidano and Liotti 1983). In other words, we create our own personal realities. According to many cognitive theorists, depressed patients construe their experience in an idiosyncratic, negative manner and construct belief structures about themselves, the world, and the future (Beck's cognitive triad) that facilitate such biased processing.

Assuming that thoughts are beliefs rather than reality, they are potentially inaccurate and falsifiable. Negative thoughts, which are problematic for depressed patients, should not be accepted as necessarily accurate accounts of reality. Instead, cognitive therapy fosters the attitude of the patient becoming a personal scientist who tests the validity of these thoughts and beliefs (Kelly 1955; Mahoney 1974). Cognitions are treated as hypotheses rather than hard truths. In discussing the role of therapists, Guidano and Liotti (1983) stated "their job is to make the patient well aware that his or her declarations concern nothing but theories and not absolute truths. This is the whole point of treatment" (p. 139). Through cognitive therapy, patients learn the impact of their thought processes on their emotional lives and well-being. Initially, they are taught this connection at a theoretical level in the context of the therapist explaining the cognitive model of depression and treatment. Later, patients become aware of this relationship between thoughts and feelings on a personal level as they explore the cognitive antecedents of their own shifts in affect. Making such connections is a vital aspect of therapy that continues throughout treatment.

Cognitive therapy suggests that these characteristic appraisals and ways of perceiving the world are learned. They are not simply a function of the event or of the person's temperament, but are styles that develop through learning principles. Most importantly, cognitive therapists traditionally assumed these thoughts and beliefs can be unlearned and changed fairly readily. From this perspective, the process of therapy involves helping patients modify their belief structures and their characteristic ways of processing information. Alternatively, some theorists (Barber and DeRubeis 1989; Hartlage 1993; S. Hartlage et al., unpublished data, 1996) argue that cognitive therapy does not initially modify people's long-standing negative beliefs. Instead, they postulate that cognitive therapy teaches patients to intentionally counteract negative thoughts with more adaptive cognitions after they occur.

In contrast to other forms of therapy, such as psychodynamic approaches, cognitive therapy more directly targets maladaptive thoughts and behaviors.

Symptoms are not viewed as symbols for some underlying, intrapsychic pathology. Likewise, conscious thoughts are not seen as disguised representations of unconscious conflicts. Also in contrast to other approaches, patients are treated as active collaborators in their therapy and are expected to complete assignments between sessions. These assignments help assess and modify maladaptive cognitive-affective behavior cycles that are maintaining their depression.

Although correcting maladaptive misrepresentations of reality (cognitive distortions) is an important goal of cognitive therapy, such rehabilitation also will have significant consequences for feelings about the self. Many of the negative cognitive biases in depression revolve around themes of self-deprecation (Pietromonaco and Markus 1985), such that altering these themes will enhance one's self-evaluations. A recent review suggests that difficulties in regulating and maintaining stable levels of self-esteem are an important vulnerability factor for depression and that psychological treatments should be geared to improving these deficits (Roberts and Monroe 1994).

In addition to feeling worthless, depressed patients often feel helpless and powerless. Cognitive therapy attempts to modify these biased and unrealistic beliefs about self-efficacy. Cognitive therapy also can be seen as teaching patients greater self-control by regulating their thoughts, feelings, and behavior. Patients learn to recognize how their characteristic processing styles affect their feelings, to be aware when they enact such processes, and to restructure their thinking to feel less miserable. They learn strategies and techniques involved in self-control and self-regulation, which increase feelings of self-efficacy (Bandura 1977). The development of greater self-control and self-regulation can be viewed as a major goal and central mechanism in cognitive therapy (see Rehm 1988).

Case Example

Susan is a 34-year-old, single mother of three children. She was laid off a year ago and has a hard time making ends meet. Susan sought outpatient psychotherapy after increased feelings of depression, apathy, and fatigue. She had little appetite and lost 15 lbs. over the past month. She complained of early morning awakening and a worse mood in the morning. Susan became depressed after her boyfriend of several years left her for another woman. Susan has been uninterested in seeing her friends, going to church, or performing household chores. She said she does not have the energy to do these things and she would probably feel more depressed if she interacted with cheerful people. Susan also believed that she would never develop another relationship because she was less attractive and charming than other women and was anxious about her finances. Finally, she believed that she needed to be liked by everyone she met or she would be unpopular and alone.

Therapeutic Techniques

Although many have warned that cognitive therapy is much more than a sterile and mechanistic technology, it is often misperceived as such by novice therapists. Cognitive techniques are most effective when employed by a sensitive and skilled therapist in a flexible manner within a trusting and supportive relationship. There is a specific correspondence between therapeutic goals and techniques based on cognitive theories of depression. Interventions are strategically incorporated to understand the patient's idiosyncratic thought processes, to help the patient evaluate their validity and emotional impact, and modify or counteract maladaptive cognitions. Novel techniques, not typically associated with cognitive therapy, may be used to elicit or correct cognitive schemata. For example, Safran and Segal (1990) describe using Gestalt two chair techniques to help a patient access underlying beliefs about interpersonal relationships. Such techniques are judiciously selected based on the patient's specific treatment plan. Table 14–1 lists and briefly describes some of the standard techniques in cognitive therapy for depression.

The relative balance between more direct, behavioral interventions (e.g., having the patient schedule pleasurable activities) and more exploratory, hypothesis framing and testing (cognitive) interventions (e.g., recording thoughts and identifying cognitive distortions) depends on the severity of the depression and stage of treatment. Generally, treatment of severe cases begins with a more behavioral focus and becomes more cognitive as the depression abates. Figure 14–1 is a common representation of how the balance of cognitive and behavioral interventions shift during treatment. However, treatment is conceptualized cognitively even when using behavioral interventions. The goal is to use behavioral strategies to alter negatively biased information processing and cognitive representations of self (e.g., self as incompetent, lazy, unworthy, unlovable). Changes in behavior can be a powerful source of disconfirming information.

Activity Scheduling

Scheduling activities is a simple yet powerful intervention used during the early stages of therapy with patients with more severe depression. These patients frequently feel overwhelmed and typically experience inertia. Becoming more active allows depressed patients to see themselves as more effective and to obtain positive reinforcement (i.e., rewarding experiences) from the environment. Patients can benefit from obtaining greater structure by keeping a written schedule of activities for the days between sessions. The therapist and the patient create this schedule together, and the patient rates each completed activity for its degree of pleasure and mastery.

Table 14–1.   Standard therapeutic techniques

Activity scheduling: The patient increases the frequency of mastery-related and pleasurable events. These in turn tend to boost feelings of self-efficacy and mood.

Graded task assignments: Complicated tasks are broken down into simpler, concrete steps as a means of making them less overwhelming. Long-range goals are decomposed into shorter-range goals. The patient is taught to self-reinforce after completing each step.

Self-monitoring: The patient keeps track of thoughts, behaviors, and situations related to mood. These can be recorded informally in a notebook or on structured rating sheets (e.g., the Daily Dysfunctional Thoughts Record). "Thought catching" automatic negative thoughts is a critical skill in cognitive therapy that patients develop with practice.

Cognitive restructuring: Maladaptive thought processes are modified or challenged through Socratic dialogue, thought stopping (i.e., mentally saying "No!" after a negative thought), thought substitution (i.e., replacing a negative thought with a more adaptive and realistic thought), and behavioral experiments (personal experiments designed to test the validity of the patients' beliefs).

Challenging dysfunctional assumptions: The therapist uses consequential analysis (i.e., exploring the meaning of disturbing automatic thoughts) to uncover underlying beliefs that render patients vulnerable to depression. These underlying assumptions often are generated from nonconscious, tacit beliefs that only can be subject to reality testing after they are articulated.

Relapse prevention: The therapist helps patients modify dysfunctional assumptions, counteract negative thoughts when they occur, and identify high risk situations in which they are more likely to become depressed. Strategies are developed to avoid or cope with these potentially problematic situations.

As a consequence of increased activity, depressed patients often experience some improvement in their moods. Patients may see themselves as more competent, particularly as they perform mastery activities (i.e., activities that patients rated high on mastery). Also, activities distract patients from ruminative thoughts that help maintain depression (Nolen-Hoeksema 1987) and provide the opportunity for significant others to give positive feedback. Finally, patients may begin to enjoy these activities (Beck 1976).

As shown in Hartlage and Clements' chapter in this book, clinical depression is associated with a loss of positive reinforcement (see also Lewinsohn et al. 1979). Therefore, encouraging patients to monitor and schedule pleasurable activities should increase their rewarding experiences. If the patient has

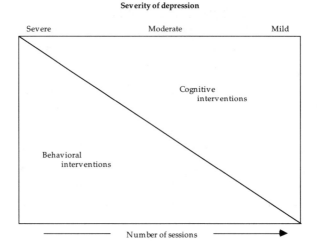

Figure 14–1.   Relative proportion of cognitive and behavioral techniques used as a function of stage in therapy and/or severity of depression. *Source.*   Adapted from Williams et al. 1989.

difficulty spontaneously recalling enjoyable activities, there is a comprehensive inventory that may help. The Pleasant Events Schedule lists 320 events rated pleasurable by diverse samples of people (MacPhillamy and Lewinsohn 1982). Although developed as a research tool, it can be useful in helping patients monitor positive life experiences and activities, and serve as a menu for scheduling new ones.

Graded Task Assignments

To facilitate success, patients are initially asked to perform easy mastery related tasks in which they are very likely to succeed. For example, Susan was asked to vacuum her living room carpet after she complained that she had no energy to do *any* household chores. As her depression remitted, she completed increasingly difficult household projects.

It is often useful to break down complex activities into their subcomponents. Although a large task taken as a whole might seem overwhelming, the patient is more likely to successfully negotiate it one step at a time. For example, Susan wanted to become a nurse, but had no education beyond high school. In therapy, she listed the basic steps to achieve this long-range goal, beginning with returning to school at night. This initial step was broken down and concretized into calling a community college for information about course offerings and registration. Susan was taught to self-reinforce, either mentally (e.g., silently praising herself for a good job) or behaviorally (e.g., engaging in a pleasurable activity such as telephoning a friend), after completing each step. Such competency building experiences are important because they provide powerful disconfirming evidence of the patient's negative beliefs.

Self-Monitoring

Cognitive therapy is critically dependent on the patient's ability to carefully monitor thoughts, feelings, and the situations in which they arise. Such monitoring not only provides the "grist" for therapy (learning connections between thoughts and feelings), but also begins to challenge some of the patient's dysfunctional thinking. For example, after keeping a diary of her feelings for a week, Susan learned (contrary to her belief) that she was not sad and depressed 100% of the time and that there were times when she felt better. This realization gave her hope that her depression would remit and motivated her to collaborate with her therapist to understand the factors related to feeling better or worse.

Helping the patient uncover relationships between particular core thought patterns and feelings is not a rudimentary skill achieved simply by asking patients to report their thoughts. Rather, it is a clinical skill that often requires a great deal of sophistication. The therapist must be aware of the implied meanings and the subtext of the patient's speech. This point is especially true when nonconscious thoughts and memories are involved (Brewin 1989; Teasdale and Barnard 1993). Such thoughts can be heavily defended against (Bowlby 1980) and result from a dysfunctional core cognitive organization (Guidano 1987; Guidano and Liotti 1983). This uncovering process is known as guided discovery.

Depressed patients are taught to "thought catch" their automatic negative thoughts and images. These cognitions are assumed to mediate between an experience and an emotional reaction. Such automatic thoughts may come in such a rapid succession and an effortless stream that the patient is not aware of having them (Hartlage et al. 1993). For example, when Susan was asked to monitor her automatic thoughts during the week, she reported that it would be too difficult, and that she did not think she could do a good job with the assignment. The therapist pointed out that she just stated two automatic thoughts. Generally, patients are instructed to recall the thoughts or images that run through their heads between the occurrence of an event and a strong emotional reaction. Key automatic thoughts fill this gap. The sensitive clinician inquires about such thoughts and images during the therapy session when the patient's affect shifts or his or her speech becomes hesitant. In our case example, Susan identified automatic thoughts better when the therapist asked her to picture herself in situations that preceded emotional distress. Role playing also can be used to access "hot cognitions" (i.e., core thoughts related to strong affect) in the session. For example, when role-playing a confrontation with her mother, a stream of Susan's negative automatic thoughts came to the surface (e.g., "I'm not good enough to deserve my mother's love and respect"; "Mom will reject me if I disagree with her").

The Daily Record of Dysfunctional Thoughts (DRDT) is a frequently used method for helping patients self-monitor between sessions (Beck et al. 1979). Figure 14–2 is an adaptation of the DRDT with a sample entry. The DRDT has columns for recording: particular situations in which strong emotions arise, type and degree of emotion, automatic thoughts that preceded the emotion and degree of belief in them, rational responses and degree of belief in them, and outcome in terms of degree of subsequent emotion. Rational responses to automatic thoughts are discussed later under the topic of cognitive restructuring.

Self-monitoring typically leads to distancing and decentering. These processes introduce a gap between patients' reactions to events (cognitive and emotional) and the events themselves. Patients begin to experientially realize the constructive process that occurs when they respond to events and situations in their lives (i.e., how they create meaning out of the world). They learn to view their thoughts more objectively as beliefs rather than as irrefutable facts. Consequently, these thoughts carry less emotional punch and become more open to challenge (Beck 1976; Safran and Segal 1990). In addition, self-monitoring provides the patient and therapist with important information about thoughts and behaviors that seem to be maladaptive and emotionally disturbing.

Cognitive Restructuring

A fundamental aspect of cognitive therapy involves helping patients challenge and correct maladaptive beliefs about themselves, significant others, and the world. The first step in this process is to identify these beliefs. Beck uses a method of Socratic dialogue that gently leads patients to explore and articulate basic assumptions and rules by which they live (Beck et al. 1979). Patients begin to examine the validity of their beliefs through such exploration or guided discovery. Patients are asked to generate alternative explanations or ways of thinking and to evaluate their degree of belief in each alternative. They are asked questions such as, "What is your evidence for this belief?" "What are some

SITUATION	EMOTION(S)	AUTOMATIC THOUGHTS	RATIONAL RESPONSES	OUTCOME
Briefly describe the actual event leading to the unpleasant emotion	1. Type of emotion (e.g., sad, angry) 2. Degree of emotion, 1%–100%	1. Write automatic thoughts that accompany the emotion 2. Rate degree of belief in automatic thoughts, 0%–100%	1. Write rational response(s) to the automatic thoughts. 2. Rate degree of belief in rational response(s), 0%–100%	Specify and rate subsequent emotion, 0%–100%
Friend turns down my invitation to go to the movies, saying she was too tired and wanted to go to bed early.	Sad, 85% Lonely, 95% Rejected, 95%	1. She obviously has better things to do than spend time with me, 90% 2. No one likes me, 90% 3. I'll have nothing to do and will end up sitting in my apartment feeling awful, 100%	1. She really has been putting in long hours at work and is tired, 95% 2. I do have several friends who tell me that they care about me and enjoy my company, 90% 3. I can invite someone else to go to the movie or I could even go by myself and still have a good time, 85%	Sad, 40% Lonely, 60% Rejected, 30% Hopeful, 60%

Figure 14-2. The Daily Record of Dysfunctional Thoughts (DRDT) partially completed by Susan (adapted from Beck AT, Rush AJ, Shaw BF, et al: *Cognitive Therapy of Depression.* New York, Guildford, 1979).

alternative explanations?" "Even if this were true, are the consequences really so dire?" Such approaches help patients reframe their experiences in more adaptive and less depressogenic ways. Beck also recommends using behavioral experiments to disconfirm negative beliefs. For example, Susan believed that if she disagreed with anyone, even on small points, that person would reject her. Her therapist asked her to poll friends about whether they had acquaintances who disagreed with them on any issue and about how such disagreements affected their relationships. Susan was surprised to find out that almost everyone had differences with friends and that these differences typically did not lead to rejection.

Thought stopping and thought substitution also are used to help patients modify their dysfunctional thinking. Thought stopping involves recognizing negative thought patterns and saying to oneself "No!" as a means of shutting down these cognitions. For example, Susan mentally shouted to herself "No!" whenever the thought that she was unlovable popped into her head. This distraction interrupted the chain of negative automatic thoughts that would otherwise follow. Thought substitution involves having the patient mentally say a more adaptive statement after the negative thought. For example, after Susan had the automatic thought "I'm not good enough", she said to herself "I am worthwhile. I am not perfect, but I am good enough." Negative automatic thoughts tend to have a snowballing effect. There can be a cognitive avalanche after the first few thoughts pop into the depressed person's head. Thus, it is important for patients to learn to use thought stopping and thought substitution early in the cascade of negative cognitions while they have greater control. Patients are instructed to note the first signs of an impending avalanche and to respond immediately.

The cognitive model of depression suggests that there are common types of cognitive distortions that contribute to the maintenance of the patient's negative beliefs, several of which are described in Table 14–2 (Beck 1967; Burns 1980). One of the most frequent and pernicious of these distortions is dichotomous or black and white thinking. Patients have difficulty seeing gray areas and immediately jump to the extreme negative pole. For example, when Susan did not do a perfect job on a task she often thought, "I didn't do as well as I could have, so I did terribly." It is helpful to provide patients with a list of these distortions (as found in Burns 1980) to facilitate self-monitoring. The process of beginning to recognize these errors frequently leads to the patient challenging them. In turn, challenging and correcting these cognitive distortions facilitates the modification of underlying dysfunctional beliefs.

Table 14–2.   Common cognitive distortions in depression

Dichotomous thinking: Things are seen as black or white with no shades of gray in between. For example, Susan believed, "I need to be liked by everyone or I'm unpopular."

Overgeneralization: A specific negative event is seen as characteristic of life in general. Susan saw the breakup with her boyfriend as evidence that no man would want a relationship with her.

Selective abstraction: A single, negative detail becomes the focus of attention to the exclusion of all other aspects of the situation. For example, Susan focused on a dinner companion's passing comment that she preferred her vegetables steamed as opposed to boiled. She ignored the many compliments about dinner and ruminated about this comment instead.

Mind reading: The person assumes that others are reacting negatively to him or her without any evidence and without checking out this belief. Susan thought that the dinner companion must think that she is either an incompetent cook or just did not care enough to prepare a "nice" meal.

Fortune-telling: The person's negative expectations about future events are treated as established facts. After dinner, Susan thought that her friend would never want to come to her place again, and acted as if this belief was true.

Disqualifying the positive: Positive experiences are rejected by declaring that they "don't count." In Susan's case, she believed that her friend made compliments about the dinner only to be nice.

Catastrophizing: The importance of negative events is exaggerated. Susan inflated the importance of her friend enjoying dinner and believed that if she did not, it meant that the friendship was in jeopardy.

Minimization: The importance of positive characteristics or experiences is treated as insignificant. For example, Susan said that it did not matter that she was a "snazzy" dresser because she did not have a boyfriend.

Emotional reasoning: Feelings are thought to reflect the true situation. Susan felt alone and abandoned and assumed that meant that she really was alone.

"Should" statements: Should and must statements are used for self-motivation and to self-control behavior. Susan thought she should not ever get mad at her parents and felt guilty whenever she did.

Labeling: Rather than referring to specific actions or characteristics, the person describes his or her total self using global labels. Instead of saying, "I made a mistake about dinner," Susan said to herself, "I'm stupid and a failure."

Personalization: The patient assumes that she or he is the cause of some event when other factors were responsible. When a friend declined an invitation to go to the movies, Susan immediately thought this woman did not want to spend time with her, when she was simply tired from a hard day at work.

Source.   Adapted from Beck AT: *Depression: Clinical, Experimental and Theoretical Aspects.* New York, Harper & Row, 1967 and Burns DD: *Feeling Good.* New York, Signet, 1980.

Underlying Dysfunctional Assumptions

Beck (1976) and others (Guidano 1987; Guidano and Liotti 1983) conceptualize automatic negative thoughts (e.g., "I'm a bad person," "things never go right") as arising from underlying assumptions or cognitive schemata. Although there tend to be a few general themes, dysfunctional attitudes are idiosyncratic to the individual. Examples of such cognitive structures might include the belief that "everyone must like me or I'm no good" and "I must do everything perfectly or I'm a failure." These underlying beliefs have been conceptualized as "dysfunctional contingencies of self-worth" (Kuiper and Olinger 1986). Those vulnerable to depression maintain a rigid self-contract concerning what makes them feel worthy and good. For example, Susan equated her self-worth with being liked by others. Beck and his colleagues (1979) argued that the patient might relapse unless these schemata are modified. The patient would remain vulnerable because these depressogenic schemata could be reactivated later by stressful life events.

To uncover underlying assumptions, therapists listen for the patient's use of the verbs "should," "must," and "ought." Using these verbs and expressing unusually strong affect can indicate the influence of dysfunctional schemata. Next, the therapist engages in *consequential analysis,* asking the patient "What if _____ were true? What would that mean?" or "What would be so upsetting about _____ for you?" These questions can be pursued until core beliefs are uncovered. For example, when Susan became teary while stating that she could not express her political opinions to her neighbor "because he might disagree with them," the therapist asked what would be so bad if he disagreed. Susan said the neighbor might think she is stupid and reject her. When pushed about the consequences and meaning of such rejection, Susan stated that "if he thinks I'm stupid and rejects me, other people will too. I'll be all alone and lonely." When asked about the meaning of such isolation, Susan stated that "it would mean that I was so worthless and unlovable that no one would want to be friends with me." As a result of this belief structure, Susan's self-esteem was threatened by any sign of social friction or rejection even from people she did not know well.

Schemata also can be inferred from the clustering of negative automatic thoughts into particular content themes. For example, Susan's automatic negative thoughts frequently dealt with fear of social rejection and loneliness. The Dysfunctional Attitude Scale (Weissman and Beck 1978; printed in an abbreviated form in Burns 1980) is a self-report inventory that also can be helpful in identifying the patient's particular assumptions. Patients rate their degree of agreement with attitudes associated with depression (e.g., people will probably think less of me if I make a mistake).

Once these beliefs are made explicit they can be subjected to reality testing. They can be challenged in many of the same ways that automatic thoughts are. Patients might be asked questions such as, "What's your evidence for this belief?", "What are some alternative ways of looking at it?", "How can you test this belief?" Furthermore, patients are encouraged to engage in a cost-benefit analysis of maintaining their underlying beliefs. They evaluate and weigh the costs relative to the benefits of their beliefs. For example, Susan recognized that her belief that she would be rejected, scorned, and abandoned if she expressed her opinions was partially adaptive in that it protected her from potential rejection. She never risked going out on a social limb and never acted overbearing. However, she also came to see that the costs of this belief dwarfed its benefits. This belief made her feel anxious, intimidated, and stifled in many of her relationships.

Relapse Prevention

Unveiling and modifying the underlying belief structure that makes certain people vulnerable to depression and learning to counteract automatic negative thoughts may be key elements in relapse prevention. It is believed that cognitive therapy is superior to other interventions, such as pharmacotherapy, in terms of being more likely to prevent or postpone relapse and recurrence (Beck et al. 1979). Patients leave treatment with a set of new skills for coping with difficulties that otherwise might lead to subsequent depressive episodes. Furthermore, in many cases, underlying dysfunctional attitudes are modified, which is thought to decrease risk for future depression

The final sessions of treatment explicitly focus on relapse prevention, often borrowing from Marlatt and Gordon's (1985) model developed in the treatment of addictions. When using relapse prevention, patients identify high risk situations (i.e., circumstances in which emotional difficulties may appear) and develop plans about how they might avoid or cope with these situations. For example, Susan recognized that dateless weekend evenings were a high risk situation. Consequently, she developed a number of alternative strategies, including inviting a girlfriend to the movies, to cope with this particular type of situation. Patients also are given the expectation that they are likely to have periods of mild dysphoria. Obviously, sadness is a normal human emotion that we all experience. Recovered depressed patients, however, may have the unrealistic expectation that they will never feel sad or blue again. Such expectations can set them up for relapse should they criticize themselves for becoming dysphoric or believe that such feelings mean that they are becoming depressed again. They learn not to become depressed about being sad. Finally, as with most approaches to psychotherapy, patients are told that returning to treatment in the future does not mean that they have failed. In fact, "booster sessions" are encouraged.

Nature of the Therapeutic Relationship

Within traditional cognitive therapy for depression, the therapeutic relationship is seen as a means of facilitating client experimentation with new techniques and behaviors. These latter techniques and behavioral changes are viewed as the "active ingredient" of successful treatment. A climate of *collaborative empiricism* is established in which therapists help patients clarify and test hypotheses about themselves and their circumstances, and teach them skills to defeat the cognitive-affective behavior cycles that maintain their depression (Beck et al. 1979). A problem-solving orientation is embraced in which the patient and therapist are working together against the depression. The therapist may be viewed as a psychoeducator teaching the patient new coping skills (Lewinsohn and Hoberman 1982). In this role, the therapeutic relationship itself is of little importance, except to the extent that problems in it may interfere with treatment.

Recent movements in cognitive therapy show a trend away from this rather neutral stance on the therapeutic relationship. Safran and Segal (1990) are pioneers in this line of clinical theory. In their hybrid of cognitive and interpersonal approaches, Safran and Segal articulate a much stronger role for the therapeutic relationship. They believe that much significant dysfunctional thinking is embedded in an interpersonal context (also see Horowitz 1991). Such thinking may become activated, primed, and affectively charged only within the confines of a relationship that focuses on affect and process. Furthermore, with its emphasis on cognitive relativism, cognitive therapy is inherently a phenomenological approach. Therefore, it is essential that the therapist understand the patient's idiosyncratic cognitive processes and affective experience as completely as possible. Therapists constantly must ask what various cognitions mean for patients and not assume that they understand underlying connotations. "Because cognition and affect are inseparable, empathy is simultaneously a cognitive and affective process. The therapist must not only get the 'idea' of patients' inner experiences, but also the 'feel' for subtle nuances of those experiences, which the patients may not have articulated for themselves" (Safran and Segal 1990, p. 85).

Safran and Segal (1990) use the therapeutic relationship as a laboratory to explore the patient's maladaptive beliefs and thoughts. In this regard, the therapist's own internal reactions are valuable data. Safran and Segal encourage the therapist to take the stance of a participant-observer and to be constantly attuned to the thoughts, feelings, and images that are aroused within herself or himself during the therapeutic encounter. Effective therapy is predicated on such internal awareness within the therapist. In some cases, the therapist's thoughts and feelings may be disclosed to generate discussion of the patient's impact on others and to clarify the nature of the interaction (Safran and Segal 1990).

Similar to the role of the parent in attachment theory, the therapeutic relationship provides a secure base for patient exploration (Guidano and Liotti 1983). The relationship also can be used as to identify and challenge dysfunctional cognitive-interpersonal cycles. Cognitive structures can be inferred from the way in which patients direct and maintain their relationship with the therapist (Guidano and Liotti 1983). Because the therapist serves as a model for vicarious learning, it is sometimes helpful for the therapist to talk aloud while thinking through problems to subtly teach coping skills (Mahoney 1974). Patients also learn self-acceptance by witnessing the therapist acknowledge and take ownership of negative feelings generated within the therapeutic encounter, e.g., frustration over feeling unable to help the patient (Safran and Segal 1990).

Rather than treatment obstacles, therapeutic impasses and resistances can be reframed as golden opportunities to help the patient understand critical interpersonal beliefs and assumptions. Transference (and counter transference) reactions are treated similarly. "Because alliance ruptures often occur when the therapeutic intervention activates an important interpersonal schema, the constructive resolution of a rupture provides an ideal opportunity to explore that interpersonal schema and also modify it" (Safran and Segal 1990, p. 158). Within such a framework, therapy becomes more process oriented than traditional cognitive approaches with their focus on the happenings of the previous week.

Life Stress, Depressive Realism, and Self-Esteem

Many clinicians first learning cognitive therapy for depression ask about the patient who has good reason to be depressed because of a miserable life situation (e.g., extreme poverty or a chronic, deteriorating medical condition). Where are the cognitive distortions here? In fact, some theorists view nondepressed individuals as having unrealistic, positive biases or illusions (Taylor and Brown 1988) and depressed persons as having more accurate appraisals of the world, a phenomenon termed depressive realism (Alloy and Abramson 1988). In our case example, environmental adversity and life stress were large contributors to Susan's depression. In fact, empirical studies indicate that environmental stressors trigger most episodes of major depression (Brown and Harris 1978; Monroe and Simons 1991). Is there an important role for cognitive processes in treating depression when reality does not appear to be negatively distorted?

Two possible roles for cognitive therapy have been suggested, regardless of life circumstances. First, because of cognitive therapy's problem-solving focus, it helps patients better cope with substantial stress in their lives. Cognitive therapy helps patients identify problems related to their dysphoric affect and teaches them skills to deal more effectively with these difficulties (see Hawton and Kirk 1989). For example, graded task assignments help patients negotiate complex tasks by breaking them down into manageable chunks. Cognitions that might otherwise interfere with adaptive coping are identified and challenged. In Susan's case, she believed that not receiving a job interview for every position to which she applied meant that she was a failure and that she was totally rejected. Her attempts to complete job applications were paralyzed until this cognition was recognized and challenged. Susan's poverty was real and psychologically draining, but her cognitive style interfered with overcoming it.

Second, cognitive therapy may prevent people from becoming clinically depressed in response to real losses and deprivations, although they may develop healthy sadness (i.e., depressed affect that does not include vegetative and cognitive symptoms). Hard line cognitivists (Burns 1980) argue that people's thinking makes them clinically depressed, no matter how harsh the reality. Within this perspective, depressed patients distort the importance of their privation, viewing it as an insurmountable roadblock to happiness and allowing it to affect their self-worth. Why might some objectively negative experiences and circumstances get magnified such that the person feels worthless and believes the future holds no happiness? Recent theory and research suggest that some people are vulnerable to loss of self-esteem and feelings of hopelessness as a result of matching particular areas of cognitive sensitivity with particular forms of life stressors (Beck 1983; Blatt and Zuroff 1992; Hammen 1992; Kuiper and Olinger 1986; Nietzel and Harris 1990). Major life events appear most relevant to depression if they affect people's central goals and aspirations, i.e., their sources of self-definition and self-esteem (Oatley and Bolton 1985; Pyszczynski and Greenberg 1987; Roberts and Monroe 1994). Such unfortunate matching results in loss of a clear sense of identity and decreased self-worth. For example, Susan based her worth as a person primarily on maintaining social relationships and therefore was sensitive to threats within this domain. Yet, threats within other life domains (e.g., career) had less impact on her because they were not as important.

This perspective implies that people do not become depressed in response to major stressful life events in general, but in response to the particular experiences to which they are sensitive. It also implies that those at risk for depression have fewer sources of self-worth that could lead to temporally unstable self-esteem (Roberts and Monroe 1992, 1994). Cognitive therapy teaches patients to protect their self-worth during stressful experiences so that it is less prone to oscillate with the ups and downs of life. A major part of Susan's treatment involved helping her find alternative sources of self-worth and exploring the developmental roots of her self-esteem contingencies. Susan needed to develop a more flexible foundation of self-evaluation and learn to value other qualities within herself. Many of the techniques and practices discussed earlier (e.g., cognitive restructuring; identifying cognitive distortions) were targeted at Susan's self-evaluations. For example, she learned how she tended to minimize many of her positive qualities.

Furthermore, depression-prone individuals do not appear to automatically take credit for positive things that happen to them. These patients need to be trained to effortfully make such attributions (Hartlage S, Alloy LB, Arduino: Depression, attributional vulnerability to depression, and automatic processing of attributional inferences. Unpublished data, 1996). Susan had difficulty recruiting positive images and memories during the dysphoria associated with loss. Therefore, her sense of positive self-worth was less readily accessible in regulating negative affect and buffering herself from life's vicissitudes. Given that life stress and lack of social support may contribute to depression by continuously activating painful nonconscious thoughts and memories (Brewin 1989), depressed patients may be in special need of such buffering. Susan needed to consciously practice recalling positive thoughts and memories of herself as a means of coping with dysphoric feelings.

Efficacy of Cognitive Therapy of Depression

There have been a number of outcome studies of cognitive therapy for depression comparing it with no treatment and placebo controls, other forms of psychotherapy, and pharmacotherapy. Several studies have examined the issue of relapse after successful treatment with these interventions. We briefly review the results of these investigations and address which patients may (or may not) benefit from cognitive therapy.

Early research suggested that cognitive therapy is a highly effective treatment for depression with effects that might exceed pharmacotherapy. For example, Rush et al. (1977) found that cognitive therapy led to remission in 79% of cases, whereas pharmacotherapy (imipramine) led to remission in only 23%. Furthermore, there were fewer premature terminations in the cognitive therapy group. Patients in this study generally had chronic or intermittent depression with a first onset 8.8 years before the study. Twenty-two percent had previous psychiatric hospitalizations and 12.2% had a history of suicide attempts. More recent studies also have found that cognitive therapy is at least equal to pharmacotherapy in achieving remission (Beck et al. 1985; Blackburn et al. 1981; Hollon et al. 1992; Murphy et al. 1984), although this finding is not universal

(Elkin et al. 1989). Several of these studies suggest that there is a substantially reduced risk of relapse after successful treatment with cognitive therapy when compared with pharmacotherapy without prophylactic continuation (Evans et al. 1992; Simons et al. 1986). Although a meta-analytic review found that cognitive therapy was somewhat more effective than no treatment, behavioral therapy, and pharmacotherapy (Dobson 1989), another recent review was somewhat more cautious (Hollon et al. 1991). Hollon et al. warned that the quality of pharmacotherapy is suspect in many of these studies (Hollon et al. 1991). For example, medication dosage was often lower than that of typical clinical practice.

Cognitive therapy has been seen as a potentially effective treatment for mild to moderately severe cases of nonendogenous depression. It was assumed that more severe cases, as well as those with an endogenous symptom profile (e.g., early morning awakening, anhedonia), would be better treated with pharmacotherapy. Although it is true that cognitive therapy is less successful with severe cases than with milder depression (Elkin et al. 1989; Thase et al. 1991), there also is evidence that pharmacotherapy is less effective with such cases (Thase and Kupfer 1987). The rate of symptomatic improvement appears to be equivalent in the severe and less severe groups treated with cognitive therapy, suggesting that more severe cases simply require a longer course of treatment (Thase et al. 1991).

Additionally, cognitive therapy has proven successful in the treatment of patients meeting Research Diagnostic Criteria for endogenous major depression, even when the diagnosis is accompanied by shortened REM latency (a traditional marker of "biological depression"). In one study, 57% of these patients (selected for endogeneity) fully remitted after 20 sessions of cognitive therapy, whereas an additional 32% partially remitted (Simons and Thase 1992). There was no difference in remission between those with shortened REM latency and those without. Another study also found that endogenous features did not interfere with cognitive therapy (Blackburn et al. 1981). Results from additional studies show that cognitive therapy and pharmacotherapy have equivalent effects on biological and cognitive outcome variables (Imber et al. 1990; Simons et al. 1984). Specific treatment effects have been difficult to demonstrate.

A recent article from the Collaborative Study of Depression examined the issue of differential predictors of treatment response among cognitive therapy, interpersonal therapy, and pharmacotherapy. Somewhat paradoxically, this study found that cognitive therapy was most effective with patients with little cognitive dysfunction, whereas interpersonal therapy was most effective with patients with the least social dysfunction (Sotsky et al. 1991). These data suggest that psychotherapy is most effective when it builds on the patient's strengths.

Summary

Cognitive therapy is a structured, short-term therapy based on the cognitive model of depression. Theoretically, its mode of action is through correcting the cognitive distortions and maladaptive thoughts associated with depression. Changes in these cognitions presumably lead to mood improvement. However, the cognitive model does not deny that mood can be improved by other means. Recent formulations suggest that cognition is but one "port of entry" into a multi-determined, multi-faceted disorder that also can be accessed and treated through other ports, such as biological and interpersonal systems. Within this perspective, cognition, mood, social functioning, and biology are reciprocally related and equally important in depression (Beck 1983; Teasdale and Barnard 1993; Wright and Thase 1992). Cognitive therapy may lead to changes in both biology and cognition; whereas pharmacotherapy may improve certain cognitive deficits (e.g., negative automatic thoughts), as well as alter biochemical mechanisms underlying depression.

Although cognitive therapy for depression is a relative newcomer, there is good evidence that it is an effective treatment for depression. Importantly, there is mounting evidence that cognitive therapy delays or diminishes likelihood of relapse. Although the integrative position just mentioned suggests that the combination of cognitive therapy and pharmacotherapy would be superior to either approach individually, there is little empirical evidence for such additive effects (Hollon et al. 1991). More research needs to be conducted to better determine who will most benefit from cognitive therapy for depression, and whether certain patients respond better to combined treatment.

References

Alloy LB, Abramson LY: Depressive realism: four theoretical perspectives, in Cognitive Processes in Depression. Edited by Alloy LB. New York, Guilford, 1988, pp 223–265

Bandura A: Self-efficacy: toward a unifying theory of behavioral change. Psychol Rev 84:191–215, 1977

Barber JP, DeRubeis RJ: On second thought: where the action is in cognitive therapy for depression. Cognitive Therapy and Research 13:441–457, 1989

Beck AT: Depression: Clinical, Experimental and Theoretical Aspects. New York, Harper & Row, 1967

Beck AT: Cognitive Therapy and the Emotional Disorders. New York, International Universities Press, 1976

Beck AT: Cognitive therapy of depression: new perspectives, in Treatment of Depression: Old Controversies and New Approaches. Edited by Clayton PJ, Barrett JE. New York, Raven Press, 1983, pp 265–284

Beck AT, Rush AJ, Shaw BF, et al: Cognitive Therapy of Depression. New York, Guilford, 1979

Beck AT, Hollon SD, Young JE, et al: Treatment of depression with cognitive therapy and amitriptyline. Arch Gen Psychiatry 42:142–148, 1985

Berger PL, Luckman T: The Social Construction of Reality. New York, Anchor Press, 1966

Blackburn IM, Bishop S, Glen AIM, et al: The efficacy of cognitive therapy in depression: a treatment trial using cognitive therapy and pharmacotherapy, each alone and in combination. Br J Psychiatry 139:181–189, 1981

Blatt SJ, Zuroff DC: Interpersonal relatedness and self-definition: two prototypes for depression. Clinical Psychology Review 12: 527–562, 1992

Bowlby J: Loss: Sadness and Depression. New York, Basic Books, 1980

Brewin CR: Cognitive change processes in psychotherapy. Psychol Rev 96: 379–394, 1989

Brown GW, Harris T: Social Origins of Depression. New York, Free Press, 1978

Burns DD: Feeling Good. New York, Signet, 1980

Dobson KS: A meta-analysis of the efficacy of cognitive therapy for depression. J Consult Clin Psychol 57:414–419, 1989

Elkin I, Shea MT, Watkins JT, et al: NIMH treatment of depression collaborative research program, I: general effectiveness of treatments. Arch Gen Psychiatry 46: 971–982, 1989

Ellis A: Reason and Emotion in Psychotherapy. New York, Lyle Stuart, 1962

Evans MD, Hollon SD, DeRubeis RJ, et al: Differential relapse following cognitive therapy and pharmacotherapy for depression. Arch Gen Psychiatry 49:802–808, 1992

Feyerabend P: Against Method. London, Verso, 1975

Guidano VF: Complexity of the Self: A Developmental Approach to Psychopathology and Therapy. New York, Guilford, 1987.

Guidano VF, Liotti G: Cognitive Processes and the Emotional Disorders. New York, Guilford, 1983

Hammen C: Life events and depression: the plot thickens. Am J Community Psychol 20:179–193, 1992

Hartlage S: Automatic processing paradigms and assessing cognitive vulnerability to depression. Paper presented at the meeting of the American Psychological Association, Toronto, Ontario, August 1993

Hartlage S, Alloy LB, Vazquez CV, Dykman BM: Automatic and effortful processing in depression. Psychol Bull 113:247–278, 1993

Hawton K, Kirk J: Problem-solving, in Cognitive Behaviour Therapy for Psychiatric Problems. Edited by Hawton K, Salkovskies PM, Kirk J, et al. New York, Oxford University Press, 1989, pp 347–369

Hollon SD, Shelton RC, Loosen PT: Cognitive therapy and pharmacotherapy for depression. J Consult Clin Psychol 59:88–99, 1991

Hollon SD, DeRubeis RJ, Evans MD, et al: Cognitive therapy and pharmacotherapy for depression: singly and in combination. Arch Gen Psychiatry 49:774–781, 1992

Horowitz MJ: Person Schemas and Maladaptive Interpersonal Patterns. Chicago, IL, University of Chicago Press, 1991

Imber SD, Pilkonis PA, Sotsky SM, et al: Mode-specific effects among three treatments for depression. J Consult Clin Psychol 58:352–359, 1990

Kelly GA: The Psychology of Personal Constructs, Vol 1 & 2. New York, Norton, 1955

Klerman GL, Rounsaville B, Chevron E, et al: Interpersonal Psychotherapy of Depression. New York, Basic Books, 1984

Kuiper NA, Olinger LJ: Dysfunctional attitudes and a self-worth contingency model of depression. Advances in Cognitive-Behavior Research and Therapy 5:115–142, 1986

Lazarus RS: Cognition and motivation in emotion. Am Psychol 46: 352–367, 1991

Lewinsohn PM, Hoberman HM: Depression, in International Handbook of Behavior Modification and Therapy. Edited by Bellack AS, Hersen M, Kazdin AE. New York, Plenum, 1982, pp 397–431

Lewinsohn PM, Youngren MA, Grosscup SJ: Reinforcement and depression, in The Psychobiology of the Depressive Disorders: Implications for the Effects of Stress. Edited by Depue RA. New York, Academic Press, 1979, pp 291–316

MacPhillamy DJ, Lewinsohn PM: The pleasant events schedule: studies on reliability, validity, and scale intercorrelation. J Consult Clin Psychol 50: 363–380, 1982

Mahoney MJ: Cognition and Behavior Modification. Cambridge MA, Ballinger, 1974

Marlatt GA, Gordon JR: Relapse Prevention. New York, Guilford Press, 1985

Meichenbaum D: Cognitive-Behavior Modification: An Integrative Approach. New York, Plenum, 1977

Monroe SM, Simons AD: Diathesis-stress theories in the context of life stress research: implications for the depressive disorders. Psychol Bull 110: 406–425, 1991

Murphy GE, Simons AD, Wetzel RD, et al: Cognitive therapy singly and together in the treatment of depression. Arch Gen Psychiatry 41:33–41, 1984

Nietzel MT, Harris MJ: Relationship of dependency and achievement/autonomy to depression. Clinical Psychology Review 10:279–297, 1990

Nolen-Hoeksema S: Sex differences in depression. Psychol Bull 101:259–282, 1987

Oatley K, Bolton W: A social-cognitive theory of depression in reaction to life events. Psychol Rev 92:372–388, 1985

Pietromonaco PR, Markus H: The nature of negative thoughts in depression. J Pers Soc Psychol 48:799–807, 1985

Pyszczynski T, Greenberg J: Self-regulatory perseveration and the depressive self-focussing style: a self-awareness theory of reactive depression. Psychol Bull 102:122–138, 1987

Rehm LP: Self-management and cognitive processes in depression, in Cognitive Processes in Depression. Edited by Alloy LB. New York, Guilford, 1988, pp 143–176

Roberts JE, Monroe SM: Vulnerable self-esteem and depressive symptoms: prospective data comparing three alternative conceptualizations. J Pers Soc Psychol 62:804–812, 1992

Roberts JE, Monroe SM: A multidimensional model of self-esteem in depression. Clinical Psychology Review 14:161–181, 1994

Rush AJ, Beck AT, Kovacs M, et al: Comparative efficacy of cognitive therapy and pharmacotherapy in the treatment of depressed outpatients. Cognitive Therapy and Research 1:17–37, 1977

Safran JD, Segal ZV: Interpersonal Process in Cognitive Therapy. New York, Basic Books, 1990

Simons AD, Thase ME: Biological markers, treatment outcome, and 1 year follow-up in endogenous depression: electroencephalographic sleep studies and response to cognitive therapy. J Consult Clin Psychol 60:392–401, 1992

Simons AD, Garfield SL, Murphy GE: The process of change in cognitive therapy and pharmacotherapy for depression. Arch Gen Psychiatry 41:45–51, 1984

Simons AD, Murphy GE, Levine JE, et al: Cognitive therapy and pharmacotherapy for depression: sustained improvement over one year. Arch Gen Psychiatry 43:43–49, 1986

Sotsky SM, Glass DR, Shea MT, et al: Patient predictors of response to psychotherapy and pharmacotherapy: findings in the NIMH treatment of depression collaborative research program. Am J Psychiatry 148:997–1008, 1991

Taylor SE, Brown JD: Illusion and well being: a social psychological perspective on mental health. Psychol Bull 103:193–210, 1988

Teasdale JD, Barnard PJ: Affect Cognition and Change. Hillsdale, NJ, Lawrence Erlbaum, 1993

Thase ME, Kupfer DJ: Characteristics of treatment resistant depression, in Treating Resistant Depression. Edited by Zohar J, Belmaker RH. New York, PMA Publishing, 1987, pp 23–45

Thase ME, Simons AD, Cahalane J, McGeary J, Harden T: Severity of depression and response to cognitive behavior therapy. Am J Psychiatry 148: 784–789, 1991

Weissman AN, Beck AT: Development and validation of the dysfunctional attitude scale: a preliminary investigation. Paper presented at the meeting of the American Education Research Association, Toronto, Ontario, November 1978

Williams JMG, Moorey S: The wider application of cognitive therapy: the end of the beginning, in Cognitive Therapy in Clinical Practice. Edited by Scott J, Williams JMG, Beck AT. New York, Routledge, 1989, pp 227–250

Wright JH, Thase ME: Cognitive and biological therapies: a synthesis. Psychiatric Annals 22:451–458, 1992

Part IV

Practical Issues in Cognitive Rehabilitation

Chapter 15

The Cognitive Exoskeleton: Environmental Interventions in Cognitive Rehabilitation

Robert K. Heinssen, Ph.D.

The Cognitive Exoskeleton: Environmental Interventions in Cognitive Rehabilitation

The goal of psychiatric rehabilitation is to establish an optimal balance between personal capabilities and environmental features (Anthony 1979; Anthony and Liberman 1986, 1992). In theory, deficient behavior can be corrected through several methods, including coping skills training, environmental management, or some combination of these approaches (Anthony et al. 1983; Liberman and Evans 1985; Livneh 1984). In actual practice, however, rehabilitation programs tend to emphasize individual treatments more than environmental interventions (Dauwalder and Hoffman 1992; Sommers 1988). This trend is particularly true in the field of cognitive rehabilitation, where the remediation of patients' deficient processing skills is the dominant treatment strategy.

Although milieu-based treatments often assume a secondary role in cognitive rehabilitation, environmental interventions offer important advantages. First, the effectiveness of remediation programs might be increased if environmental conditions were arranged to facilitate the patient's attention, concentration, and memory. Adapting the environment to offset internal deficiencies could enhance the patient's capacity for new learning. Second, skills training might further progress if external supports and demands were continuously adjusted to match the patient's cognitive resources. This would maintain the

This work was supported in part by a Young Investigator Award to Dr. Heinssen from the National Alliance for Research on Schizophrenia and Depression. The author thanks Katherine Dunbar, Lawrence Conroy, Brian Victor, Dr. Dexter M. Bullard, Jr., and the staff of the Chestnut Lodge Research Institute for their support in the writing of this chapter.

patient's motivation for treatment by reducing problems attributable to boredom and/or overstimulation. In the event that new processing strategies cannot be acquired, environmental interventions offer a technology for managing permanent cognitive disabilities. Theoretically, prosthetic supports could be erected around the patient to form an "exoskeleton" for regulating information processing artificially.

Given the potential importance of environmental interventions to cognitive rehabilitation, any discussion of cognitive treatment must include an analysis of environmental issues. The current chapter examines how environmental factors affect the cognitive rehabilitation process. The theoretical basis of the environmental perspective is described followed by a review of the environmental strategies used in cognitive rehabilitation. Environmental interventions are considered first as an auxiliary component in cognitive remediation, and then as a prosthetic element in milieu-based rehabilitation programs. Several case reports will illustrate the application of environmental concepts in inpatient psychosocial treatment programs. The chapter concludes by proposing a broader conceptual framework for the contemporary model of cognitive rehabilitation.

Environmental Complexity and Cognitive Processing

Adaptive behavior is based on the ability to filter environmental input and to detect relevant situational cues. Competent individuals can scan their milieu, focus attention selectively, and ignore extraneous elements in the stimulus field. The prototypic example of this process is the cocktail party where many conversations occur simultaneously, but the listener attends to only one (Green et al. 1992). Organismic and environmental factors interact to determine competence on these cognitive operations (Green 1992). Perceptual problems, attention deficits, and memory impairments can hinder an individual's ability to screen out extraneous stimuli and identify relevant data. Environmental conditions also affect signal detection accuracy, either by masking existing cognitive disabilities or accentuating information processing deficits.

Results from laboratory tests of signal detection and selective attention indicate that cognitive efficiency deteriorates when the complexity of experimental tasks exceeds information processing capacity (Kahneman 1973; Nuechterlein and Dawson 1984). This relationship is illustrated in Figure 15–1. Most individuals have no trouble detecting target stimuli when these signals are unambiguous and stand out prominently from other elements in the stimulus array (i.e., a low complexity environment). Cognitive deficits, if they exist, may be concealed in this instance by an advantageous signal-to-noise ratio. The filtering

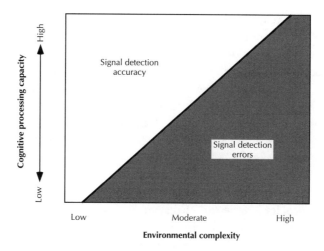

Figure 15–1. The relationships among cognitive capacity, environmental complexity, and signal detection accuracy.

task becomes much harder, however, when "clutter" is introduced into the stimulus field by degrading signals or magnifying ambient noise. Additional cognitive resources are necessary to interpret informationally complex environments, and processing differences among subjects become apparent when target stimuli are less distinct. Cognitive limitations, which may go otherwise unnoticed, are exposed when experimental conditions push the processing burden beyond the individual's capacity to cope.

Similar relationships among cognitive capabilities and environmental conditions probably operate in natural settings. In social and work situations, for example, a person must scan his or her surroundings repeatedly to ascertain the signal/noise attributes of competing stimuli. Uncontrolled settings are more "noisy" than laboratory environments, and even mild cognitive impairment could cause an individual to miss important environmental cues or to misinterpret irrelevant signals as meaningful. It is conceivable, however, that features of the real-world milieu affect social processing in the same way that laboratory conditions influence the detection of visual or auditory targets. Presumably, environments characterized by discrete discriminative stimuli (i.e., unambiguous cues that prompt specific behaviors) will present fewer cognitive challenges and will be more easily negotiated than less structured settings. Consequently, a person with cognitive impairments might appear more effective in a highly structured setting where orienting stimuli are distinct and numerous.

The workplace is one example of a natural setting that generally provides structure, consistency, and multiple orienting stimuli. The regimentation of the work setting reduces cognitive processing demands by 1) dictating when certain activities begin; 2) identifying which tasks need to be completed; 3) specifying what procedures are to be followed; and 4) determining when activities cease (Sullivan et al. 1989). Discriminative stimuli are usually plentiful on the job site and may include features such as time clocks, uniforms, posted instructions, motivational posters, and job specific materials. These elements provide contextual cues for instrumental activity and channel behavioral options into specific pathways (e.g., "I'm in the wood shop with my tools so I guess I should be working"). Thus, the workplace contains an abundant array of environmental "triggers" that facilitate adaptive responses.

The work milieu similarly structures social interactions by providing a well defined protocol for interpersonal behavior. For example, the business-like atmosphere of the workplace restricts social encounters to a set of clearly defined, job related scenarios. Social behavior is further regulated by hierarchical relationships (e.g., labor versus management), time schedules (e.g., work periods, coffee breaks), and contrasting work roles (e.g., mechanics versus secretaries). These environmental features narrow the range of possible social interactions and highlight cues for appropriate interpersonal behavior. Theoretically, these characteristics (i.e., high signal, low noise) should decrease information processing demands and allow even cognitively impaired persons to function productively in the workplace.

Social and instrumental adaptation might deteriorate, however, if external structures are weakened and/or discriminative stimuli become less distinct. For example, the person who functions adequately in a well-regulated work environment might flounder in settings where interpersonal and job boundaries become blurred, or when control stimuli cannot be easily distinguished from competing signals. These conditions necessitate greater effort to ascertain task demands (e.g., "What is it that am I supposed to do here?"), and a larger proportion of cognitive resources will be allocated to screening and attention functions. This leaves fewer cognitive assets for other endeavors (e.g., problem-solving, decision making, behavioral responding), and could result in less effective overall functioning.

When a client is confronted by an overwhelmingly "noisy" environment, the rehabilitation clinician must choose between two treatment options: either improve the patient's capacity to detect and process social and instrumental cues (i.e., the cognitive remediation approach) or manipulate situational elements to amplify control stimuli (i.e., the environmental engineering or "compensation" perspective). Specific remediation procedures will not be discussed because they are reviewed in other chapters of this book by Goldberg and Cook (Chapter 13) and by Storzbach and Corrigan (Chapter 11). Instead, the next two sections examine environmental interventions as they are implemented in cognitive rehabilitation programs.

Environmental Engineering in Cognitive Remediation Programs

Although certain environmental features can augment cognitive functioning, others present obstacles to effective information processing. This concept has influenced both treatment planning and service delivery in cognitive remediation programs (Abreu and Toglia 1987; Hayden and Hart 1986; Heinssen and Victor 1994; Henry 1983), and a variety of strategies have been proposed for achieving optimal training conditions. These tactics usually involve the manipulation of one or more of these environmental features: 1) therapist characteristics; 2) motivational factors; 3) temporal and structural elements; and 4) the physical features of the treatment setting. It is hypothesized that these variables can be adjusted to favorably balance a patient's cognitive resources against the demands of the training situation.

Therapist Characteristics

Patients referred for cognitive retraining display problems including deficits in attention, concentration, memory, and decision making. These disabilities limit the patient's comprehension of the rehabilitation process and often curb enthusiasm for treatment. It falls on the clinician to perform organizational and motivational functions on the patient's behalf. Because of these "executive" duties, the rehabilitation therapist represents the most important element in the patient's treatment.

The clinician's primary duties in cognitive remediation are to 1) protect the patient from stimulus overload; and 2) remove external obstacles that could hinder recovery. The therapist must tailor task demands to match the patient's level of understanding and then manipulate environmental stimuli (e.g., cues and distractors) to conserve the patient's cognitive resources (Freeman 1989; Tankle 1988). Since patients often are unable to judge their own capacities, the therapist usually has to regulate the intensity and difficulty of treatment, considering both the patient's emerging assets and vulnerability to relapse (McGlashan et al. 1990).

Of equal importance to treatment organization is the clinician's ongoing emotional support. The patient's initial confusion and despair may lessen after the therapist provides a rationale for treatment and explains the incremental process of retraining. This exchange sets the emotional tone for the

training experience and often is the first step in creating hope and collaboration. As treatment proceeds, the therapist reinforces these conditions by setting realistic expectations, correcting the patient's misattributions, and
attributing progress to the patient's efforts and skill (Heinssen and Victor 1994).
Other therapist characteristics such as respect, tolerance, flexibility, and opti-
mism strengthen the therapeutic alliance and bolster the patient's performance
when emotional resources are low (McGlashan et al. 1990). These "person variables" lie at the core of the therapeutic relationship and may determine the
success or failure of the retraining experience.

Maintaining a positive therapeutic relationship is made difficult, however,
by the communication problems related to cognitive impairments. The therapist should, therefore, be prepared to modify his or her communication style
according to the specific disabilities of the patient. Brenner (1987) noted that
verbal communication with cognitively impaired schizophrenic patients should
be conducted in a calm, slow, and quiet manner. He recommended paring down
speech to the bare necessities, while restricting gestures, the use of objects, and
excessive voice modulation. Brenner also advised therapists to use the same
words and tone whenever speech is repeated. These accommodations seem reasonable for any situation where communication is compromised by the patient's
limited processing capacity.

Motivational Climate

Motivational deficits, a lack of purpose, and anhedonia are negative symptoms
associated with cognitive impairment (Goldberg and Cook, Chapter 15). These
features, left unchecked, can undermine cognitive retraining by limiting
a patient's initiative and curtailing interest in rehabilitation. Motivational variables
represent a second important element in the patient's treatment environment.

Jeffrey (1981) suggests that the best method for boosting a patient's motivation for rehabilitation is to introduce "cognitive clarity" into the treatment process. He reasons that long-term goals may seem so complex and far
removed that they overwhelm the patient and undermine initiative. Jeffrey
recommends partitioning overarching treatment goals into smaller, more
easily managed tasks and then highlighting for the patient a systematic and
attractive progression from one subgoal to another. By clarifying the path to
treatment goals, the therapist reduces the complexity of the training process,
minimizes the patient's confusion and uncertainty, and fosters motivation
for achievement. An outgrowth of this incremental treatment strategy is "success momentum" and positive expectations concerning future training endeavors (Heinssen and Victor 1994).

When specific training goals are identified, differential reinforcement may provide further incentive for active treatment participation. Given patients' poor attention and memory skills, the importance of immediate, specific, and positive performance feedback is clear (Benedict 1989; Liberman et al. 1982, 1986; Pollack et al. 1984). In addition to verbal praise, concrete rewards also may be motivational catalysts. Consistent application of primary and secondary reinforcers, for example, can reestablish the connection between personal effort and environmental consequences, thereby combatting learned helplessness and depression (Hayden and Hart 1986). Not surprisingly, contingency management procedures have improved motivation and persistence in cognitively impaired patients (e.g., Godfrey and Knight 1987; Incagnoli and Newman 1985), and should be considered when motivational deficits present an obstacle to treatment.

Temporal/Structural Elements

Patients with information processing deficits are fatigued by the intellectual, emotional, and physical demands of treatment. To accommodate patients' limited endurance, it may be necessary to manipulate the frequency and length of therapy sessions and the difficulty of training tasks. The temporal and structural features of the therapy session represent a third critical component of the patient's treatment environment.

Several authors suggest decreasing the duration and increasing the frequency of treatment sessions when working with cognitively impaired patients (Liberman et al. 1982, 1986). At the very least, these variables should be adjusted to match the client's span of attention and concentration as well as physical stamina. Theoretically, brief and repetitious sessions, spaced evenly throughout the day, should reduce patients' distractibility, focus attentional resources, and promote overlearning of training tasks (Liberman et al. 1986). This format also allows the patient to temporarily escape from the demands of the training program, thus averting stimulus overload and physical or emotional exhaustion (Liberman et al. 1982).

The patient's cognitive resources can be further preserved by regulating the complexity of training tasks. Because cognitive resources are presumably lowest when treatment starts, initial assignments should be conceptually clear and uncomplicated. Coaching and prompting by treatment personnel play an important role in this phase of cognitive retraining. These activities focus attentional resources and help to keep the patient "on task." Information processing demands can be gradually increased until they approximate conditions found in the natural environment (Abreu and Toglia 1987; Bottcher 1989;

Hayden and Hart 1986; Henry 1983; Pollack et al. 1984). Supportive structures such as external cues and prompts can then be withdrawn, but at a pace that corresponds to the patient's rate of cognitive recovery (Glisky and Schacter 1988; Henry 1983). The complexity of training tasks always is calibrated to stimulate the patient's growth, but not at the cost of overwhelming stress. In this manner an optimal tension state is achieved that preserves the patient's motivation and minimizes frustrating experiences.

The Physical Setting

Certain features of the training setting can be distracting to patients referred for cognitive retraining (Linn et al. 1980). Art work, ambient noise, and other people may compete for a patient's limited attention, particularly if the training task is difficult or frustrating. It may be necessary to manipulate features of the physical environment to create a favorable rehabilitation climate.

When possible, the therapist should choose a private, quiet training location that is uncluttered and rich in task relevant, discriminative stimuli. Taking a somewhat extreme position, Diamant (1986) proposes that training should begin in the protected environment of the neuropsychological laboratory. At the very least, the physical characteristics of the training site should be constant during the early stages of treatment to minimize distraction (Bottcher 1989). To highlight control stimuli, Liberman and his colleagues (Liberman et al. 1982) recommend posting graphic charts in the training area for visual cuing of cognitive strategies. These and other prosthetic instruments (e.g., video-taped feedback) may focus attention, augment memory, and facilitate complex cognitive functions such as problem solving and decision making.

Features of the physical environment should be diversified during treatment to include "real-world" distractors such as visual diversions, background noise, and activity. These extraneous features exercise attention and concentration under more demanding processing conditions, thereby challenging and sharpening the patient's emerging cognitive skills (Hayden and Hart 1986; Kreutzer et al. 1989). Eventually, the training site's physical aspects should resemble the natural milieu in terms of ambient stressors and information processing requirements (Diamant 1986). At this point the focus of treatment shifts from skills acquisition proper to practicing new cognitive strategies at home and on the job (Hayden and Hart 1986; Namerow 1987; Westling and Floyd 1990).

Summary

The recommendations presented in this chapter are based on the hypothesis that cognitive functioning is influenced by surrounding environmental conditions. Settings that are highly structured, devoid of distracting elements, and

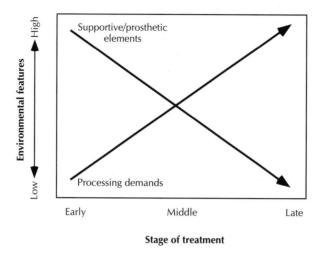

Figure 15–2.   Person-environment matching in cognitive remediation.

rich in discriminative stimuli presumably foster more efficient information processing than "noisy" or "cluttered" situations. Based on this premise, environmental engineering has emerged as an integral component in cognitive remediation programs. As the preceding review suggests, it is common for clinicians to advocate tailoring characteristics of the treatment setting to meet the patient's specific needs and capacities. This often involves orchestrating many environmental elements including the therapists' behavior, the motivational climate, the training sessions' structure, and the treatment settings' physical features.

Figure 15–2 illustrates how this "matching" concept has been applied in cognitive retraining. Most authors agree that external conditions should be arranged early to protect the patient from information overload. At this juncture, the training setting emphasizes supportive elements and downplays confusing and/or distracting features. External cues, systematic prompting, immediate reinforcement, and brief but frequent training sessions exemplify prosthetic elements that augment the patient's fragile cognitive repertoire. As recovery proceeds the informational characteristics of the treatment setting slowly change. Prosthetic elements are gradually withdrawn and training tasks become increasingly complex. Processing demands expand steadily until conditions in the treatment setting mirror those of the natural milieu. By the end of therapy, supportive features are virtually absent and the patient is expected to manage processing requirements through newly acquired cognitive strategies.

Although the model portrayed in Figure 15–2 appears conceptually sound, many of the treatment recommendations derived from this framework are vague. Few of the reports cited offer sufficient detail to determine how informational complexity was regulated during therapy. It is usually impossible to determine how specific interventions affected short-term clinical response or how environmental manipulations contributed to overall treatment outcome. This ambiguity presents a significant obstacle for those who wish to replicate another clinician's treatment procedures or to evaluate the impact of specific environmental interventions on the retraining process.

Greater methodological precision would help to illuminate the role of environmental variables in remediation programs. In most instances this could be achieved by providing fuller descriptions of the patient, milieu, and procedural variables that define the various phases of treatment. For example:

1. Which cognitive operations are necessary to succeed in each treatment setting? Are these elementary or executive functions?
2. What is the patient's level of information processing? Do cognitive resources correspond to processing requirements, or do discrepancies exist?
3. What is the relationship between external supports and task demands? Are discriminative stimuli numerous and unambiguous, or does "noise" dominate the milieu?
4. How frustrating or exhausting is the training program? Are patients allowed respites from therapy, or are training intervals constant and highly regimented?

Answers to questions such as these would clarify how personal competencies, environmental features, and retraining procedures are balanced at successive stages of therapy. Each phase would emerge as a unique combination of variables, making it possible to monitor the impact of specific manipulations on the rehabilitation process. To perform this level of analysis, however, would require that a patient's functioning be evaluated at each stage of rehabilitation and not just at the start and close of treatment. This type of "follow along" assessment strategy offers clear advantages to clinicians and researchers. Clinicians would acquire greater control of the treatment process because optimal therapeutic conditions could be identified and exploited at intermediate stages of therapy. Researchers would gain new techniques for interpreting the heterogeneous results often observed in cognitive retraining programs.

It is clear that a different type of research design is required for studying person/environment interactions in cognitive remediation. The next section presents one possible method for examining the role of environmental factors in the cognitive rehabilitation process. The matching model is operationalized in this example by ordinally ranking the informational complexity of five distinct training environments and by evaluating treatment outcome through a longitudinal assessment strategy.

A Process Analysis of Cognitive Rehabilitation

The Sullivan House Rehabilitation Program at Chestnut Lodge Hospital (Rockville, MD) offers comprehensive psychosocial treatment to schizophrenic patients. The treatment regimen at Sullivan House addresses the needs of severely mentally ill individuals who exhibit multiple impairments in self-care skills, interpersonal functioning, and vocational performance. Most patients display cognitive difficulties, which range from mild problems in attention and memory to gross impairments in abstractive and executive functions. While social learning and operant principles structure the treatment milieu (Paul and Lentz 1977), cognitive remediation techniques have been incorporated to augment traditional skills training procedures.

The influence of the cognitive framework is clearest in the program's vocational training module, an organic gardening business. In describing this project, Heinssen and Victor (1994) delineate several strategies for integrating cognitive remediation and behavioral treatment techniques. These include 1) comprehensive analysis of the cognitive and motoric operations involved in gardening; 2) functional assessment of these skills in the workplace; 3) neuropsychological testing to determine the frequency, duration, and complexity of training sessions; and 4) continuity of training procedures (i.e., modeling, coaching, shaping, and reinforcement) across cognitive and behavioral targets. The resulting therapy program emulates the matching paradigm in Figure 15–2. Skills training occurs in incremental stages within settings designed to regulate environmental complexity.

Ranking the Informational Characteristics of Treatment Settings

Table 15–1 provides an overview of the organic gardening program and depicts one method for ranking the informational complexity of different treatment settings. Five training environments are described, each characterized by a unique blend of cognitive demands, external supports, and training techniques. The least complicated scenario appears in Stage 1, which features a discrete work task (column 2), narrow processing demands (column 3), numerous prosthetic elements (column 4), and continuous support from clinicians (column 5). Conditions in this stage are designed to facilitate concentration and to protect patients from stimulus overload. This is accomplished by incorporating many of the concepts described in the previous review: 1) a clear and uncomplicated training task; 2) emphasis on subgoal completion; 3) brief but frequent training sessions; 4) continuous modeling, coaching, and prompting from clinicians; 5) immediate feedback and reinforcement; 6) sequestered

Table 15–1. Environmental complexity in a vocational rehabilitation program: defining cognitive demands, external supports, and skills training techniques

Treatment stage	Work task(s)	Requisite skills
I. (Lowest complexity)	1. Identify plants in the protected training area that need watering.	1. Sustained attention 2. Perceptual discrimination 3. Conceptual sorting 4. Decision making
II.	1. Identify plants in the general work area that need watering. 2. Observe and learn proper watering technique.	1. Sustained *and* selective attention 2. Perceptual discrimination 3. Conceptual sorting 4. Decision making
III. (Moderate complexity)	1. Water plants in the general work area with correct technique. 2. Appropriate interpersonal behavior with co-workers.	1–4. Cognitive skills from Stage II 5. Motor responding 6. Social skills

Environmental conditions	Training methods	Mastery criteria
Protected training site inside the greenhouse characterized by privacy, numerous orienting stimuli, and stable climatic conditions. Instructional posters are prominently placed. Tools are limited, clearly labeled, and immediately available. Continuous 1:1 supervision. Limited social contact with other patients.	Clinicians 1) model perceptual discrimination, concept sorting, and decision making operations; 2) prompt these skills during practice trials; and 3) provide corrective feedback and verbal reinforcement to highlight accurate patient responses. Continuous supervision during twice daily, 10-minute training sessions.	1. 90% accuracy on two consecutive visual sorting trials. 2. 90% accuracy on two consecutive tactile sorting trials. 3. 90% accuracy on two consecutive decision-making trials (i.e., "water" or "don't water").
Training sessions move to the general work area of the greenhouse. This expands the stimulus field to include extraneous, competing stimuli. Instructional posters recede into the background. Tools are stored in a centrally located cabinet and are not immediately available. Continuous 1:1 supervision. Presence of co-workers who attend to various greenhouse tasks.	Clinicians provided prompting, corrective feedback, and verbal reinforcement while patients practice perceptual discrimination, concept sorting, and decision-making skills. Clinicians then model required motor responses (i.e., watering greenhouse plants). Continuous supervision during twice daily, 10-minute training sessions.	1. 90% accuracy on several consecutive decision-making trials, (i.e., "water" or "don't water").
Same background features as Stage 2, but patients work in pairs. Interpersonal demands therefore increase. Supervision decreases as the clinician splits his or her attention between the two patients.	Same as Stage 2, but clinician also shapes behavioral responses. Verbal prompts are gradually faded as the patient demonstrates mastery. Frequency and duration change to a single 20-minute training session.	1. Twenty consecutive instances of appropriate judgment (i.e., "water" or "don't water") coupled with proper behavioral technique. 2. Ability to work cooperatively with co-workers.

(continued)

Table 15–1.   Environmental complexity in a vocational rehabilitation program: defining cognitive demands, external supports, and skills training techniques *(continued)*

Treatment stage	Work task(s)	Requisite skills
IV.	1. Water plants in the general work area with correct technique. 2. Refill empty containers. 3. Identify leaves that need pruning. 4. Appropriate interpersonal behavior with co-workers.	1–6. Cognitive-behavioral skills from Stage III 7. Cooperation with co-workers 8. Self-direction and initiative
V. (Highest complexity)	1. Water and prune in the outdoor garden. 2. Weed outdoor flower beds. 3. Harvest ripe vegetables. 4. Develop greater physical stamina. 5. Appropriate interpersonal behavior with co-workers and spectators.	1–7. Cognitive-behavioral skills from Stage IV 8. Planning, memory, and problem-solving operations

Environmental conditions	Training methods	Mastery criteria
Same background features as Stage 2, but patients are now given individual work assignments. Task demands now emphasize greater initiative and autonomy. Less supervision from clinicians increases the potential for peer interaction.	Shaping activities continue. Supervision and reinforcement schedules, however, change from continuous to intermittent. Length of session increases to 45 minutes.	1. Consistently appropriate judgments and behavioral responses. 2. Initiative and perseverance on work tasks. 3. Ability to work cooperatively with co-worker.
Work activities shift to an outdoor garden. The stimulus field expands to include variable climatic conditions as well as contact with spectators. Instructional posters are now absent. Tools and work materials are stored off-site.	Clinicians model the planning, problem solving, and behavioral operations necessary for outdoor gardening. Prompting helps to focus patient's attention. Verbal and concrete reinforcers shape task appropriate responses. Supervision is on an intermittent schedule.	1. Consistently appropriate judgments and behavioral responses. 2. Initiative and perseverance on work tasks. 3. Appropriate social skills with co-workers and spectators. 4. Expressed interest in other hospital- or community-based vocational endeavors.

training areas; and 7) instructional posters to foster attention and reduce memory requirements.

These conditions enable patients with pronounced attentional deficits to learn the sequential operations in watering greenhouse tomato plants (see Heinssen and Victor 1994, for a complete description of training procedures). Patients are taught to gather perceptual data ("Look at the soil"), to perform visual and tactile discrimination trials ("Is it light or dark? Moist or dry?"), and then to decide on appropriate behavioral responses ("Water it or walk away"). Proficiency at each skill is evaluated daily. When a patient reaches mastery criteria (column 6), he or she graduates to the next level of training.

The mix of external supports and distractors is modified in Stage 2 by relocating training sessions to the richer environment of the greenhouse open work area. This broadens the patient's stimulus field to include the presence of other workers and the noise and commotion they generate. The patient is required to exercise sustained and selective attention during decision-making exercises. Because instructional posters concurrently shift to the background, a more challenging learning atmosphere results.

Informational complexity is increased in subsequent stages by further altering the balance of supportive features and processing demands. In Stages 3–5, for example, work tasks become more complicated, social pressures intensify, and training sessions lengthen. At the same time prosthetic elements subside, supervision is curtailed, reinforcement lessens, and instructional posters disappear. Environmental complexity is high by the final stage of treatment and patients are required to sustain cognitive and behavioral performance in the relative chaos of an outdoor vegetable garden. If all goes well, the patient handles this novel milieu by applying newly acquired information processing and behavioral response skills.

Assessing the Impact of Environmental Interventions

Environmental conditions were arranged in the organic gardening program to regulate informational complexity over successive stages of treatment. The impact of these manipulations on patients' functioning is depicted in Figure 15–3. Outcome data were obtained from rehabilitation clinicians who rated each patient's work performance ("poor," "fair," or "good") on a variety of cognitive, behavioral, and social skills dimensions. Although the figure presents performance data for only three patients, it reflects prototypical variations in treatment response observed among the 38 alumni of the gardening project.

Baseline assessment indicated meager vocational assets for Mr. A., Mr. B., and Ms. C. All three had problems with routine gardening tasks such as soil mixing, seed planting, watering, leaf spraying, weeding, and pruning. Cognitive deficits also were common, although each person displayed a unique pattern of disability. Mr. A., a 29-year-old man, was the least impaired. His intelligence was in the low/average range, but poor concentration and idiosyncratic logic interfered with new learning. Mr. B., a 39-year-old man, possessed more serious cognitive limitations. His problems included perceptual difficulties, attentional deficits, restricted short-term memory, and concrete thinking. The third patient, a 34-year-old woman, fell between the extremes of Mr. A. and Mr. B. Although capable of learning new skills, Ms. C. displayed an impulsive response style that frequently spoiled her independent work efforts.

The performance data presented in Figure 15–3 indicates that all three patients progressed through the first three stages of treatment. Interestingly, each individual initially "slipped" in Stages 2 and 3 before targeted skills were mastered. This pattern of regression followed by accommodation most likely

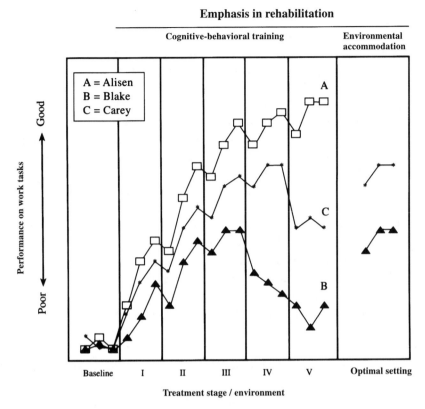

Figure 15–3. Performance data for patients Mr. A., Mr. B., and Ms. C. across five stages of vocational rehabilitation.

signals that an optimal balance was achieved between personal competencies and task demands. It is hypothesized that this particular profile identifies situations in which treatment conditions have been calibrated to stimulate growth, but not at the cost of debilitating stress.

The trajectories of the three patients begin to diverge in Stage 4. Mr. A. continues on a steady course of improvement and eventually attains all of the social and instrumental skills necessary to work in a horticultural setting. This individual's course represents the classic conceptualization of positive therapeutic outcome. Although significantly compromised before treatment, Mr. A. mastered a variety of cognitive and behavioral skills and used them productively in increasingly complicated work environments. By the end of therapy this patient focused his attention selectively, followed complicated directions, applied problem-solving strategies, and maintained his concentration for extended periods of time. Mr. A.'s ability to work independently in the outdoor garden demonstrated his readiness for further challenges. His vocational options included additional cognitive-behavior training in a more demanding setting or supported employment in the community. Approximately one-fifth (18%) of the patients enrolled in the organic gardening program have attained an outcome similar to Mr. A. and have pursued other vocational goals.

Unfortunately, such positive results are not universal, and many patients plateau before the final stage of treatment. Mr. B. and Ms. C. fall within this category and illustrate the phenomenon of partial therapeutic response. Mr. B., for example, mastered several processing challenges in Stages 1–3, including 1) the transition to a less structured work area; 2) a lengthened training session; and 3) the presence of a work partner. Performance did not decline until Stage 4, when supervision shifted to an intermittent schedule and the length of treatment sessions increased to 45 minutes. This suggests that environmental demands exceeded the patient's coping resources when prompting, encouragement, and social reinforcement from clinicians became less dependable and when greater endurance was required. Under these conditions Mr. B. was unable to focus on work tasks, to handle independent job assignments, or to work collaboratively with others. Given this patient's reliance on external structure, it is not surprising that deterioration continued in Stage 5, where situational demands necessitated an even greater degree of cognitive autonomy. Mr. B.'s profile of early plateau and subsequent deterioration has been observed for approximately one-quarter (26%) of the patients enrolled in the gardening project.

Similar ceiling effects were noted for Ms. C., but at a later point in rehabilitation. Ms. C. also advanced through the first three training environments, but contrary to Mr. B., she adjusted to the novel requirements of Stage 4. This person learned to 1) work on assigned tasks independently (e.g., "Water the plants in this section by yourself"); 2) coordinate her activities with co-workers ("Bring the empty water containers to Ellen so she can refill them"); and 3) move from task to task independently ("When you finish watering these plants, move on to the next section"). These accomplishments, however, were attained in the predictable environment of the greenhouse and did not generalize to the less structured conditions of the outdoor garden. Because executive operations could not be applied outside of the sheltered setting, it is surmised that Ms. C.'s processing threshold was surpassed by the multiple distractors of the Stage 5 milieu. This suggests that further vocational training with Ms. C. should occur in an environment similar to Stage 4. Ms. C. requires a rehabilitation setting that fosters self-directed behavior but limits input to a set of well-defined, predictable stimuli. More than one-half of the patients referred to the organic gardening program (55%) achieve outcomes that are similarly situation-specific.

Interpreting Heterogeneous Results in Retraining Programs

The significance of clinical case reports must be evaluated with caution, particularly when experimental controls are lacking. However, data from clinical trials often suggest interesting hypotheses that can guide subsequent empirical investigation. It is in this spirit that the accomplishments of Mr. A., Mr. B., and Ms. C. will be compared and implications will be drawn for contemporary models of cognitive rehabilitation.

The results obtained for the three patients reflect the diversity of outcome that is common among individuals who undergo cognitive retraining. Findings as disparate as these are perplexing and interpretation depends to a great extent on the reader's theoretical perspective. If one adheres to the cognitive remediation framework, these findings may prove disappointing because the majority of patients in therapy failed to achieve complete recovery. Only one individual mastered each of the skills in treatment. One could conclude that cognitive and behavior retraining was of limited value to most of the patients in the vocational rehabilitation program. Further analysis of outcome data suggests, however, that such a conclusion is premature and that all three patients represent varying degrees of treatment success.

To advocates of the environmental perspective, the findings reported in Figure 15–3 are intriguing. Overall, they are consistent with the hypothesis that adaptive behavior results when personal competencies and situational requirements are balanced. Mr. A., who possessed the most intact cognitive apparatus before treatment, was the only individual to move successfully through each stage of the training program. Mr. A.'s superior processing resources enabled him to learn new strategies for organizing information, resulting in steady progress through a series of challenging, but not overwhelming, learning situations. His outcome was clearly positive because he was able to combine new schemata and behavioral skills to form a more efficient vocational repertoire.

Of greater interest, however, are the accomplishments of Mr. B. and Ms. C., who registered therapeutic gains under specific environmental conditions. Progress for these individuals continued uninterrupted as long as personal competencies were equal to situational demands, but halted when environmental circumstances surpassed processing resources. Mr. B., who displayed the greatest degree of initial impairment, crested earliest in therapy. Ms. C. also displayed situation-specific competencies, although her relatively superior talents permitted treatment to progress. For both patients, however, therapeutic gains were related to external circumstances and achievements disappeared when environmental complexity increased beyond a tolerable level. Taken together, these results illustrate that treatment success often hinges on circumstances in the training milieu, particularly when environmental features are compensating for internal processing deficiencies.

It was proposed earlier that a "follow along" assessment strategy would allow clinicians greater control of the treatment process. In the present case this involves returning each patient to the training environment best matched to his or her capacities. Mr. B. would resume the continuous supervision provided in Stage 3, and Ms. C. would return to the protected indoor milieu of Stage 4. The results associated with these environmental interventions are presented in the final column of Figure 15–3, which illustrates the impact of reestablishing optimal therapeutic conditions on patients' functioning in the organic gardening program. In both instances performance rebounds soon after the patient returns to the training environment that is best suited to individual needs.

Once the patient is returned to the optimal learning situation, rehabilitation can follow either of two courses: 1) remediation procedures can be reinstituted in the hope that additional training will stimulate further improvement, or 2) environmental supports can be established to compensate for specific processing deficits. In the first category, environmental conditions could be adjusted to cushion the transition between treatment phases. Mr. B., for example, might progress further in vocational training if treatment settings were established to bridge the environmental conditions present in Stages 3 and 4. Such "micro adjustments" would reestablish the fit between personal competencies and training demands, thereby minimizing information overload and opening a broader window for the acquisition of internal structures.

While this strategy may be effective in some cases, in other instances cognitive problems will prove to be treatment refractory. For patients in this second category, the emphasis of rehabilitation must eventually shift from skills development to an environmental accommodation for chronic processing deficits. This tactic represents the second major approach to cognitive rehabilitation, that of environmental management to offset enduring cognitive limitations.

Establishing a Cognitive Exoskeleton

When cognitive retraining fails to promote full recovery, or when functioning plateaus at a suboptimal level, therapeutic efforts must shift from direct remediation to compensation for lost functions. The treatment goal becomes one of long-term support and containment in environments that minimize informational complexity and direct residual cognitive resources toward adaptive behavior. Because of the patient's limited internal capacity, processing requirements must be lessened in the areas of attention, planning, memory, and decision making. The milieu should be rearranged to execute these operations externally, thereby creating a cognitive exoskeleton that organizes behavior through prosthetic interventions.

The program that best operationalizes external information management is the social-learning system pioneered by Paul and Lentz (1977) for the rehabilitation of chronically ill schizophrenic patients. Those authors reported that persons with numerous cognitive deficits responded positively to a highly structured environmental treatment. Consequently, we launch our discussion of milieu-based interventions by analyzing the social-learning model advanced by Paul and colleagues.

The Social-Learning Milieu

Although the methods of social-learning programs have been described in detail (see Glynn and Mueser 1986, 1992 for excellent reviews), the value of this approach for cognitively impaired patients has not been fully recognized. The social-learning paradigm offers the best hope for establishing living and working environments that compensate for enduring cognitive disabilities. This is achieved through methods that continuously specify for patients what needs to be done, how tasks are to be accomplished, and when it is time to "shift gears" for new assignments.

Social-learning programs create facilitative processing conditions mainly by amplifying the environmental cues that promote adaptive behavior. This process begins by explicitly defining for patients expectations regarding social and work performance and the consequences for actions. This information is conveyed throughout the milieu by posting rules and guidelines in conspicuous places and by distributing concrete and social reinforcers contingently. A highly regimented schedule further highlights discriminative stimuli by specifying the time, the place, and the content of daily activities. In combination, external structures such as rules, schedules, and contingent reinforcement simplify information processing by 1) automatically screening information for patients; 2) narrowing the range of response options; and 3) providing clear incentives for adaptive functioning. There is little ambiguity in a social-learning program regarding appropriate behavioral responding.

The training methods and therapeutic interventions used in this system also help to conserve patients' cognitive resources. First, mastery opportunities are offered throughout the day at a steady, but not overwhelming, pace. This averts problems attributable to boredom and/or overstimulation. Second, target responses are divided into constituent elements to reduce the complexity of training tasks. This enables patients to apply their full concentration to smaller, more manageable challenges. Third, the moment-to-moment prompting and coaching provided by treatment personnel helps patients to focus attention, remember instructions, solve problems, and shift concentration to new tasks. The consistent responses of treatment personnel (who receive formal training in the principles and procedures of social-learning theory) reduce social processing demands. These features, taken together, help to allocate the patient's cognitive assets more efficiently, resulting in more effective information processing and behavioral output.

The features of the social-learning milieu combine to reduce patients' cognitive burdens by clarifying behavioral expectations, enriching discriminative stimuli, controlling situational demands, and regulating the actions of caretakers. The constancy of treatment activities and therapeutic interventions creates a stable, predictable environment that is ideally suited for patients with limited cognitive abilities (Sullivan et al. 1989). Paul and Lentz (1977) reported that social-learning procedures improved the cognitive, social, and instrumental responses of severely ill schizophrenic patients, resulting in increased functioning and greater levels of autonomy. Similarly organized programs have reported comparable results with other groups of mentally ill and cognitively impaired persons (Baker et al. 1977; Fullerton et al. 1978; McCreadie et al. 1978; Stoffelmayr et al. 1979; Turner and Luber 1980; Wong et al. 1986; Woods et al. 1984).

While the effectiveness of the social-learning approach is well documented, more than two decades have passed since Paul and Lentz formulated their particular rehabilitation model. Considerably more is known today about cognitive factors in human learning. Advances in computer and communication technology make therapeutic interventions possible that were unimaginable 20 years ago. Given these developments, it is likely that the prosthetic features of the social-learning milieu can be improved by augmenting traditional techniques with contemporary information management strategies. The following case example illustrates how this might be accomplished in an inpatient treatment setting.

Prosthetic Interventions in an Inpatient Milieu

Ms. J. is a 43-year-old woman with a diagnosis of chronic, undifferentiated schizophrenia. She became ill in her early 20s, having completed high school and one year of junior college. Her illness has been characterized by periodic episodes of psychosis and significant decline in social and instrumental functioning. She has never married or held a job. Ms. J.'s deteriorating course has necessitated many hospitalizations, frequently for long periods. At her most recent hospital admission she was underweight, disheveled, largely incoherent, and unable to perform basic self-care functions.

Because of her disorganized behavior, Ms. J. was admitted to an inpatient social-learning program. Neuroleptic medications were introduced to suppress psychotic symptoms and cognitive and behavioral competencies were assessed when hallucinations had abated. Neuropsychological evaluation revealed profound deficits in attention, memory, and abstract concept formation. Ms. J.'s only observed strength was understanding simple language, particularly written material. She performed best when directions were simple, when instructions were printed, and when tasks involved structured, concrete responses.

Based on these data, a rehabilitation plan was developed to accommodate Ms. J.'s numerous cognitive impairments. A program was initiated that reduced information processing demands, starting with a revised strategy for cultivating waking, washing, and dressing skills. A series of prosthetic interventions were introduced to structure Ms. J.'s responses, including prompts from staff members, external memory aids, and pre-recorded audiotaped instructions.

Each evening at 10 P.M. a staff member cued Ms. J to prepare for the next day's activities. She was escorted to her room and directed to the "Evening Routine" poster that listed a series of simple, concrete instructions. First, Ms. J. selected a clean set of clothes and laid them out in a prominent location. Coordinating her outfits was simplified by having color coded tags sewn into each piece of clothing. She was encouraged to "match the bars" when choosing the next day's garments.

Ms. J. and the staff member then set up her cassette recorder alarm clock. She was helped to load and rewind a pre-recorded "wake up tape" and to program the alarm mechanism. The staff member briefly reviewed what would transpire the next morning: "Ms. J., the alarm will go off at 7:15 and a taped message will instruct you to get up, wash your face, comb your hair, and then to put on these clean clothes. These instructions will be repeated every 30 seconds for 10 minutes. As soon as you've followed all of the directions you can go to the nursing office and turn in these tokens for your morning soda. But you have to be ready by 7:30, or else you'll lose the chance to get the soda." Ms. J. was then rewarded for her efforts and encouraged to shower and change into bedtime clothing. She was oriented to the "Independent Grooming Poster" in her bathroom and was reminded to complete each step in the personal hygiene program. Thirty minutes later, a staff member checked her progress and disbursed reinforcers for completed tasks. The wake up message was delivered approximately 9 hours after this final exchange of the day.

Concrete reinforcers were delivered contingently by day shift personnel who coupled verbal praise and encouragement with directions to proceed to breakfast.

Ms. J. was slow to establish a consistent morning routine. The taped message initially held little meaning for her and several weeks passed before preparatory activities were controlled by the alarm clock. It was necessary to use both associative learning and shaping procedures to establish the alarm clock as a reliable discriminative stimuli. In the early stages a staff member was positioned outside of her door with a soda. After the audiotaped message started, the staff member would enter Ms. J.'s room, make sure her eyes were open, and then disburse the soda: "You see, Ms. J., the tape went off and you woke up. So you've earned this soda as a reward. Now let's follow the instructions on the tape and get ready for the day." As Ms. J. slowly responded to this intervention, more effort was required of her before the soda was delivered. By using a strategy of successive approximation, the taped message gained the power to cue all three desired behaviors (i.e., waking, grooming, and dressing).

Although Ms. J. responded positively to this intervention, she did not complete wake up activities when audiotaped instructions were discontinued. Her performance rebounded when the taped message was re-introduced, suggesting that the pre-recorded directions compensated for internal deficits, most likely by highlighting discriminative stimuli, reducing memory requirements, and specifying a concrete plan of action. Similar environmental interventions were incorporated into other areas of Ms. J.'s rehabilitation program.

After breakfast, cues for adaptive behavior were delivered through various sources, including prompts from treatment personnel, a pocket calendar, and a programmable watch. Ms. J. organized her activities during a morning planning meeting where group leaders helped her to list appointments and responsibilities in a day calendar. Approximately eight training sessions were scheduled each day, along with individual self-care projects, interpersonal functioning, and vocational performance. Attendance at assigned activities was facilitated by a watch that produced an audible hourly signal (Sullivan et al. 1989). Ms. J. was taught to check her day calendar when she heard the tone and then proceed to her next designated activity. In the event that this process failed, staff members intervened with verbal prompts and instructions. Group leaders reinforced punctuality by providing immediate rewards or corrective feedback, depending on Ms. J.'s performance. Through these interventions, Ms. J. eventually attained an acceptable "on time" record (85%) for activities assigned to her in the rehabilitation program.

The schedule of well-defined activities helped to improve Ms. J.'s interpersonal performance by setting the time, the place, and the content of social interactions (Abreu and Toglia 1987). Group leaders preserved conceptual clarity during training sessions by rewarding patients who remained "on task" and censoring those who drifted from identified topics. Ms. J. benefited from this structured approach and became more communicative during group meetings. Her verbal responses became better organized, but remained so only as long as the conversational topic was clearly defined. Group leaders reported that Ms. J. relied on posters and verbal prompts to maintain her concentration and that her interpersonal performance suffered whenever these "props" were removed. External supports proved particularly important in the vocational setting, where Ms. J. was easily distracted by the activities of co-workers. Performance was assisted in this instance by designing a separate work cubicle that featured posted instructions, concrete tasks, and intermittent reinforcement from supervisors.

After 1 year in treatment Ms. J. had noticeably improved. She could groom herself, care for her room, clean her laundry, and cook a simple meal. She enrolled in a sheltered vocational training program and mastered several simple jobs related to furniture repair. However, her achievements were related to the prosthetic features of the social-learning environment and her performance declined whenever independent planning and self-direction were required. She quickly deteriorated in these situations, which suggested a continued need for externally organizing systems.

Like Ms. J., many patients with enduring cognitive limitations require long-term support in institutional programs that regulate behavior through external means. Environmental interventions, characterized by an enriched system of cognitive props, enable these individuals to achieve a level of functioning that would otherwise be impossible. More self-sufficient patients may show a similar reliance on information processing aids to remain independent in the community. The prosthetic features of inpatient social-learning programs may be transferred to halfway houses, group homes, or private apartments to sustain patients' adaptive functioning.

Conclusions

The results achieved by these four Chestnut Lodge patients illustrate the heterogeneity of outcome that characterizes cognitive rehabilitation. Like Mr. A., (Figure 15–3) certain patients respond well to remediation efforts and learn to compensate for cognitive difficulties with new strategies for organizing and processing information. Accumulating data suggest, however, that such positive results are not universal and that certain cognitive deficits do not respond to remediation procedures (Butler and Namerow 1988; Miller 1992; Tankle

1988). For patients in this category, environmental interventions offer an alternate method for managing cognitive limitations. Rather than change the person, environmental treatments facilitate information processing by modifying features of the milieu. The results obtained by Ms. J. illustrate that such interventions offer long-term benefits to patients who experience permanent cognitive disabilities.

The mixed results of remediation programs, combined with the clinical cases presented in this chapter, argue for a broader conceptualization of cognitive rehabilitation. As the clinical data for Mr. A., Mr. B., and Ms. C. demonstrate, remediation procedures and environmental interventions are not antithetical treatments. Cognitive skills training and environmental engineering represent complementary strategies in a "stage model" of rehabilitation. According to this scheme, remediation procedures receive greater emphasis early in treatment because more effective cognitive functioning augurs for better overall adjustment. Environmental interventions are used in this phase to calibrate processing demands to match the patient's limited endurance. As treatment proceeds, environmental manipulations help to sharpen the patient's emerging cognitive skill and to determine the extent of recovery. In the final stages of rehabilitation, environmental treatments supplant remediation procedures as the focus of rehabilitation shifts from skills acquisition to long-term management of chronic processing deficits.

For patients who require ongoing cognitive support, containment in a well-regulated environment is the best therapeutic alternative. Asylum may be forever necessary for these severely impaired individuals. This does not mean, however, that asylum must assume the quality of custodial care. Although deficits may be irreversible, treatment remains active, with the goal of increasing the patient's autonomy within the protective milieu. Creating an environment that adapts to the patient's deficiencies can liberate what functional capacities do exist and allows the patient to experience further change and growth. As a result, the cognitive exoskeleton better prepares individuals to care for themselves and to interact with others with self-respect and dignity. The satisfaction in regaining even some lost ground can improve the quality of life not only for patients, but also for those who live and work with them.

References

Abreu BC, Toglia JP: Cognitive rehabilitation: a model for occupational therapy. Am J Occup Ther 41:439–448, 1987

Anthony WA: Principles of Psychiatric Rehabilitation. Baltimore, MD, University Park Press, 1979

Anthony WA, Liberman RP: The practice of psychiatric rehabilitation. Schizophr Bull 12:542–559, 1986

Anthony WA, Liberman RP: Principles and practice of psychiatric rehabilitation, in Handbook of Psychiatric Rehabilitation. Edited by Liberman RP. New York, Macmillan, 1992, pp 1–29

Anthony WA, Cohen M, Cohen B: The philosophy, treatment process and principles of the psychiatric rehabilitation approach. New Dir Men Health Serv 17:67–79, 1983

Baker R, Hall JK, Hutchinson K, et al: Symptom changes in chronic schizophrenic patients on a token economy: a controlled experiment. Br J Psychiatry 131:381–393, 1977

Benedict RHB: The effectiveness of cognitive remediation strategies for victims of traumatic head-injury: a review of the literature. Clinical Psychology Review 9:605–626, 1989

Bottcher SA: Cognitive retraining: a nursing approach to rehabilitation of the brain injured. Nurs Clin North Am 24:193–208, 1989

Brenner HD: On the importance of cognitive disorders in treatment and rehabilitation, in Psychosocial Treatment of Schizophrenia: Multidimensional Concepts, Psychological, Family, and Self-Help Perspectives. Edited by Strauss JS, Boker W, Brenner HD. Toronto, Ontario, Huber, 1987, pp 136–151

Butler RW, Namerow NS: Cognitive retraining in brain-injury rehabilitation: a critical review. Journal of Neurologic Rehabilitation 2:97–109, 1988

Dauwalder JP, Hoffman H: Ecological vocational training. New Dir Ment Health Serv 53:79–86, 1992

Diamant JJ: Specific features of cognitive rehabilitation of psychiatric patients. Cognitive Rehabilitation 4:12–16, 1986

Freeman, H. Relationship of schizophrenia to the environment. Br J Psychiatry 155: 90–99, 1989

Fullerton DI, Cayner JJ, McLaughlin-Reidel T: Results of a token economy. Arch Gen Psychiatry 35:1451–1453, 1978

Glisky EL, Schacter DL: Acquisition of domain-specific knowledge in patients with organic memory disorders. J Learn Disabil 21:333–351, 1988

Glynn SM, Mueser KT: Social learning for chronic mental inpatients. Schizophr Bull 12:648–668, 1986

Glynn SM, Mueser KT: Social-learning programs, in Handbook of Psychiatric Rehabilitation. Edited by Liberman RP. New York, Macmillan, 1992, pp 127–152

Godfrey HPD, Knight RG: Interventions for amnesics: a review. Br J Clin Psychol 26:83–91, 1987

Green MF: Information processing in schizophrenia, in Schizophrenia: An Overview and Practical Handbook. Edited by Kavanagh D. London, Chapman & Hall, 1992, pp 45–58

Green MF, Nuechterlein KH, Gaier DJ: Sustained and selective attention in schizophrenia, in Progress in Experimental Personality and Psychopathology Research. Edited by Walker EF, Dworkin RH, Cornblatt BA. New York, Springer, 1992, pp 290–313

Hayden ME, Hart T: Rehabilitation of cognitive and behavioral dysfunction in head injury. Adv Psychosom Med 16:194–229, 1986

Heinssen RK, Victor BJ: Cognitive-behavioral treatments for schizophrenia: evolving rehabilitation techniques, in Cognitive Technology in Psychiatric Rehabilitation. Edited by Spaulding W. Lincoln, University of Nebraska Press, 1994, pp 159–181

Henry K: Cognitive rehabilitation and the head-injured child. Journal of Children in Contemporary Society 16:189–205, 1983

Incagnoli T, Newman B: Cognitive and behavioral rehabilitation interventions. International Journal of Clinical Neuropsychology 7:173–182, 1985

Jeffrey DL: Cognitive clarity: key to motivation in rehabilitation. J Rehabil 47:33–35, 1981

Kahneman D: Attention and Effort. Englewood Cliffs, NJ, Prentice-Hall, 1973

Kreutzer JS, Gordon WA, Wehman P: Cognitive remediation following traumatic brain injury. Rehabilitation Psychology 34:117–130, 1989

Liberman RP, Evans CC: Behavior rehabilitation for chronic mental patients. Journal of Clinical Psychopharmacology 5:8S–14S, 1985

Liberman RP, Nuechterlein KH, Wallace CJ: Social skills training and the nature of schizophrenia, in Social Skills Training: A Practical Handbook for Assessment and Treatment. Edited by Curran JP, Monti PM. New York, Guilford, 1982, pp 5–56

Liberman RP, Mueser KT, Wallace CJ, et al: Training skills in the psychiatrically disabled: learning coping and competence. Schizophr Bull 12:631–647, 1986

Linn MW, Klett CJ, Caffey EM: Foster home characteristics and psychiatric patient outcome. Arch Gen Psychiatry 37:129–132, 1980

Livneh H: Psychiatric rehabilitation: a dialogue with Bill Anthony. Journal of Counseling and Development 63:86–90, 1984

McCreadie RG, Main CJ, Dunlap RA: Token economy, pimozide, and chronic schizophrenia. Br J Psychiatry 133:179–181, 1978

McGlashan TH, Heinssen RK, Fenton WS: Psychosocial treatment of negative symptoms in schizophrenia, in Modern Problems in Pharmacopsychiatry: Vol 24 Schizophrenia: Positive and Negative Symptoms and Syndromes. Edited by Andreasen NC. Basel, Switzerland, Karger, 1990, pp 175–200

Miller E: Psychological approaches to the management of memory impairments. Br J Psychiatry 160:1–6, 1992

Namerow NS: Cognitive and behavioral aspects of brain-injury rehabilitation. Neurol Clin 5:569–583, 1987

Nuechterlein K, Dawson M: Information processing and attentional functioning in the developmental course of schizophrenic disorders. Schizophr Bull 10:160–203, 1984

Paul GL, Lentz R: Psychosocial Treatment of Chronic Mental Patients. Cambridge, MA, Harvard University Press, 1977

Pollack IW, Kohn H, Miller MH: Rehabilitation of cognitive function in brain-damaged persons. J Med Soc N J 81:311–315, 1984

Sommers I: The influence of environmental factors on the community: adjustment of the mentally ill. J Nerv Ment Dis 176:221–226, 1988

Stoffelmayr BE, Faulkner GE, Mitchell WS: The comparison of token economy and social therapy in the treatment of hard-core schizophrenic patients. Behavior Analysis and Modification 3:3–17, 1979

Sullivan MJL, Dehoux E, Buchanan DC: An approach to cognitive rehabilitation in multiple sclerosis. Canadian Journal of Rehabilitation 3:77–85, 1989

Tankle RS: Application of neuropsychological test results to interdisciplinary cognitive rehabilitation with head-injured adults. Journal of Head Trauma Rehabilitation 3:24–32, 1988

Turner SM, Luber RF: The token economy in day hospital settings: contingency management or information feedback. J Behav Ther Exp Psychiatry 11:89–94, 1980

Westling DL, Floyd J: Generalization of community skills: how much training is necessary? Journal of Special Education 23:386–406, 1990

Wong SE, Massel HK, Mosk MD, et al: Behavioral approaches to the treatment of schizophrenia, in Handbook of Studies on Schizophrenia. Edited by Burrows GD, Norman TR, Rubenstein G. Amsterdam, The Netherlands, Elsevier Science, 1986, pp 79–100

Woods PA, Higson PJ, Tannahill MM: Token economy programmes with chronic psychiatric patients: the importance of direct measurement and objective evaluation for long-term maintenance. Behav Res Ther 22:41–51, 1984

Chapter 16

Cognitive Rehabilitation and Interactive Video

Judith Waters, Ph.D., and George Ellis, M.A.

The development of the personal computer in the late 1970s generated a vast technological revolution first in the United States and then more slowly around the world. These new compact machines offered almost the same technology that was previously only possible with the use of very large and expensive mainframe computers. Consequently, computer technology became available to many segments of the population (e.g., small businesses, educational institutions, the medical profession) whose opportunities to use its broad applications had previously been limited.

Cognitive rehabilitation specialists recognized the potential of personal computers for assisting in treatment programs. One of the first computer-assisted treatment applications was the use of interactive video games. The rationale for this approach was developed by Lynch at the Palo Alto Veterans Affairs Medical Center. He noted that video games tapped some of the same cognitive abilities that he was trying to rehabilitate in his patients by other means. Eventually Lynch (1983) devised a study to see whether playing video games aided in the remediation of cognitive deficits. Although the results of his study indicated only marginal effectiveness, Lynch's research set the stage for other studies that attempted to demonstrate the efficacy of this treatment approach (Bracy 1983; Drew and Waters 1986; Larose et al. 1989; Middleton et al. 1991; Owen 1986; Robertson et al. 1988; Ruff et al. 1989).

Several factors contributed to the proliferation of video games as a treatment tool, the first of these being their inherent motivational quality. Before video games were actually incorporated into cognitive rehabilitation programs, researchers had already found evidence that teenagers were fascinated by arcade-type video games (Loftus and Loftus 1983). It was quickly hypothesized that the intrinsic attraction might be useful for working with other populations such as elderly persons and patients with closed head injuries. When video games were first introduced into cognitive rehabilitation, it was shown that patients tended to practice more often and for longer periods than they did with other traditional therapeutic approaches. Consequently, it was expected that long-term outcomes would improve.

Another perceived advantage of incorporating interactive video games into treatment was their cost-effectiveness. For example, it was anticipated that there would be less need for clinicians to spend long periods of time instructing patients in how to play the games because video games were thought to be easy both to learn and to use. Also, the use of these games seemed to have "face validity," with both popular and professional appeal.

The first software specifically designed for cognitive rehabilitation focused on attention, reaction time, perceptual-motor skills, memory, problem solving, and reasoning (Lynch 1992). Previous cognitive rehabilitation programs frequently involved paper-and-pencil drills and practice in an attempt to restore cognitive deficits. These programs were frequently based on a *building block theory*, which postulates that an individual must begin by working on basic cognitive processes before he or she can proceed to more complex tasks.

It was thought that the skills acquired in computer-assisted cognitive rehabilitation (CACR) would generalize to specified activities of daily living (Bracy 1986). Unfortunately, because the research frequently involved a small number of subjects and lacked control groups, the outcomes were difficult to evaluate. Evidence of improvement in performance on typical daily tasks (ecological validity) was largely anecdotal or based on self-report. Although the most recent trend in thinking is away from the building block theory, there is still strong support in many quarters for the concept that many patients need to begin with simple processes that virtually guarantee success and progress to the increasingly complex tasks (see Table 16–1).

Division 40 of the American Psychological Association, which is devoted to the study and application of theory in neuropsychology, formulated a set of guidelines for the use of interactive videos in therapy. Among their prescriptions is the recognition that any form of cognitive rehabilitation must be ecologically valid (i.e., generalize to functioning in typical activities of daily living) to warrant its inclusion in a treatment plan (Matthews et al. 1991) (see Table 16–2).

Current Use of Interactive Videos in Cognitive Rehabilitation

The development of an individual program for each patient is based on the results of a neurological assessment battery. The use of selected software along with traditional training in activities of daily living should produce positive results in patients who have been evaluated as appropriate for this type of cognitive rehabilitation. Much of the currently available cognitive rehabilitation software focuses on the need to practice a variety of tasks, including reaction

Table 16–1. Building block theory of cognitive rehabilitation

1. **Accurately sense from the environmental and bodily cues.** This implies that receptors, nerve pathways and primary cortical areas are intact and functioning properly.

2. **Attend to sensory information.** Attending here refers to general awareness such as discomfort, heat, or irritation. Conscious thought might not be involved but a response may be emitted in reaction to the simulation.

3. **Focus on sensory input.** This implies an attentional focus, a more conscious process.

4. **Maintain that focus for an extended period.** Although an extremely attractive stimulus may magnetically produce sustained attention, this refers more to attention maintained by the effort of the individual.

5. **Extract detail from the information sensed.** A quantitative and qualitative analysis are implied. The entire stimulus situation provides a gestalt from which details must be discerned and processed so the information can be useful.

6. **Attach meaning to sensory input.** This infers a process of comparison of the gestalt and details of the current situation with those details experienced previously to determine novelty, familiarity, recognition, etc.; in short, perception.

7. **Attend to multiple stimuli simultaneously.** Until this point reference has been to basic processes conducted on a single stimulus. This is a giant step in that at this point events one through six are occurring simultaneously for many stimulus situations that also are constantly occurring simultaneously.

8. **Shift from detail to detail spatially.** At any one moment in time numerous stimuli are impinging on the nervous system both internally and externally. The individual must attend to the spatial gestalt formed by a particular stimulus, picking out and relating to details presented simultaneously (i.e., such as one frame of a movie film).

9. **Shift from stimulus to stimulus spatially.** This is similar to number eight but much larger in scope as the whole process must be simultaneously occurring for many simultaneously occurring stimuli.

10. **Track from detail to detail temporally.** Every detail of each stimulus is linked in time to the details of the next moment in time. The process occurring in step eight occurs at a single frozen moment. Process ten involves linking together the details of differing moments such that relationships are perceived and evolving situations are recognized.

11. **Track from stimulus to stimulus temporally.** This is a more complex process than number ten in that it involves performing those processes mentioned in ten for many stimuli, resulting in a higher level of information integration.

(continued)

Table 16–1.   Building block theory of cognitive rehabilitation *(continued)*

12. **Relate information temporally and spatially.** This is a further evolution of the last four (8–11) processes in that relationships perceived spatially and temporally are integrated.

13. **Integrate new with stored information.** This is considered a high level perception in which information currently being processed is further compared and integrated with past learning, experiences, etc. Memory skills come into play in a much greater way.

14. **Integrate different sensory input.** Processes 1–13 may be completed within single sensory areas. This process implies the combination and integration of the information from many or all of the sensory areas.

15. **Integrate perceptions.** This is a higher level process by which the perceptions formed, based upon single sensory mechanisms, are integrated to form one general gestalt encompassing the total stimulus situation.

16. **Form new concepts from analysis of current input and stored information.** This involves some level of abstraction, the ability to generate hypotheses and the ability to predict and suppose when data are not complete.

17. **Generate programs of action.** Motor programming of responses is implied. This involves preparing for both the content of the response and the motor actions necessary to convey that content.

18. **Coordinate programs temporally and execute sequentially.** Apraxic behavior would be an example of a breakdown in this process area.

19. **Control muscle activity (to initiate and inhibit).** On a basic level, this simply refers to the ability to carry out a motor action or to stop that action. On a higher level it also refers to an executive type control over whether or not what is in thought actually gets executed.

20. **Monitor behavior and compare against program.** This involves analysis of sensory input from both internal and external sources for the purpose of facilitating the execution of the motor program.

21. **Alter behavior to maintain the program.** This refers to the ability to alter a response sufficiently to keep it within the plan if the motor response being executed is deviating in any way from the planned program. The deviation could be produced by effects of environmental conditions or impaired ability to perform the planned program.

22. **Profit from feedback to maintain or alter the program.** This involves analysis and monitoring of the execution of a motor response on a higher level. The analysis determines if the response begin executed is having the desired effect on the environmental or stimulus situation. If it is not having that effect, this information is utilized to alter the motor program.

23. **Store information, program, consequences, alternatives, conclusions.** This involves organizing information, encoding it, and placing it in memory.

24. **Retrieve stored information.** This implies a higher level memory function than referred to in number 16 above. Conscious recall and the ability to verbalize past events, old information, etc., is implied.

Source. Reprinted from Bracy OL: "Cognitive Rehabilitation: A Process Approach." *Journal of Cognitive Rehabilitation* 4:10–17, 1986.

time and language, visuospatial, numerical, and reasoning skills. The efficacy of each program, however, still depends on the capability of the therapist, the quality of the tools, and the interaction of the program with specific patient variables. The therapist cannot expect positive outcomes if the patient cannot or will not sustain the effort or does not have the support of family and friends.

Lynch (1992) made a distinction between two principal models of treatment that use training tasks: the restorative model and the compensatory model. The restorative model assumes that skill improvement is derived from repeated practice with a particular type of software program. The model does not seem appropriate for all skills. For example, drill and practice alone do not constitute an effective strategy for rehabilitating memory deficits. The compensatory model is based on the premise that software should be designed to teach alternative strategies that will substitute or compensate for cognitive deficits. This model uses software to demonstrate various situations in which memory may be acquired and thus allows the patient to learn and practice memory techniques in a context bearing greater resemblance to some setting of everyday life. Unfortunately, studies of the restorative model generally yielded negative results (Lynch 1992). Because no theory is better than its implementation, we include a brief discussion of equipment next.

Discs or Tapes

Petty and Rosen (1987) evaluated the relative advantages of videodiscs versus videotapes. They came to the conclusion that the long-term advantages provided by discs outweigh the cost differential—discs being more expensive than tapes. Videodiscs have excellent image quality and the ability to hold still frames without damage to the disc itself. In addition, they have superior audio characteristics.

Lynch (1992) saw some promise in the use of the interactive videodisc for ecologically valid cognitive rehabilitation. He described the typical interactive videodisc system as a "specifically configured videodisc player, . . . a personal computer, . . . and one or two color display screens" (p. 43). Either still images or full-motion videos may be presented. The impressive storage capacity of interactive videodiscs enables the program to access 54,000 separate pictures

Table 16–2. Sample of Division 40 Guidelines for the use of computer technology in cognitive rehabilitation

---

Issue 1. Does computer-assisted cognitive rehabilitation have a role in the practice of clinical neuropsychology?

Resolutions:

1.1 Computer-assisted rehabilitation procedures appear to have a sufficient number of practical advantages and potential benefits to encourage the continued experimental investigation, further development, and empirical validation.

1.2 Appropriate clinical use of computer software in rehabilitation is dependent on maintaining a clear distinction between software being properly viewed as a component in an organized treatment program versus being improperly viewed as treatment itself.

Issue 2. What is the evidence for the efficacy of computer-assisted neuropsychological rehabilitation and cognitive remediation?

Resolutions:

2.1 In view of the absence of evidence for the efficacy of memory drills for the purpose of generalizable memory improvement, there appears to be no empirical justification for clinical use of computers to these ends.

2.2 The use of computers to teach mnemonic tasks, as external aids, and as supports for employment appears to have more realistic and promising prospects, although much more research is needed before confident deployment in the clinical realm is justified.

2.3 The efficacy of cognitive rehabilitation techniques should be evaluated in terms of the specific cognitive domains under study. Thus, negative findings in the domain of memory should not be unfairly generalized to more redeemable deficits in other areas (e.g., visuoperceptual disorders, attention). This implies that comprehensive neuropsychological examinations using reliable and valid tests at strategic points independent of training content are an essential component of such programs of development. Standardized psychological and neuropsychological tests should not be used in cognitive remediation exercises or therapy.

2.4 Results of investigations based on less ideal research designs should not be subjected to pejorative dismissal if the limitations of such designs are explicitly stated by the investigator and appropriately modest conclusions are offered. Many clinical settings and difficult clinical questions may not lend themselves to rigorous experimental research, but such considerations should not limit continuing investigation using other scientific methodologies (e.g., single case design, systematic clinical observations). At the same time, reports of efficacy based on uncontrolled case or cohort studies, testimonials, or anecdotal findings are unacceptable evidence of efficacy.

2.5 The Discussion and Resolutions offered under issue 2 should be reviewed on a regular basis (e.g., every 5 years) and updated as required, based on new research findings.

For a complete list of Division 40's guidelines for cognitive rehabilitation please see: Matthews CG, Harley JP, Malec JF: Guidelines for computer-assisted neuropsychological rehabilitation and cognitive remediation. The Clinical Neuropsychologist 5:3–19, 1991

Source. From Matthews CG, Harley JP, Malec JF: "Guidelines for Computer-Assisted Neuropsychological Rehabilitation and Cognitive Remediation." *The Clinical Neuropsychologist* 5:3–19, 1991. Reprinted with permission from Swets Publishing Service.

or frames in no more than 1 or 2 seconds. Thus, the patient or therapist can move from one sequence to another without the search lag time that occurs with videotapes.

Lynch completed an interactive videodisc prototype with the capability to assess and treat memory deficits. He wrote that the clinician can establish parameters and present environments that will require patients to use their memory skills in a more dynamic fashion than was possible with previous programs. A person can be put in a situation where he or she meets other people, orders food, or gets directions to a location. He or she can be required to recall this information immediately or after some delay. Feedback for incorrect responses includes use of graded cues, prompts, and a multiple-choice paradigm. This type of system appears to be ecologically valid not only for training but also for assessment.

Home-Based Computer-Assisted Therapy

CACR at home has distinct advantages over traditional independent therapy tasks such as notebook exercises because it can offer stimuli with various levels of difficulty in endless repetition and can provide feedback in the absence of a therapist (Purdy and Neri 1989). However, some very important considerations must be taken into account before patients can begin to use interactive videos at home. For example, the therapist must be careful to select only those patients who can benefit from the procedure and who will not be put at risk. Purdy and Neri suggested that home-based computer-assisted therapy is appropriate for individuals who are capable of relatively independent work and who can sustain attention to the tasks. The patients also must be able to learn the tasks during the therapeutic session and then transfer that learning to the home situation. The patients must be sufficiently intact to acquire the computer skills necessary to use the equipment, and they need the motor skills and the visual and auditory acuity to make the most of the process. Semi-independent patients would require assistance, such as the aid of family members, friends, or volunteers who would be willing to be responsible for the tasks that the patient cannot perform alone. The patient's assistant must be aware of the goals of the program, know how to use a computer, and be trained to support the patient as required but not to take over the tasks completely. These are not inconsequential considerations.

Bracy (1992) formulated a set of rules for the home use of therapeutic interventions. His patients are required to attend formal sessions in the clinic once a week. During those sessions, the clinicians present therapy tasks to their patients and observe their ability to perform the assignment. Clinicians then provide the patients with a home prescription written in detail and a diskette containing the exercises. The patients must, of course, have easy access to computers. Bracy expects patients to be able to complete three sessions per day (1 hour each), 7 days per week. The usual term of therapy is from 12 to 14 months. Data from home sessions are stored and analyzed to monitor the progress of the patients. Although it is reasonable to expect some schedule conflicts (e.g., vacations, visitors), strict adherence to the program is critical.

Other Qualities of Computer-Assisted Cognitive Rehabilitation

According to Le Fever (1984), well-designed CACR programs should include the following components:

1. Repeated opportunities for the patient to confront the facts of his or her disabilities, to learn in detail what they are and what they are not, and to learn what assets he or she has available for new ways of coping.
2. Opportunities to cope with numerous problems in a setting that minimizes the anxiety or frustration these problems might elicit if the patient confronted them alone.
3. Opportunities to go beyond initial emotional reactions to problems, so that the patient's own observations and experiments, assisted by sympathetic but skilled observers, will give him or her the best chance of discovering new ways of working within limitations and drawing on hidden strengths.

4. A setting in which the patient may grow, not necessarily in perceptual or cognitive abilities as strictly defined, but in ability to use what he or she has.

5. A chance for the patient to grow more competent to cope with problems because of increased self-knowledge, self-mastery, and self-confidence based on a realistic understanding of what he or she can and cannot do, with the wisdom and willingness to seek help when appropriate.

Research Problems

Early published research, including both experimental designs and single and multiple case studies, supported the contention that cognitive rehabilitation could facilitate improvement in perceptual-motor functioning in patients who had brain damage caused by accidents, strokes, or other head traumas (Lynch 1992). Many of these experiments, however, were no more than demonstrations because they did not involve appropriate control groups or random assignment of subjects. One project that did use both random assignment and a control group only had 12 subjects (Drew and Waters 1986). Trying to establish equivalent groups by matching patients or using random assignment is almost impossible in any but the largest facilities that serve brain-injured patients (e.g., Veterans Administration hospitals). Malec et al. (1984) pointed out that experimental research with brain-injured patients is particularly difficult due to the "uneven and unpredictable manner in which cognitive abilities improve during the months following brain injury" (p. 18). Even within the same individual, the various cognitive abilities recover at different rates.

Dismantling research designs should be considered, in which the relative efficacy of the various components of rehabilitation strategies is related to outcomes attributed to the total rehabilitation package. Finally, as previously stated, research must examine the generalizability of CACR to ensure that the gains observed on computerized microtasks are transferred to functions that are relevant in the real world.

Virtual Reality and Cognitive Rehabilitation

Virtual reality (VR) is a recent innovation in computer technology that may hold much promise for expanding the use of interactive videos in cognitive rehabilitation and for overcoming some of the shortcomings specified earlier. VR is a type of computer system that seems to transport people into a three-dimensional alternate environment in which they can interact freely using all of their available senses and mobility but without any physical dangers. Rheingold (1991) described the essence of VR best:

Imagine a wraparound television with three-dimensional programs, including three-dimensional sound, and solid objects that you can pick up and manipulate, even feel with your fingers and hands. Imagine immersing yourself in an artificial world and actively exploring it, rather than peering in at it from a fixed perspective through a flat screen in a movie theater, on a television set, or on a computer display. (p. 16)

Presently, VR systems use true stereoscopic three-dimensional displays and audio equipment. Specially designed gloves, head sets, and body suits allow the user to interact with the system. As Lavroff (1992) wrote, "The input devices are no longer simple joysticks or mice. Now your head, arms, and body are the input devices" (p. vi). To design an application, the programmer must compute the various positions of the head (its elevation, roll, and azimuth) and then use "changes in multiple readings to compute vectored motion and velocity for all these parts of your body" (p. vi).

VR introduces the computer as "a mediator or imagination enhancer" in that it manages data from multiple sources to create the illusion of other environments (Lavroff 1992). The individual soon feels as if he or she is actually moving within a simulated world—not merely observing it on the screen. The head-mounted display makes use of the concept of binocular disparity to establish a sense of occupying three-dimensional space.

Although this description of VR technology sounds promising, it is still in the early stages of development, and few actual applications for the field of rehabilitation have been designed and implemented. Because of this problem, most of the literature has been speculative, focusing primarily on the possible future uses of VR in rehabilitation. When this technology is fully developed, it will provide a controlled environment where patients will be able to practice various activities without endangering themselves physically or emotionally.

Research in the field of VR has been limited for several reasons. One of the problems with a VR system is its "dependence on complicated (and expensive) hardware" (Lavroff 1992, p. vii). Cognitive rehabilitation patients would most probably use a desktop system, which is basically a personal computer with specially designed hardware and software. Such a home system could cost more than $15,000. The more effective systems with head-mounted displays and glove input devices are priced higher than of $50,000. This estimate does not include the software for the rehabilitation program or the salaries of the staff needed to operate the equipment and work with the patient.

The Human Component of CACR

For the most part, the focus has been on the theories behind CACR and the development of promising systems and software, while delaying discussion of a very important element in cognitive rehabilitation—the human factor. It is now time to turn to the psychological issues associated with designing, initiating, and maintaining cognitive rehabilitation programs.

Not everyone in the field of cognitive rehabilitation has jumped on the computer bandwagon. Some therapists are as computer phobic as many members of the general population. Other clinicians feel that they do not have the time or resources for the necessary training and equipment, even if they are interested in learning the techniques. Still others maintain their faith in more traditional methods that do not incorporate CACR. There also are professionals who worry that their patients will not respond well to either the concept or the reality of CACR treatment technology. A sizable number is concerned that the human relationships that clinicians strive so hard to establish will be negatively influenced by the introduction of CACR into their treatment programs.

Summary

Despite some limitations, CACR has several benefits that, when incorporated into a well designed treatment program, should augment the rehabilitation process significantly. For example, CACR provides multiple iterations of a cognitive task in an unchanging format. CACR feedback is continuous, without contingencies changing because of fatigue. Moreover, computer-phobic therapists will find that CACR is not as threatening as they expect when they become familiar with the technology. Cost, of course, remains a serious issue.

As the end of the 20th century looms, computer technology continues to evolve at an incredible rate. Although this technology has been embraced warily by some and rejected by others, it is indisputable that the creative potential of the computer will continue to provide us with a medium to develop many types of therapeutic interventions that would not otherwise be possible. R. Gianutsos (1992) wrote:

> Technology is certain to remain important for cognitive rehabilitation, and the challenge for professionals is to harness the power it offers. Computers are the ultimate in flexibility: They are readily modifiable and completely docile. They inspire us to act to mold them to our purposes, recognizing that they may change us while we change them. (p. 68)

References

Bracy OL: Computer-based cognitive rehabilitation. Cognitive Rehabilitation 1:7–8, 18, 1983

Bracy OL: Cognitive rehabilitation: a process approach. Cognitive Rehabilitation 4:10–17, 1986

Bracy OL: My personal computer, my personal assistant. Computer Assisted Rehabilitation Therapy 1:3–6, 1992

Drew B, Waters J: Video games: utilization of a novel strategy to improve perceptual motor skills and cognitive functioning in the non-institutionalized elderly. Cognitive Rehabilitation 4:26–31, 1986

Gianutsos R: The computer in cognitive rehabilitation: it's not just a tool anymore. Journal of Head Trauma Rehabilitation 7:61–69, 1992

Larose S, Gagnon S, Ferland C, et al: Psychology of computers, XIV: cognitive rehabilitation through computer games. Percept Mot Skills 69:851–858, 1989

Lavroff N: Virtual Reality Playhouse. Corte Madera, CA, Waite Group Press, 1992

Le Fever FF: A neuropsychological look at cognitive rehabilitation, in Head Injury: Help, Hope, and Information. Albany, NY, State Head Injury Association, 1984, pp 145–172

Loftus GR, Loftus EF: Mind at Play: The Psychology of Video Games. New York, Basic Books, 1983

Lynch W: Cognitive retraining using microcomputer games and commercially available software. Cognitive Rehabilitation 1:19–22, 1983

Lynch W: Ecological validity of cognitive rehabilitation software. Journal of Head Trauma Rehabilitation 7:36–45, 1992

Malec J, Jones R, Rao N, et al: Video game practice effects on sustained attention in patients with craniocerebral trauma. Cognitive Rehabilitation 2: 18–23, 1984

Matthews CG, Harley JP, Malec JF: Guidelines for computer-assisted neuropsychological rehabilitation and cognitive remediation. The Clinical Neuropsychologist 5:3–19, 1991

Middleton DK, Lambert MJ, Seggar LB: Neuropsychological rehabilitation: microcomputer–assisted treatment of brain injured adults. Percept Mot Skills 72:527–530, 1991

Owen N: Exploratory study: effect of computer cognitive rehabilitation on visual–spatial skills of learning disabled students. Dissertation Abstracts International 47:1284A, 1986

Petty LC, Rosen EF: Computer-based interactive video systems. Behavior Research Methods, Instruments, & Computers 19:160–166, 1987

Purdy M, Neri L: Computer-assisted cognitive rehabilitation in the home. Cognitive Rehabilitation 7:34–38, 1989

Rheingold H: Virtual Reality. New York, Summit Books, 1991

Robertson I, Gray J, MacKengie S: Microcomputer-based cognitive rehabilitation of visual neglect: three multiple-baseline single case studies. Brain Inj 2:151–163, 1988

Ruff R, Baser C, Johnston J, et al: Neuropsychological rehabilitation: an experimental study with head-injured patients. Journal of Head Trauma Rehabilitation 4:20–36, 1989

Index

*Page numbers in **boldface** type refer to figures and tables.*